Navigating Knowledge Translation in Health and Care

Building on Harvey and Kitson's influential *Implementing Evidence-Based Practice in Healthcare*, this new book draws on up-to-date research to demonstrate how to navigate a knowledge translation approach.

Recognising that the process of implementation is complex and dynamic, the first section of the book explores how understandings of knowledge translation can be applied and utilised at every stage of the research process to maximise impact and research uptake in practice. The second section of the book is made up of case studies incorporating 'how-to' advice and practical insights, demonstrating how the theory from the first section can work in the real life context. The final section considers future leadership challenges.

This is an essential guide for students, academics, and clinicians with an interest in knowledge translation and implementation science in health and care.

Sarah Hunter is a Senior Research Fellow in the Caring Futures Institute, College of Nursing and Health Sciences, Flinders University, South Australia.

Michael Lawless is a Senior Research Fellow in the Caring Futures Institute, College of Nursing and Health Sciences, Flinders University, South Australia.

Alison Kitson served as inaugural Vice President and Executive Dean of the College of Nursing and Health Sciences at Flinders University, South Australia, from 2017 to 2024, and as foundational Director of the Caring Futures Institute from 2019 to 2024.

Navigating Knowledge Translation in Health and Care

Edited by Sarah Hunter, Michael Lawless, and Alison Kitson

Routledge
Taylor & Francis Group

LONDON AND NEW YORK

Designed cover image: The editors

First published 2026
by Routledge
4 Park Square, Milton Park, Abingdon, Oxon OX14 4RN

and by Routledge
605 Third Avenue, New York, NY 10158

Routledge is an imprint of the Taylor & Francis Group, an informa business

For Product Safety Concerns and Information please contact our EU representative GPSR@taylorandfrancis.com. Taylor & Francis Verlag GmbH, Kaufingerstraße 24, 80331 München, Germany.

Trademark notice: Product or corporate names may be trademarks or registered trademarks, and are used only for identification and explanation without intent to infringe.

British Library Cataloguing-in-Publication Data
A catalogue record for this book is available from the British Library

Library of Congress Cataloging-in-Publication Data
Names: Kitson, Alison L., 1956– author | Hunter, Sarah C., 1991– author |
Lawless, Michael author
Title: Navigating knowledge translation in health and care /
Alison Kitson, Sarah Hunter, Michael Lawless.
Description: Abingdon, Oxon ; New York, NY : Routledge, 2026. |
Includes bibliographical references.
Identifiers: LCCN 2025030660 (print) | LCCN 2025030661 (ebook) |
ISBN 9781032158587 hardback | ISBN 9781032158570 paperback |
ISBN 9781003245995 ebook
Subjects: LCSH: Medicine–Research–Methodology | Research teams |
Evidence-based medicine
Classification: LCC R850 .K548 2026 (print) | LCC R850 (ebook)
LC record available at https://lccn.loc.gov/2025030660
LC ebook record available at https://lccn.loc.gov/2025030661

ISBN: 9781032158587 (hbk)
ISBN: 9781032158570 (pbk)
ISBN: 9781003245995 (ebk)

DOI: 10.4324/9781003245995

Typeset in Sabon
by Newgen Publishing UK

The editors would like to dedicate this book to anyone who is stepping outside their comfort zone and taking on the challenge of integrated knowledge translation.

Contents

Figures

Tables

Boxes

About the editors

Sarah Hunter is a Senior Research Fellow in the Caring Futures Institute, College of Nursing and Health Sciences, Flinders University, South Australia. Dr Hunter is a social psychologist and implementation scientist, and she applies her knowledge translation and implementation skills to shape an evidence-informed Early Years System in Australia that engages and supports parents and caregivers. Her research focuses on understanding the complex and diverse ways in which caregivers enact child rearing, and how they navigate services and support. This program of research intersects implementation science and integrated knowledge translation as it explores facilitating and implementing evidence into complex multi-sector systems, with a focus on the contextual and recipient factors that influence success.

Michael Lawless is a Senior Research Fellow in the Caring Futures Institute, College of Nursing and Health Sciences, Flinders University, South Australia. Dr Lawless is a social psychologist and health services researcher, focusing on self-care and supporting healthy ageing in primary care. He has authored over 40 articles addressing critical issues in healthy ageing and knowledge translation. Dr Lawless investigates the intersection of transdisciplinary research collaboration and knowledge translation in order to enhance healthcare practices and outcomes, particularly in the context of community-dwelling older adults with chronic health conditions.

Alison Kitson served as inaugural Vice President and Executive Dean of the College of Nursing and Health Sciences at Flinders University, South Australia, from 2017 to 2024, and as foundational Director of the Caring Futures Institute from 2019 to 2024. In her academic and research role, she is recognised internationally as a leading research translation scientist, nurse leader, and champion of improving person-centred fundamental care research and practice. She has held several joint appointments between academia and practice in both the United Kingdom and Australia. She co-authored *Implementing Evidence-Based Practice in Healthcare* (Harvey and Kitson, 2015), has published over 300 peer reviewed articles and book chapters in top nursing and translational science journals and is ranked in the top 2% of most cited researchers in her field in the world. In 2015 she was elected a Fellow of the Australian Academy of Health and Medical Science, and in 2022 she was awarded a Distinguished Matthew Flinders Professorship from Flinders University. She has several international and Australian visiting professorships and honorary doctorates from Sweden and Denmark. In 2025 she was inducted into the Sigma Theta Tau International Research Hall of Fame for her transformational research in person-centred fundamental care and knowledge translation.

Contributors

Tiffany Conroy is Deputy Dean-Nursing Leadership for the College of Nursing and Health Sciences, and Caring Futures Institute at Flinders University and the Director of Nursing and Midwifery Research at the Southern Adelaide Local Health Network, South Australia. Having graduated from Flinders University as a Registered Nurse in 1994, Professor Conroy initially worked as a clinician, then as researcher and a nursing academic. She is a Fellow of the Australian College of Nursing and an office bearer for the International Learning Collaborative, the global representative organisation for promoting patient centred fundamental care. Professor Conroy's educational and research focus includes knowledge translation, the methodology and conduct of systematic reviews, and improving the delivery of fundamental care for all care recipients regardless of clinical setting. She has authored more than 75 journal articles and 15 book chapters including 'Chapter 12: Case study of the Signature Project- an Australian-US knowledge translation project' in *Implementing Evidence-Based Practice In Healthcare* (Harvey, G. and Kitson, A., 2015) and 'Chapter 12: Evidence based practice/knowledge translation: a practical guide' in *Transitions in Nursing; preparing for professional practice*, 6th edn, Chang, E. & Hatcher, D. (eds) (2016).

Gill Harvey is Matthew Flinders Professor of Health Services and Implementation Research in the College of Nursing and Health Sciences at Flinders University, South Australia, and Deputy Director (Knowledge Translation) in the College's Caring Futures Institute. Gill is an Adjunct Professor of Implementation Science at Queensland University of Technology, and an Affiliated Researcher at Dalarna University in Sweden. Gill has a clinical background in nursing and has held academic positions in Alliance Manchester Business School at the University of Manchester, and Adelaide Nursing School, University of Adelaide. Prior to working in academia, she was Director of the UK Royal College of Nursing's Quality Improvement Program, and Director of the National Institute for Care Excellence (NICE) National Collaborating Centre for Nursing and Supportive Care. Her research interests focus on knowledge translation and implementation science in health care.

Claire Hutchinson is a Senior Research Fellow in the Health and Social Care Group of the Caring Futures Institute, Flinders University, South Australia. Since gaining her PhD in Psychology, she has worked in many cross-disciplinary teams conducting research on the quality of life, psychosocial well-being, and lived experience of social care recipients (older adults and adults with disability). Her economic evaluation experience has been in the mixed methods approach social return on investment analysis which captures and values diverse outcomes at the personal, community, and societal level. Dr Hutchinson considers knowledge translation to be an essential component of high-quality applied research, and is crucial for research to present a good return on the investment for the time and resources involved. As a former organisational psychologist, she is committed to supporting her industry partners to translate new knowledge into meaningful organisational change and to deliver evidence-based practice.

Bo Kim is an Investigator at the United States Department of Veterans Affairs (VA) Center for Healthcare Optimization and Implementation Research, and an Assistant Professor of Psychiatry at Harvard Medical School, United States. She is a health services researcher and implementation scientist with an academic background in systems science and engineering. Her research focuses on applying interdisciplinary methodologies toward studying the quality and implementation of health and related services, such as her work in partnership with the VA Homeless Programs Office that evaluates the implementation of VA's efforts to improve access to legal services for veterans.

Rachel Milte is an Australian Research Council Early Career Fellow in the Health and Social Care Group of the Caring Futures Institute, Flinders University, South Australia. Her PhD predominantly focused on applying economic evaluation techniques alongside a clinical trial evaluating a multidisciplinary nutrition and exercise rehabilitation program for older people following hip fracture. As part of this she implemented a cost-utility analysis as part of its measurement of the benefits of a new intervention. Associate Professor Milte also evaluated a range of diverse instruments for measuring Quality of Life in older people (including those admitted from residential aged care) for their practicality, feasibility, and validity of use. Associate Professor Milte understands the critical importance of knowledge translation through experiences in her applied research which covers care across diverse sectors including hospitals, subacute care settings, aged care facilities, as well as participants homes. Experiencing all these settings in all their individual idiosyncratic glory has led her to value research which tries to engage with and capture the way organisations, context, and people all interact to support (or conversely block) the implementation of 'best practice' care.

Lily Xiao is a Matthew Flinders Professor in the Caring Futures Institute at the College of Nursing and Health Sciences, Flinders University, South Australia. She has been working in research fields of dementia care, caring for older people from culturally and linguistically diverse backgrounds, and aged care workforce development since completing her PhD 17 years ago. The care service research focus enables Professor Xiao to work with a truly multi-disciplinary team of researchers, industry partners, clinical experts, older people receiving care services, their carers, and other stakeholders in the dementia field. Professor Xiao believes that the complexity of care service research with a knowledge translation focus requires researchers to journey with all stakeholders to understand the problem in real care settings, produce rigorous research evidence to inform policy, resource and practice development, and take a collective action for uptake, scale up and sustainability of evidence-based practice in care services.

Foreword

Despite an abundance of available knowledge, applying it in practice remains a challenge – making this book a timely and valuable contribution. It presents a rich, practice-oriented perspective from the Caring Futures Institute at Flinders University in Australia, where researchers and partners are reimagining how research can extend beyond academic dissemination to create lasting impact on health, care and well-being.

What distinguishes this book is its deep engagement with the real-world complexities of applied research. It provides a nuanced exploration of integrated knowledge translation as a framework for bridging the often-cited gap between knowledge generation and implementation. Readers are invited into a reflective narrative that acknowledges both the achievements and the inherent challenges of translating research into policy and practice. With a thoughtful and engaging tone, the authors trace their journey of embedding IKT into research processes, actively involving diverse stakeholders across health and care systems.

A particular strength of this book lies in its integration of theoretical foundations with lived experience. The Knowledge Translation Complexity Network Model, introduced in these pages, draws on insights from Complexity Science, Systems Thinking, and Social Network Theory to illuminate the dynamic processes through which knowledge is co-created, adapted and applied in context-rich environments. This synthesis of theory and practice is crucial: theory explains why certain approaches succeed, while experience demonstrates how they function in real-world settings. Together, they provide a deeper and more holistic understanding.

At its core, the book argues that research must aim not only to inform but to transform. It advocates for a more engaged, relational and adaptive approach to achieving research impact. As readers progress through the chapters, they will find themselves both challenged and supported – encouraged to question their assumptions about knowledge production and to embrace the collaborative possibilities that integrated knowledge translation affords.

Per Nilsen,
Linköping University,
22 March 2025

Preface

The process of writing books happens over many years and involves many people. It is a journey that twists and turns and it gathers its own momentum often leading the editors and contributors to new insights and discoveries. This has certainly been our experience as we have navigated this exciting journey. As three editors, we started this book assuming our ideas for the ways we wanted to share our own learning journeys would be straightforward and engaging. We also wanted to practice the philosophy we were sharing in the book. In telling the story of how we established and embedded an integrated knowledge translation approach to the applied research activity of the Caring Futures Institute at Flinders University, we would be able to engage our colleagues and stakeholders in co-producing material that would help clarify many of the complex issues involved in successfully translating new evidence into practice.

Each of our own journeys has had different trajectories. Alison Kitson, one of the developers of the Promoting Action on Research Implementation in Health Services (PARIHS) and subsequently in developing the refined version – the integrated Promoting Action on Research Implementation in Health Services (i-PARIHS) has a long history in implementation research, integrated knowledge translation, executive leadership and in mentoring and supporting new academics and researchers. Her vision for transforming caring interventions led to the setting up of the Caring Futures Institute in 2019 where she was Foundational Director. She also advocated for embedding knowledge translation as the key approach within the institute. She worked with colleagues Sarah Hunter and Michael Lawless (along with many others) to shape this according to the principles embedded in integrated knowledge translation.

Sarah Hunter's journey into the world of integrated knowledge translation began as a post-doctoral researcher working with Alison Kitson in 2017. She was thrown into facilitating several pilot implementation projects, supervised by Alison, as ways to help her develop her research and facilitation skills. From those beginnings, Sarah is leading a program of work in improving child and family health and wellbeing as a joint appointment working across research, policy and practice. She continues to work with international colleagues on improving the way the i-PARIHS framework is used in research projects and is embracing a more holistic approach to understanding how integrated knowledge translation ways of thinking can speed up the spread and add to the success of getting evidence into policy and practice.

Michael came to work with Alison as part of a National Health and Medical Research Council Centre of Research Excellence grant looking at older peoples' experiences of frailty in 2017. Michael was part of the knowledge translation team in that project whose job it was to understand what frailty meant to different people – to older people, to members of the healthcare team and to the wider community. With an interest in older peoples' self-care capabilities, Michael was able to use the methodologies of integrated knowledge translation to elicit the views, opinions, concerns and hopes surrounding frailty for older people. This work was also linked to a longitudinal study of how research leaders develop an understanding of knowledge translation. Michael is also developing his practical facilitation skills working with several other research teams where he is helping them identify how best to engage with multiple partners across different parts of the research process.

As three editors our job has been to engage our colleagues in the learning journey of understanding why integrated knowledge translation matters, how it can be used as a way of thinking about getting evidence into practice and how it can generate practical tools and templates that will help guide the research and the implementation work. What we found was that everyone starts from different places and perspectives and that people don't like to have to think differently about things unless there is a practical benefit. So, our approach to the book has been to illustrate the journey of how we introduced integrated knowledge translation into the Caring Futures Institute by inviting our colleagues to share their experiences of understanding and doing integrated knowledge translation. Each chapter is peppered with real-life case studies that describe how we have all worked together to understand better some of the theoretical ideas we were developing.

Have we come to the end of the journey? And is this the definitive description of integrated knowledge translation success? Of course, not. So far, we have illustrated how the thinking around implementation science and knowledge translation have moved towards partnering at every stage of the research process and how this impacts methodological approaches to the design, testing and evaluation of future studies. Integrated knowledge translation approaches combined with complexity science thinking ought to provide more flexibility within study designs to help us describe what's happening in the real world and help us move forward more effectively and efficiently to see the changes needed in the areas where we are undertaking research.

Integrated knowledge translation involves complex, dynamic, and collaborative networks of individuals and organisations, in which both evidence producers and evidence users (and various intermediaries) work together to discuss ideas, raise questions, share knowledge, and consider the implications for everyone involved. Integrated knowledge translation is a conscious, deliberate, specific, and systematic practice aimed at increasing the likelihood that research evidence will be adopted and taken up in locally relevant, context sensitive, meaningful, and sustainable ways that will improve care and be of benefit to individuals and society.

Before this book begins, we want to take some time to reflect on some high-level learnings that influence our perspective of integrated knowledge translation:

There is increasing recognition that the problems our world faces have become more interconnected, dynamic, and harder to control. These problems are complex due to inconsistent, incomplete, and contradictory aspects that are often difficult to recognise and deal with. These types of problems are frequently called 'wicked problems'. Wicked problems do not have a single or simple solution. Further, due to interdependencies, efforts to solve wicked problems, often result in identifying or even creating more problems. In other words, these efforts create more questions rather than answers.

Despite a greater understanding of, and appreciation for complexity, working within complexity is difficult. Notions of complexity undoubtedly discourage researchers who want tools, measures, certainty, or consistency, clinicians who want guidelines and protocols that ensure high quality care and safety, and policy makers who want clear evidence to inform their decision making.

Therefore, our aim with this book is to share our learnings of undertaking and embedding integrated knowledge translation into our applied research institute, with the hope to support your integrated knowledge translation efforts. We do not expect anyone to be a master at every research methodology or integrated knowledge translation approach. Our goal instead is to equip you with the core elements required to use any method, in any context, at any time.

To keep this book accessible, we are making a commitment to minimise use of abbreviations or acronyms. The health sector and health research use abbreviations and acronyms to simplify and facilitate quicker and easier communication. However, an unintended consequence has been the proliferation of too many abbreviations and acronyms, making it more difficult to understand. This book is broken down into three key sections. The first section 1) is on starting the integrated knowledge translation journey, the second section 2) is on navigating the journey, and the third section 3) is on facilitating the integrated knowledge translation journey. This book can be read from cover to cover. However, each chapter is written to stand alone. Therefore, you can read this book sequentially or choose the chapter(s) that speaks to you. Each chapter shares where we started and our aspirations, relevant theory and background knowledge, what we have learnt, what we have applied and things to consider.

We hope that through doing this we can help others navigate their own integrated knowledge translation journey and tell their own story with joy and confidence.

Sarah Hunter, Michael Lawless, and Alison Kitson

Acknowledgements

Firstly, we acknowledge the sovereignty of the Kaurna people, the First Nations people upon whose land the Flinders University Caring Futures Institute is located and where we, the editors, live and work. We pay our respects to the Kaurna people and all Australian First Nations people, and in particular we pay our respects and continuously learn from their practices of knowledge generation, knowledge sharing, caring, and kinship.

We also want to acknowledge and thank the many colleagues that we have worked with to discuss, deliberate, share and develop the ideas that we present in this book. We thank all our colleagues who attended the early workshops we hosted to brainstorm and plan this book. We thank our colleagues who are part of the Caring Futures Institute Knowledge Translation Working Group for their feedback, input, and safe space to discuss ideas. We also thank the many individual colleagues and Higher Degree Research students who generously read chapters and provided feedback to ensure the accessibility and readability of this book. We also acknowledge and thank the many colleagues we have all worked with over the years on knowledge translation projects, our work together has shaped our understanding and learnings of doing knowledge translation which underpin what we share in this book.

We would also like to thank Reuben Gore and Sonia Zanatta from TopBunk, our Creative Communication Partner, who were instrumental in bringing our visions to life. Thanks, must also go to Taylor & Francis Group for commissioning this book and to Grace McInnes and Madii Cherry-Moreton for their support throughout the production process. Finally, a special thank you to Rebekah O'Shea for her support in bringing this book together.

Abbreviations

CFIR	Consolidated Framework for Implementation Research
COVID-19	Coronavirus Disease of 2019
DHEF	Digital Health Equity Framework
FRAME	Framework for Reporting Adaptations and Modifications to Evidence-Based Interventions
FRAME-IS	Framework for Reporting Adaptations and Modifications to Implementation Strategies
i-PARIHS	Integrated-Promoting Action on Research Implementation in Health Services framework
NASS	Non-adoption, Abandonment, Scale-Up, Spread, and Sustainability framework
PARIHS	Promoting Action on Research Implementation in Health Services framework
RE-AIM	Reach, Effectiveness, Adoption, Implementation, Maintenance
T2D	Type 2 Diabetes Mellitus
T-CAST	Theory, Model, and Framework Comparison and Selection Tool

Section I
Starting the journey

1 Book overview and setting the scene

Alison Kitson, Michael Lawless and Sarah Hunter

Introduction

This book describes an ongoing journey of how a group of applied researchers and knowledge translation experts are embedding a knowledge translation approach (called integrated knowledge translation) into research activity at the Caring Futures Institute, Flinders University, in South Australia. This story is used as a real-life case study to illustrate the learning journey of institute members and how that is helping us work with our industry and community partners to get new knowledge into policy and practice. The Caring Futures Institute is an applied research institute, working with industry including policy makers and local and national governments, community and individual partners to address issues around health, wellbeing, care, and self-care across the life course.

When you embrace knowledge translation and particularly when you take an integrated knowledge translation approach, you are expected to know how to take the research findings or evidence that you or other researchers have generated and work with partners to get that research into practice. This means that your responsibility as a researcher or clinical academic extends to your ability to understand not only how new evidence or knowledge is generated but how that new evidence or knowledge effectively finds its way to being used by the people who need to adopt and apply it in policy and practice. We will go into more detail about what knowledge translation and integrated knowledge translation mean later in this introductory chapter as well as subsequent chapters. At this point, all that is necessary to remember is that knowing how to get new evidence and knowledge into policy and practice is a fundamental skill set for applied researchers and their collaborators, and this book will help you develop those insights and skills.

In this first chapter we set the scene, tell you about what applied research institutes do, and as part of the case study, what the Caring Futures Institute does. Then we introduce you to knowledge translation ways of thinking which includes a brief outline of where knowledge translation and integrated knowledge translation ideas emerged and how they can be used. We finish off the chapter by outlining what else is in the book, and how you can use it to help you understand how to do integrated knowledge translation.

Who the book is for

The contents of this book should be useful to the following groups:

- **Early and mid-career researchers** working in applied research institutes/academic departments who are responsible for doing health and care services research, clinical

DOI: 10.4324/9781003245995-2

trials, population and public health research as well as economic and other types of evaluations and implementation research. In other words, researchers and research teams whose job it is to make a difference in the real world and are increasingly expected to know how to get their research evidence into policy and practice – in other words, to have an impact.

- **Practitioners/clinicians/academics** in positions who are embedded in industry, and community partners with an interest in, or indeed are expected to know how, to embed new knowledge/research findings/clinical guidelines or other types of evidence into practice (and policy). Put simply, those who want to have an impact on the ground and whose job it is to be able to do this.
- **Senior researchers** who are leading teams and working in applied research centres or institutes who want to learn from the experiences of one research institute's journey – successes and challenges – and the learnings from this to optimise the impact their research can have on policy and practice.
- **Students** enrolled in research degrees working in applied research settings who may be exploring the language and ideas of knowledge translation for the first time.
- **Service users or consumers** who want to be more engaged in research and knowledge translation activities and who need to understand some of the theory, methods and language.

This book has been co-designed and developed by a range of early, mid and senior researchers within the Caring Futures Institute, local and international partners, and many other key partners. Several real-life case studies are used to illustrate how researchers, who are at various stages in their knowledge translation journey, can learn by doing. This means that there will be examples where things did not go according to plan and critical reflections as to why things did not work as much as understanding why things did work as expected. The style of the book is exploratory, story-driven, and reflective, rather than a structured recipe for successful knowledge translation. Through these descriptions we hope you will recognise some of the important self-reflective and growth points in your own journey of understanding the contribution of knowledge translation to improving the use of new knowledge in practice.

What applied research institutes and centres do

But first, let's think about what applied research is and what applied research institutes do.

In the research world, there are two major types of research – basic or discovery research (pure and strategic) and applied research. Table 1.1 summarises the ways we use and define terms such as research, basic and applied research and the underlying worldviews about how new knowledge is created.

Basic research covers the types of investigations focused on improving our understanding of a particular phenomenon, or law of nature. It seeks to explain why and how things work. Think about the discovery work involved in connecting the human papilloma virus with cervical cancer (zur Hausen, 1976, 1977) or making the connection between stomach or gastric ulcers and infection with the Heliobacter pylori bacterium (Marshall & Warren, 1984; Warren & Marshall, 1983).

Information from basic research often creates a foundation for applied research. This has been the case for the two breakthrough discoveries mentioned above. The scientists involved in the basic human papilloma virus cancer-related research and development

Table 1.1 Research definition and types of research activity

Research activity	Definition
Research	The creation of new knowledge and/or the use of existing knowledge in a new and creative way to generate new concepts, methodologies, inventions and understandings. This could include synthesis and analysis of previous research to the extent that it is new and creative. (National Health and Medical Research Council, 2018)
Pure Basic Research	Research carried out for the advancement of knowledge, without seeking long-term economic or social benefits or making any specific or conscious effort to apply the results to practical problems or to transfer the results to sectors responsible for their application. (Australian Bureau of Statistics, 2020)
Strategic Basic Research	Experimental and theoretical research undertaken to acquire new knowledge directed into specified broad areas in the expectation of practical discoveries. (Australian Bureau of Statistics, 2020)
Applied Research	Original research undertaken to acquire new knowledge. It is, however, directed primarily towards a specific, practical aim or objective. (Australian Bureau of Statistics, 2020)

of an effective vaccine initially encountered resistance to their ideas (Matson, 2022) but those discoveries have resulted in a World Health Organisation global strategy – that 90% of girls under 15 years of age are fully vaccinated with the Human Papillomavirus vaccine by the year 2030 (World Health Organization, 2020). Findings from a recent United Kingdom study support the dramatic impact that Human Papillomavirus vaccination at an early age can have on reducing cervical cancer rates (Falcaro et al., 2021). Being able to bring new paradigms and ways of thinking to health problems and linking the basic and applied research with policy and community needs, has been the basis for such significant steps forward in public health.

Applied research therefore tackles problems in the real world and works with partners in the community, industry and organisations to find practical ways to solve problems or gain deeper insight as to why problems have occurred. The types of research methodologies or approaches typically found in such applied research organisations include empirical or experimental methods to check whether a new approach to solving the problem is more effective than the current way of doing things. Methods may include, but are not limited to, co-design approaches (e.g. experience-based co-design), participatory action research (e.g., community workshop approaches), mixed methods in terms of combining experimental and participatory action research approaches together to understand some of the complex interrelationships happening between knowledge producers and knowledge users, and increasingly more innovative approaches to getting different partners involved in the research process such as arts-based and other exploratory ways to elicit peoples' views (e.g. visual elicitation, photovoice).

Some examples of the sorts of applied research undertaken by teams across the Caring Futures Institute include promoting the voices of people in Aged Care through production of relevant quality of life measurement tools (see Chapter 6); improving the support carers of people with dementia get in Australia and in China (see Chapter 7); helping families prevent childhood obesity (see case study 1 in Chapter 3 and case study 2 in Chapter 5); understanding how to improve cancer survivorship experiences by introducing new navigator roles (see case study 6 in Chapter 5 for more on this) and many, many more.

What connects these examples and the ways that we are engaging with partners is that they are complex, i.e. the new evidence or knowledge that has been co-designed is being introduced into complex systems with a range of partners who may or may not be interested in the proposed change. That means there are rarely single elements of the intervention that you can test independently because you cannot control for all the other bits in the situation or context. You have to understand the nature of the thing you are introducing (the intervention), either to test its effectiveness (does it do what it is supposed to do in real life settings to a range of ordinary patients and people), or to test how you have actually managed to successfully get it into practice.

The guidance from the Medical Research Council on complex interventions acknowledges these contextual and intervention complexities. The Medical Research Council framework highlights the importance of an applied and flexible approach to complex interventions (Craig et al., 2006; Skivington et al., 2021). It emphasises that the phases of intervention development and implementation require engagement of partners, consideration of contextual factors, and continual refinement of both the logic model and the intervention itself (Skivington et al., 2021).

In summary, people do research to generate new knowledge that can be used to solve problems. In health and care research we know that problems are complex, wicked even, because they not only deal with basic scientific matters (such as how viruses can cause cancer) but they need to take account of the social, behavioural and contextual dimensions of how people and systems respond to new knowledge (such as why people choose to get vaccinated or not).

Knowledge translation – what it is and where it came from

When knowledge translation started to emerge as a way of thinking, it was in direct response to the gaps created between research and practice. So, knowledge translation was seen as a step in the research process which is why it is often viewed as a linear or bridging process as seen in Figures 1.1 and 1.2.

The Institute of Medicine in the United States, launched an approach that looked at the traditional research pipeline and identified the specific gaps that needed to be addressed (Sung et al., 2003). They described these gaps as similar to roadblocks – blockages in the movement of knowledge between pure science to clinical trials (T1) (Sung et al., 2003); blockages from clinical trials to everyday practice (T2); and within organisations (T3) (Woolf, 2008). By 2010, two additional blockages had been identified – one from the practitioner to the patient (T4) and the other relating to population health (T0) (Khoury et al., 2010). These roadblocks or gaps, T1, T2, T3, T4 and T0, and the approach taken by the Institute of Medicine was to invest in intervention studies focusing on overcoming each of the identified roadblocks.

At the same time, the Canadian Institutes of Health Research was developing its approach to knowledge translation, which was markedly different. They defined knowledge translation as:

"A dynamic and iterative process that includes the synthesis, dissemination, exchange and ethically-sound application of knowledge to improve the health of [people], provide more effective health services and products, and strengthen the health care system".

(Canadian Institutes of Health Research, 2016)

The 'Pipeline' Model of Getting Research into Evidence-Based Practice and Policy

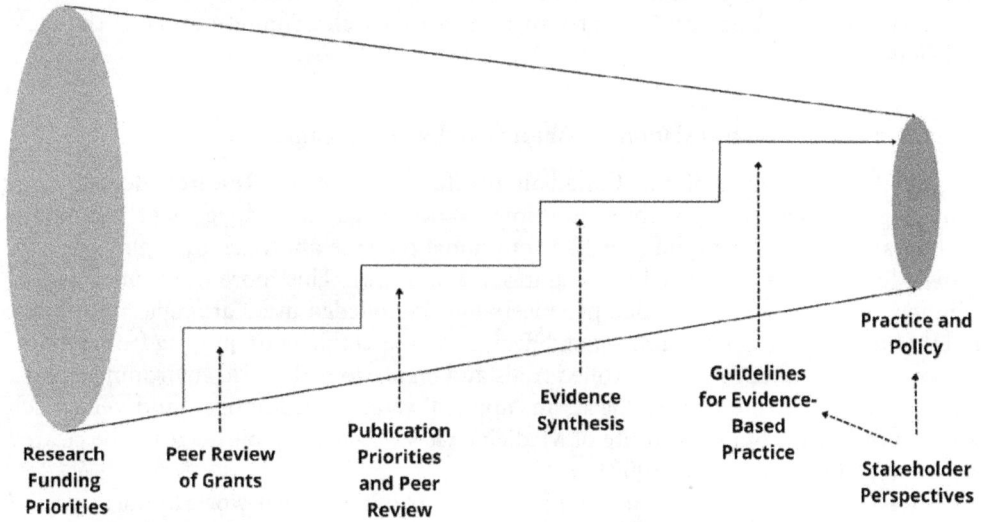

Research Funding Priorities

Peer Review of Grants

Publication Priorities and Peer Review

Evidence Synthesis

Guidelines for Evidence-Based Practice

Stakeholder Perspectives

Practice and Policy

Figure 1.1 The 'pipeline' model showing a linear stepwise progression from funding priorities through to application.

Source: https://doi.org/10.25451/flinders.29192228.v1

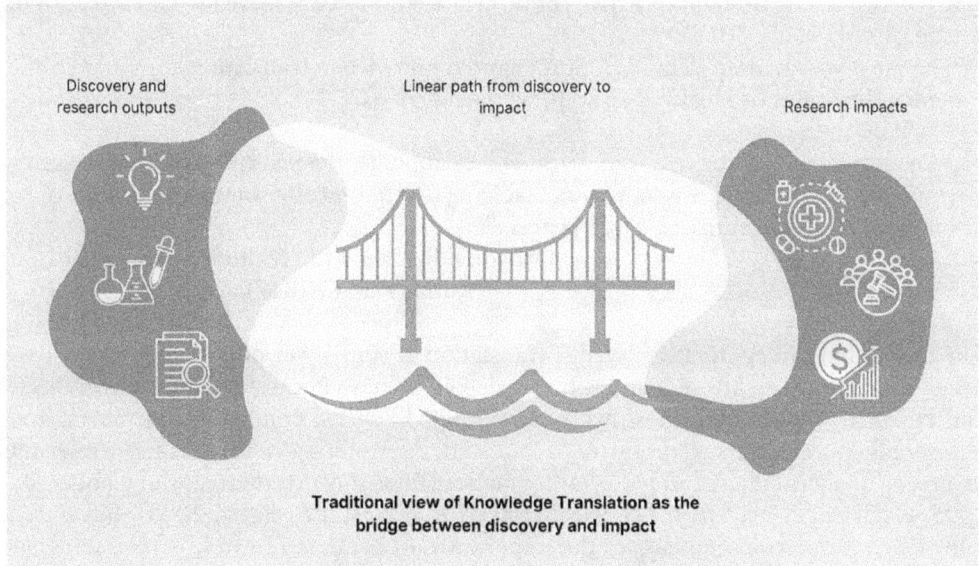

Discovery and research outputs

Linear path from discovery to impact

Research impacts

Traditional view of Knowledge Translation as the bridge between discovery and impact

Figure 1.2 Bridging the gap between research knowledge and real-world impact.

Source: https://doi.org/10.25451/flinders.29192570.v1

This definition of knowledge translation did not take a pipeline or linear approach. Unlike the United States approach, the Canadian definition of knowledge translation has its roots in social movements and innovation (Ryan & Gross, 1943). The Canadian Institutes of Health Research popularised knowledge translation, with Governments and funding bodies now taking interest in knowledge translation principles (Lucylynn et al., 2025). The Canadian Institutes of Health Research definition remains the most widely used.

Integrated knowledge translation – what it is and where it came from

Despite the dominance of the Canadian Institutes of Health Research definition of knowledge translation highlighting the importance of partner engagement and multi-method approaches, there did prevail a traditional pipeline approach to explaining how knowledge translation worked (see Figures 1.1 and 1.2). This more traditional way of thinking assumes that knowledge producers and knowledge users are separate groups, and that translation follows a rational, linear, and predictable path, moving from laboratory research to randomised controlled trials and finally to real-world environments (i.e., from 'bench to bedside', from 'basic' to 'applied' research traditions), and very much reflected the United States Institute of Medicine view of gaps and blockages to be cleared along a pipeline (Sung et al., 2003)

However, this view does not account for the complexities of real-world application and the adaptive nature of knowledge within social systems as articulated in applied research, the Canadian Institutes of Health Research knowledge translation definition, or indeed in the Medical Research Council Complex Intervention guidance (Campbell et al., 2000; Craig et al., 2008; Skivington et al., 2021). The shift to a more integrated approach, drawing on complexity and systems thinking, occurred as researchers, practitioners, and policymakers recognised the need for effective, context-sensitive methods to bridge the 'gaps' between research and practice (Braithwaite et al., 2018; Greenhalgh et al., 2004; Kitson, Brook, et al., 2018).

The most widely used definition of integrated knowledge translation comes from the Canadian Institutes of Health Research, who define it as:

> "An approach to doing research that involves applying the principles of knowledge translation (synthesis, dissemination, exchange, and ethically sound application of knowledge) to the **entire research process**"
>
> (Canadian Institutes of Health Research, 2015;
> Kothari et al., 2017). (emphasis added)

The idea behind integrated knowledge translation is simple yet powerful: when knowledge producers (i.e., those responsible for creating new knowledge, like researchers) and knowledge users (i.e., those who use it, like clinicians, community members, and policy-makers) work in collaborative partnership, the resulting research is more relevant and more likely to be used in policy and practice (Bowen & Martens, 2006; Choi et al., 2005; Gagliardi et al., 2017; Gagliardi et al., 2015; Kitson & Bisby, 2008). Integrated knowledge translation emphasises the importance of genuine research partnerships, as opposed to one-off engagement or consultation (Gagliardi et al., 2017; Nguyen et al., 2020). It champions problem-focused, collaborative research, moving away from the traditional, academic-driven, 'top-down' approach (Kothari et al., 2017; Straus et al., 2013) to a more collaborative and engaged approach.

Integrated knowledge translation – the Caring Futures Institute approach

The perspective we are adopting in the Caring Futures Institute underscores the importance of employing integrated knowledge translation approaches, fostering collaboration, forming partnerships, and paying close attention to contextual factors. Importantly, it combines a collaborative, participatory approach (Graham et al., 2018; Nguyen et al., 2020) with a more explicit acknowledgement of the way that complexity theory (Kitson, Brook, et al., 2018) can help us understand the ways we can work together with key partners to solve real world problems.

This viewpoint aligns with the broader trend of recognising healthcare as a 'complex adaptive system' (Braithwaite et al., 2018; Greenhalgh & Papoutsi, 2018; May et al., 2016; Plsek & Greenhalgh, 2001). Complexity emerges through the interactions between elements within a system, such as the staff and clients in an organisation, as well as between the system and its external environment. This dynamic interplay can lead to ripple effects, where the actions of one part of the system impact other parts, but in unpredictable ways.

This means that as well as embracing a collaborative approach to knowledge translation we are taking account of the contextual factors – systems, processes, cultures, behaviours, relationships and power dynamics to name but a few – that need to be considered when it comes to understanding how knowledge is translated into policy and practice. By combining integrated knowledge translation ways of thinking with complexity science thinking we can begin to describe the many factors that will come into play when we want to introduce new knowledge into systems.

Knowledge translation researchers (Damschroder et al., 2022; Harvey & Kitson, 2016; Squires et al., 2019) have long acknowledged the impact that contextual factors have on the success or otherwise of getting new knowledge adopted into systems. As research teams have explored this, they have moved more to understanding the dynamic nature of systems.

So, how we approach research in the Caring Futures Institute is to combine two traditions – integrated knowledge translation and complexity thinking – to help us more effectively navigate the multiple complex systems we work in and the relationships we manage within them. This means that our own knowledge of mechanisms that change the way systems and people work needs to be quite extensive. So, we need to know something about complex adaptive systems, systems thinking, how organisations learn and use that learning to improve, and how people connect and network within systems and what impact such relationships have on the way knowledge moves within and across systems and between people.

To simplify this, we have generated a table of some of the main terms that people use when they talk about integrated knowledge translation and complexity, see Table 1.2.

Understanding the basics of complexity thinking is helpful for creating a more nuanced understanding of how, why, and under what conditions a particular knowledge translation strategy might be effective in practice. It essentially involves being mindful of the elements (e.g., people, organisations, technologies), relationships, and dynamics within complex social systems such as healthcare. This involves developing a practical

Table 1.2 Key terms for integrated knowledge translation and complexity science

Term	Definition
Integrated knowledge translation (Esmail et al., 2020)	An approach where researchers and partners (such as policymakers, practitioners, and community members) collaborate throughout the **entire research process**. This partnership ensures that the research is relevant, co-created, and more likely to be effectively applied in real-world settings, potentially leading to greater impact.
Complexity science (Plsek & Greenhalgh, 2001)	The study of complex systems, where numerous interconnected parts interact in ways that can lead to unpredictable and emergent behaviours. It focuses on understanding how these interactions within systems, such as eco-systems, economies, or healthcare systems, produce outcomes that cannot be easily predicted by analysing individual components alone.
Complex adaptive systems (Kitson, Brook, et al., 2018)	Systems composed of multiple interconnected components that interact and adapt to changes in their environment. These systems are characterised by their ability to evolve, learn, and self-organise, leading to emergent behaviours that are often unpredictable.
Systems thinking (Arnold & Wade, 2015)	An approach to understanding complex systems by examining the relationships, interactions, and patterns among their components. It involves looking at the whole system rather than focusing on individual parts, recognizing that changes in one part of the system can impact the entire system in unpredictable ways.
Learning health system (World Health Organization et al., 2021)	Healthcare systems designed to continuously improve by integrating data, research, and clinical practice. Such systems use real-time data and feedback, and generate new insights, implement changes, and rapidly apply what is learned to enhance patient care, outcomes, and system efficiency.
Social network theory (Krause et al., 2007)	The study of how individuals or entities are connected through relationships, and how these connections influence behaviour, information flow, and social dynamics. It examines the structure of networks, including nodes (individuals or groups) and ties (relationships), to understand how social interactions shape outcomes within communities, organisations, and societies.

understanding of organisational practices within specific contexts, being intellectually open and curious, building authentic relationships, and engaging in deliberative dialogue and negotiation (Mallidou et al., 2018). Incorporating complexity thinking and an integrated knowledge translation approach can support the development of more effective and responsive strategies. We will return to the concepts of integrated knowledge translation and complexity thinking in more detail in Chapter 4.

Introducing the Knowledge Translation Complexity Network Model

Our discussions with colleagues in the Caring Futures Institute while writing this book have focused on ways to refine and operationalise our shared approach to integrated knowledge translation. These conversations have been guided by the Knowledge Translation Complexity Network Model, which several of us have been involved in developing and refining (Brook et al., 2016; Kitson, Brook, et al., 2018; Kitson, O'Shea, et al., 2018). The model was co-created with research partners. It combines ideas from integrated knowledge translation with complexity science. The model emphasises the dynamic interactions between individuals in various sectors. Unlike models that see 'knowledge producers' and 'knowledge users' as separate entities to be bridged, the Knowledge Translation

Complexity Network Model views them as part of a dynamic process of interaction and collaboration. Another important point about the Knowledge Translation Complexity Network Model is that it recognises that we are not just working in one complex adaptive system called healthcare delivery. In fact, every human system we work in is a complex adaptive system. That means the research organisation you work in, the health system or government departments you work in or with, all operate as complex adaptive systems. Imagine you are learning how to waltz, and you are part of a large set of dancers circulating around the room – you need to get into the rhythm not just with your partner but with everyone else on the dance floor. So, with integrated knowledge translation, we need to be in sync with our partners as we work together on a common goal.

This means that in our pursuit to understand how to more effectively generate co-designed and co-produced solutions for practical problems, we will have to learn how to look at issues from multiple perspectives and generate multiple potential ways of solving the problem(s) in ways that can be analysed and, if successful, scaled across policy and practice. Such novel ways of thinking are both scary and exciting in equal measure but there are lots of practical tips and tricks we can share with you that will make your journey exciting, enjoyable and rewarding.

The Knowledge Translation Complexity Network Model integrates five key research processes. These five processes are: Problem Identification, Knowledge Creation, Knowledge Synthesis, Implementation, and Evaluation. Figure 1.3 provides an updated representation of the model from its representation in the original article it was published in (Kitson, Brook, et al., 2018) and Table 1.3 summarises these research processes that inform knowledge translation activity.

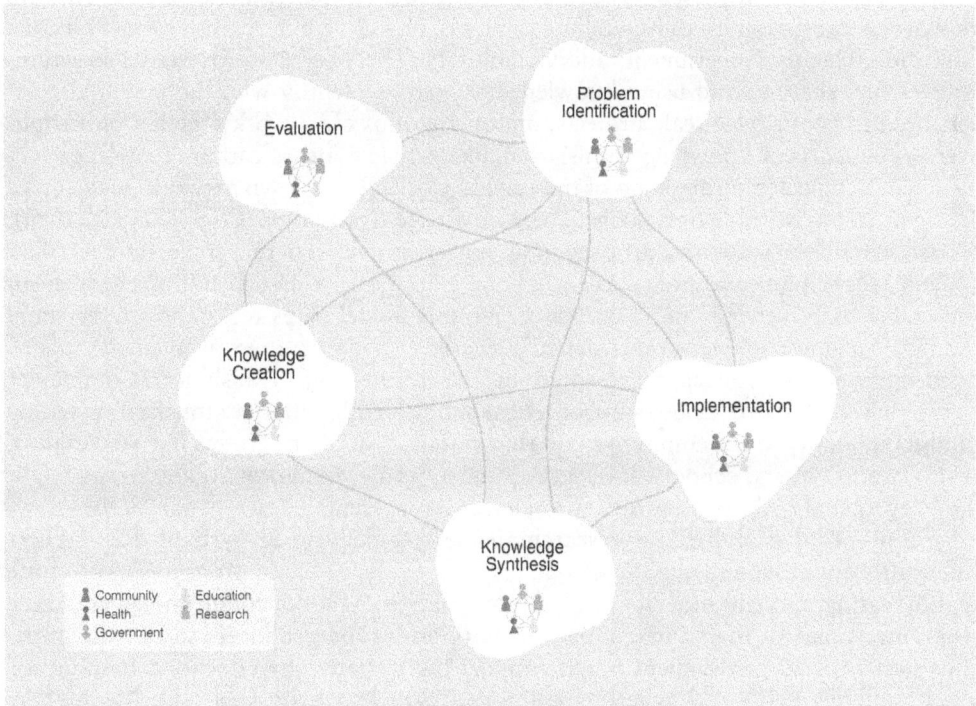

Figure 1.3 The Knowledge Translation Complexity Network Model.
Source: https://doi.org/10.25451/flinders.29192585.v1

Table 1.3 Key terms used within the Knowledge Translation Complexity Network Model

Term	Definition
Knowledge Translation Complexity Network Model	A model that views knowledge translation as a dynamic, interconnected process involving multiple partners across various sectors. Instead of a linear approach, this model emphasizes the complex interactions and networks that shape how knowledge is generated, shared, adapted, and applied in real-world contexts. It highlights the importance of collaboration, adaptability, and the consideration of contextual factors in effectively translating knowledge into practice.
Problem Identification	The process of defining research problems systematically, serving as an initial step for formulating and shaping research questions for comprehensive collaborative investigation.
Knowledge Creation	The generation of new knowledge to address specific research questions and bridge identified gaps in our understanding.
Knowledge Synthesis	The systematic identification, appraisal, and synthesis of knowledge to create tools, products, or interventions designed for application designed for application in policy and practice.
Implementation	The rigorous application of knowledge into policy and practice, guided by relevant theories and tailored strategies.
Evaluation	The systematic review of intervention processes and outcomes with the goal of ensuring ongoing use and sustainability.

Source: Kitson, Brook, et al. (2018).

In addition, and in keeping with complexity science thinking, the Knowledge Translation Complexity Network Model brings together different sectors involved in knowledge translation in health and care systems, including but not limited to Research, Education, Health, Government, and Community. These sectors provide the structures for creating, sharing, and using knowledge as well as identify who the potential partners need to be. In large-scale projects, multiple groups often work together on various overlapping parts of knowledge translation, like problem identification, knowledge synthesis, and implementation. Each of these areas works like its own network, made up of different groups with shared goals. The Knowledge Translation Complexity Network Model sees these networks as part of a bigger system where people interact, link up, and adapt. It proposes that success in knowledge translation depends on engagement and connectivity between these groups. Using this model helps researchers understand and improve how knowledge gets shared and used to solve complex problems.

To unpack the concepts presented in the Knowledge Translation Complexity Network Model, let's consider a hypothetical public health initiative aimed at preventing childhood obesity in the community. In this initiative, different groups like researchers, healthcare providers, schools, local government, and community organisations might come together to address the problem. Each sector represents a different part of the knowledge translation as well as the research and service delivery ecosystems. Researchers and healthcare providers might focus on creating evidence-based programs to promote healthy eating and physical activity among children. Schools could implement these programs as part of their curriculum and work with food producers to provide nutritious meals. Local government might support the initiative by allocating funding for sports facilities and parks where children can play and exercise safely. Meanwhile, community organisations could organise community events and workshops to raise awareness about the importance of healthy lifestyles for children, parents, and the whole community.

In this scenario, the research team, healthcare providers, schools, local government, food producers and community organisations form 'networks' working together as part of a collective effort. Each of them operates as complex adaptive systems independently but when they choose to come together to solve commonly recognised problems, they create new networks and connections that enable movement of knowledge and uptake of new ideas and actions. This means that each group involved in the initiative initially functions independently, like their own complex adaptive systems, meaning that they have their own structures, processes, and ways of working. When these groups collaborate to tackle shared issues (like childhood obesity), they form new connections and networks. These networks then can facilitate the sharing of insights, and the adoption of new ideas and practices across all involved groups, making their efforts more effective than if each group worked in isolation (see Figure 1.4).

Each of the different groups collaborate and interact to address childhood obesity from different angles, sharing knowledge, resources, and expertise, thereby enriching the

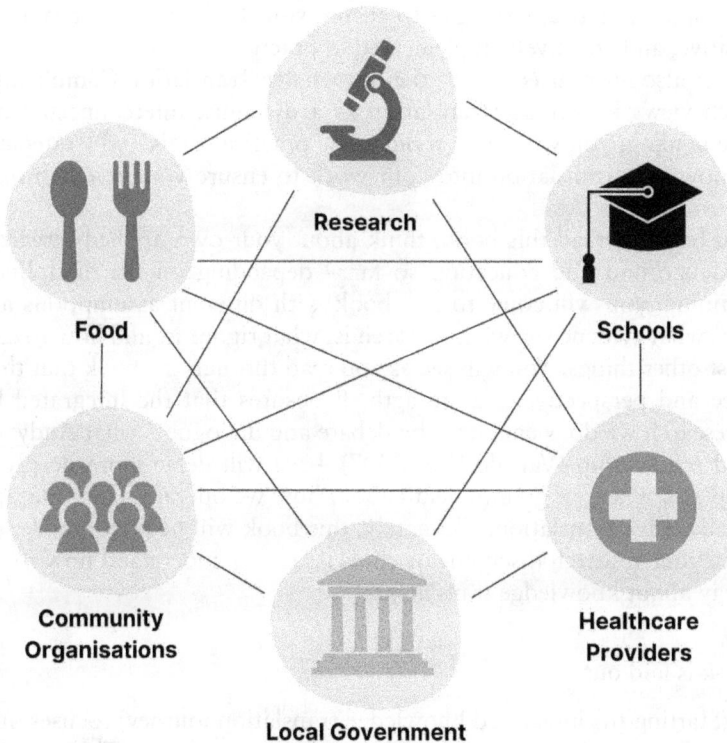

Figure 1.4 Cross-sector collaboration in childhood obesity prevention initiative.
Source: https://doi.org/10.25451/flinders.29192594.v1

shared understanding of, and knowledge about, the causes of childhood obesity, which in turn promotes more effective interventions that can be trialled and tested by the engaged partners. The success of the initiative relies on effective communication and coordination between these sectors to create a holistic approach to addressing the problem. Through this collaborative effort, the community can develop more effective and sustainable solutions to combat childhood obesity and improve public health and wellbeing. And it is the job of the integrated knowledge translation experts to know how to get all these pieces of the jigsaw puzzle working together.

Starting your own integrated knowledge translation journey

This chapter has provided a starting point to understanding why knowledge translation is an essential part of the research process and why integrated knowledge translation together with complexity science principles help us to understand how new knowledge can more effectively be used in policy and practice. We discussed the difference between basic and applied research. While basic research generates important foundational knowledge, applied research focuses on finding practical solutions. At the Caring Futures Institute, we are using integrated knowledge translation to understand and solve complex health and care challenges by working in partnership throughout the entire research process. In this book, you will learn how to move beyond traditional research methods and mindsets and apply practical strategies to ensure your findings are relevant, co-created, context-sensitive, and effectively implemented in practice.

This chapter also introduced you to the Knowledge Translation Complexity Network Model, which views knowledge translation as a dynamic, interconnected process. As you continue reading, you will learn about some practical tools and strategies to weave integrated knowledge translation into your work to ensure your research makes a real difference.

So, as you begin to read this book, think about your own applied research journey, your own background and education so far – depending on the discipline, research methods, training, you will come to this book with different assumptions about what knowledge is, what evidence is, what research is, what rigour is, and how to engage partners, amongst other things. You will see as you read through the book that this diversity of experience and perspective is a strength. It ensures that the integrated knowledge translation research we do is enhanced by debate and dialogue – what Andy Van de Ven calls engaged scholarship (Van de Ven, 2007) – we will delve more deeply into these ideas in Chapter 4 when we go into detail about how we operationalise our approach to integrated knowledge translation. Ultimately, this book will help you move from where you started in your research discipline or clinical area to understand how to think in an integrated way about knowledge translation.

How the book is laid out

- **Section I** (Starting the integrated knowledge translation journey) focuses on the background and theoretical underpinnings of knowledge translation. This section includes:
  - **Chapter 2** delves into implementation science and the phases of implementation, including pre-implementation planning, implementation designs, evaluation, and sustainability.

- **Chapter 3** explores working in partnership, discussing how to identify and involve different individuals or groups of individuals at various research stages to enhance successful uptake and use.
- **Chapter 4** introduces more integrated ways of conducting knowledge translation and learning how to use complexity science principles to help guide integrated knowledge translation processes and methods.
- **Section II** (Navigating the integrated knowledge translation journey) is more practical as it provides guidance through case studies and checklists. This section includes:
  - **Chapter 5** provides seven short and diverse case studies from across the Caring Futures Institute to illustrate our approach to undertaking integrated knowledge translation.
  - **Chapters 6 and 7** provide detailed case studies written by research teams within the Caring Futures Institute to demonstrate how they have undertaken integrated knowledge translation.
  - **Chapter 8** introduces what we believe are the core elements to undertaking integrated knowledge translation and provides a distilled guide to developing your own integrated knowledge translation plan.
- **Section III** (Facilitating the integrated knowledge translation journey) looks at leadership within integrated knowledge translation. This section includes:
  - **Chapter 9** explores how to champion integrated knowledge translation as a research leader.
  - **Chapter 10** reflects on the key challenges and issues that remain in the field of integrated knowledge translation and looks to the future.

References

Arnold, R. D., & Wade, J. P. (2015). A definition of systems thinking: A systems approach. *Procedia Computer Science, 44*, 669–678. https://doi.org/10.1016/j.procs.2015.03.050

Australian Bureau of Statistics. (2020). *Australian and New Zealand Standard Research Classification (ANZSRC). A statistical classification used for the measurement and analysis of R&D in Australia and New Zealand.* Australian Bureau of Statistics. Retrieved 29 August from www.abs.gov.au/statistics/classifications/australian-and-new-zealand-standard-research-classification-anzsrc/latest-release

Bowen, S., & Martens, P. J. (2006). A model for collaborative evaluation of university-community partnerships. *Journal of Epidemiology and Community Health (1979), 60*(10), 902–907. https://doi.org/10.1136/jech.2005.040881

Braithwaite, J., Churruca, K., Long, J. C., Ellis, L. A., & Herkes, J. (2018). When complexity science meets implementation science: A theoretical and empirical analysis of systems change. *BMC Medicine, 16*(1), 63–63. https://doi.org/10.1186/s12916-018-1057-z

Brook, A. H., Liversidge, H. M., Wilson, D., Jordan, Z., Harvey, G., Marshall, R. J., & Kitson, A. L. (2016). Health research, teaching and provision of care: Applying a new approach based on complex systems and a knowledge translation complexity network model. *International Journal of Design & Nature and Ecodynamics, 11*(4), 663–669. https://doi.org/10.2495/DNE-V11-N4-663-669

Campbell, M., Fitzpatrick, R., Haines, A., Kinmonth, A. L., Sandercock, P., Spiegelhalter, D., & Tyrer, P. (2000). Framework for design and evaluation of complex interventions to improve health. *British Medical Journal, 321*(7262), 694–696. https://doi.org/10.1136/bmj.321.7262.694

Canadian Institutes of Health Research. (2015). *Guide to knowledge translation planning at CIHR: Integrated and end-of-grant approaches.* https://cihr-irsc.gc.ca/e/45321.html

16   *Navigating Knowledge Translation in Health and Care*

Canadian Institutes of Health Research. (2016). *Knowledge translation: Definition.* Canadian Institutes of Health Research. Retrieved 22 August 2022 from https://cihr-irsc.gc.ca/e/29418.html#1

Choi, B. C. K., Pang, T., Lin, V., Puska, P., Sherman, G., Goddard, M., Ackland, M. J., Sainsbury, P., Stachenko, S., Morrison, H., & Clottey, C. (2005). Can scientists and policy makers work together? *Journal of Epidemiology and Community Health (1979), 59*(8), 632–637. https://doi.org/10.1136/jech.2004.031765

Craig, P., Dieppe, P., Macintyre, S., Michie, S., Nazareth, I., & Petticrew, M. (2006). *Developing and evaluating complex interventions.* Medical Research Council.

Craig, P., Dieppe, P., Macintyre, S., Michie, S., Nazareth, I., Petticrew, M., & Medical Research Council, G. (2008). Developing and evaluating complex interventions: The new Medical Research Council guidance. *BMJ, 337,* a1655. https://doi.org/10.1136/bmj.a1655

Damschroder, L. J., Reardon, C. M., Widerquist, M. A. O., & Lowery, J. (2022). The updated consolidated framework for implementation research based on user feedback. *Implementation Science: IS, 17*(1), 1–75. https://doi.org/10.1186/s13012-022-01245-0

Esmail, R., Hanson, H. M., Holroyd-Leduc, J., Brown, S., Strifler, L., Straus, S. E., Niven, D. J., & Clement, F. M. (2020). A scoping review of full-spectrum knowledge translation theories, models, and frameworks. *Implementation Science: IS, 15*(1), 11–11. https://doi.org/10.1186/s13012-020-0964-5

Falcaro, M., Castañon, A., Ndlela, B., Checchi, M., Soldan, K., Lopez-Bernal, J., Elliss-Brookes, L., & Sasieni, P. (2021). The effects of the national HPV vaccination programme in England, UK, on cervical cancer and grade 3 cervical intraepithelial neoplasia incidence: A register-based observational study. *The Lancet, 398*(10316), 2084–2092. https://doi.org/10.1016/S0140-6736(21)02178-4

Gagliardi, A. R., Kothari, A., & Graham, I. D. (2017). Research agenda for integrated knowledge translation (IKT) in healthcare: What we know and do not yet know. *Journal of Epidemiology and Community Health (1979), 71*(2), 105–106. https://doi.org/10.1136/jech-2016-207743

Gagliardi, A. R., Webster, F., & Straus, S. E. (2015). Designing a knowledge translation mentorship program to support the implementation of evidence-based innovations. *BMC Health Services Research, 15*(1), 198. https://doi.org/10.1186/s12913-015-0863-7

Graham, I. D., Kothari, A., Alvarez, G., Banner, D., Botti, M., Bucknall, T., Botting, I., Considine, J., Duke, M., Dunn, S., Dunning, T., Gagliardi, A., Gainforth, H., Gifford, W., Harlos, K., Horsley, T., Hutchinson, A., Kastner, M., Kreindler, S., ... Tetroe, J. (2018). Moving knowledge into action for more effective practice, programmes and policy: Protocol for a research programme on integrated knowledge translation. *Implementation Science, 13,* 22. https://doi.org/10.1186/s13012-017-0700-y

Greenhalgh, T., & Papoutsi, C. (2018). Studying complexity in health services research: Desperately seeking an overdue paradigm shift. *BMC Medicine, 16*(1), 95–95. https://doi.org/10.1186/s12916-018-1089-4

Greenhalgh, T., Robert, G., Macfarlane, F., Bate, P., & Kyriakidou, O. (2004). Diffusion of innovations in service organizations: Systematic review and recommendations. *The Milbank Quarterly, 82*(4), 581–629. https://doi.org/10.1111/j.0887-378X.2004.00325.x

Harvey, G., & Kitson, A. (2016). PARIHS revisited: From heuristic to integrated framework for the successful implementation of knowledge into practice. *Implementation Science: IS, 11*(1), 33–33. https://doi.org/10.1186/s13012-016-0398-2

Khoury, M. J., Gwinn, M., & Ioannidis, J. P. A. (2010). The emergence of translational epidemiology: From scientific discovery to population health impact. *American Journal of Epidemiology, 172*(5), 517–524. https://doi.org/10.1093/aje/kwq211

Kitson, A., & Bisby, M. (2008). *Speeding up the spread: Putting KT research into practice and developing an integrated KT collaborative research agenda.* Alberta Heritage Foundation for Medical Research.

Kitson, A., Brook, A., Harvey, G., Jordan, Z., Marshall, R., O'Shea, R., & Wilson, D. (2018). Using complexity and network concepts to inform healthcare knowledge translation.

International Journal of Health Policy and Management, 7(3), 231–243. https://doi.org/10.15171/ijhpm.2017.79

Kitson, A., O'Shea, R., Brook, A., Harvey, G., Jordan, Z., Marshall, R., & Wilson, D. (2018). The knowledge translation complexity network (KTCN) model: The whole is greater than the sum of the parts – A response to recent commentaries. *International Journal of Health Policy and Management*, 7(8), 768–770. https://doi.org/10.15171/ijhpm.2018.49

Kothari, A., McCutcheon, C., & Graham, I. D. (2017). Defining integrated knowledge translation and moving forward: A response to recent commentaries. *International Journal of Health Policy and Management*, 6(5), 299–300. https://doi.org/10.15171/ijhpm.2017.15

Krause, J., Croft, D. P., & James, R. (2007). Social network theory in the behavioural sciences: Potential applications. *Behavioral Ecology and Sociobiology*, 62(1), 15–27. https://doi.org/10.1007/s00265-007-0445-8

Lucylynn, L., Zoe, J., Ecushla, L., & Craig, L. (2025). Concept analysis of health research translation nomenclature. *BMJ Open Quality*, 14(1), e002904. https://doi.org/10.1136/bmjoq-2024-002904

Mallidou, A. A., Atherton, P., Chan, L., Frisch, N., Glegg, S., & Scarrow, G. (2018). Core knowledge translation competencies: A scoping review. *BMC Health Services Research*, 18(1), 502–502. https://doi.org/10.1186/s12913-018-3314-4

Marshall, B. J., & Warren, J. R. (1984). Unidentified curved bacilli in the stomach of patients with gastritis and peptic ulceration. *Lancet*, 1(8390), 1311–1315. https://doi.org/10.1016/s0140-6736(84)91816-6

Matson, L. (2022). *Into the archives: The story of HPV and cervical cancer*. Cancer Research UK. Retrieved 2 September from https://news.cancerresearchuk.org/2022/11/21/into-the-archives-the-story-of-hpv-and-cervical-cancer/

May, C. R., Johnson, M., & Finch, T. (2016). Implementation, context and complexity. *Implementation Science: IS*, 11(1), 141–141. https://doi.org/10.1186/s13012-016-0506-3

National Health and Medical Research Council. (2018). *Australian code for responsible conduct of research*. Commonwealth of Australia. www.nhmrc.gov.au/guidelines/publications/r41

Nguyen, T., Graham, I. D., Mrklas, K. J., Bowen, S., Cargo, M., Estabrooks, C. A., Kothari, A., Lavis, J., MacAulay, A. C., MacLeod, M., Phipps, D., Ramsden, V. R., Renfrew, M. J., Salsberg, J., & Wallerstein, N. (2020). How does integrated knowledge translation (IKT) compare to other collaborative research approaches to generating and translating knowledge? Learning from experts in the field. *Health Research Policy and Systems*, 18(1), 35–35. https://doi.org/10.1186/s12961-020-0539-6

Plsek, P. E., & Greenhalgh, T. (2001). Complexity science: The challenge of complexity in health care. *BMJ*, 323(7313), 625–628. https://doi.org/10.1136/bmj.323.7313.625

Ryan, B., & Gross, N. C. (1943). The diffusion of hybrid seed corn in two Iowa communities. *Rural Sociology*, 8(1), 15–24.

Skivington, K., Matthews, L., Simpson, S. A., Craig, P., Baird, J., & Blazeby, J. (2021). A new framework for developing and evaluating complex interventions: Update of Medical Research Council guidance. *BMJ*, 374, n2061.

Squires, J. E., Graham, I., Bashir, K., Nadalin-Penno, L., Lavis, J., Francis, J., Curran, J., Grimshaw, J. M., Brehaut, J., Ivers, N., Michie, S., Hillmer, M., Noseworthy, T., Vine, J., Demery Varin, M., Aloisio, L. D., Coughlin, M., & Hutchinson, A. M. (2019). Understanding context: A concept analysis. *Journal of Advanced Nursing*, 75(12), 3448–3470. https://doi.org/10.1111/jan.14165

Straus, S. E., Tetroe, J., & Graham, I. D. (2013). *Knowledge translation in health care: Moving from evidence to practice* (2 ed.). Wiley.

Sung, N. S., Crowley, W. F., Genel, M., Salber, P., Sandy, L., Sherwood, L. M., Johnson, S. B., Catanese, V., Tilson, H., Getz, K., Larson, E. L., Scheinberg, D., Reece, E. A., Slavkin, H., Dobs, A., Grebb, J., Martinez, R. A., Korn, A., & Rimoin, D. (2003). Central challenges facing the national clinical research enterprise. *JAMA: The Journal of the American Medical Association*, 289(10), 1278–1287. https://doi.org/10.1001/jama.289.10.1278

Van de Ven, A. H. (2007). *Engaged scholarship: A guide for organizational and social research.* Oxford University Press.

Warren, J. R., & Marshall, B. (1983). Unidentified curved bacilli on gastric epithelium in active chronic gastritis. *Lancet, 1*(8336), 1273–1275.

Woolf, S. H. (2008). The meaning of translational research and why it matters. *JAMA: The Journal of the American Medical Association, 299*(2), 211–213. https://doi.org/10.1001/jama.2007.26

World Health Organization. (2020). *Global strategy to accelerate the elimination of cervical cancer as a public health problem.* www.who.int/publications/i/item/9789240014107

World Health Organization, Sheikh, K., Abimbola, S., Alliance for Health, P., & Systems, R. (2021). *Learning health systems: Pathways to progress: Flagship report of the Alliance for Health Policy and Systems Research.* World Health Organization. https://iris.who.int/handle/10665/344891

zur Hausen, H. (1976). Condylomata acuminata and human genital cancer. *Cancer Research, 36*(2 pt 2), 794.

zur Hausen, H. (1977). Human papillomaviruses and their possible role in squamous cell carcinomas. *Current Topics in Microbiology and Immunology, 78*, 1–30. https://doi.org/10.1007/978-3-642-66800-5_1

2 Integrated implementation science

Sarah Hunter and Bo Kim

Introduction

When researchers come across knowledge translation it is generally because they are seeking guidance and support on how they can best get their evidence or innovation into the real-world, as they believe they can make a difference. Alternatively, practitioners and clinicians come across knowledge translation as they have identified a problem or have an idea for improvement in their practice, and they want guidance and support on how they can find and implement evidence-based solutions. Whether you come to knowledge translation from a solution- or problem-oriented starting point, your key goal is to get a 'thing' into practice (Curran, 2020). Implementation science is a specific field of research that aims to provide that guidance and support by developing and testing scientific methods that promote the uptake and sustained use of evidence-based innovations in routine practice.

Therefore, implementation science is considered the rigorous approach to reducing the 'evidence to practice gap'. It is commonly viewed as a linear process or a step that fits within the research process. From a researcher perspective, Figure 2.1 depicts a simplified representation of how implementation science fits into the research process.

From a practitioner or clinician perspective, Figure 2.2 depicts a simplified representation of how implementation science fits into the quality improvement process.

In the Caring Futures Institute, we take a different approach to implementation science. In Chapter 1, we introduced integrated knowledge translation and how we are embedding it into the Caring Futures Institute. We discussed our perspective of integrated knowledge translation and the Knowledge Translation Complexity Network Model which involves us adopting a complexity-informed approach to doing knowledge translation. We recognised that our ultimate goal of embedding integrated knowledge translation within the Caring

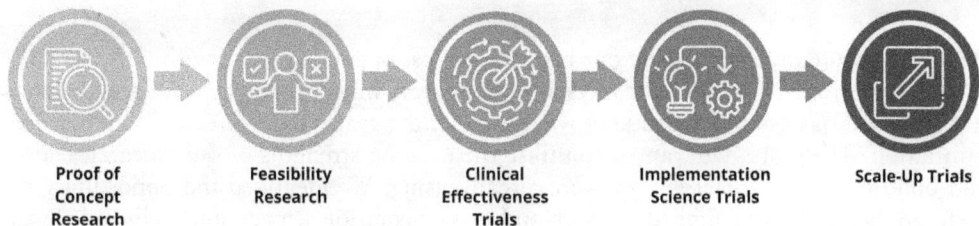

| Proof of Concept Research | Feasibility Research | Clinical Effectiveness Trials | Implementation Science Trials | Scale-Up Trials |

Figure 2.1 Implementation science within the research process from a researcher perspective.
Source: https://doi.org/10.25451/flinders.29192609.v1

DOI: 10.4324/9781003245995-3

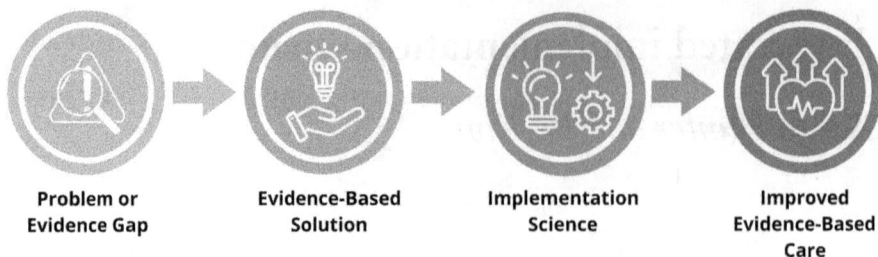

Figure 2.2 Implementation science within the research process from a clinician perspective.
Source: https://doi.org/10.25451/flinders.29192612.v1

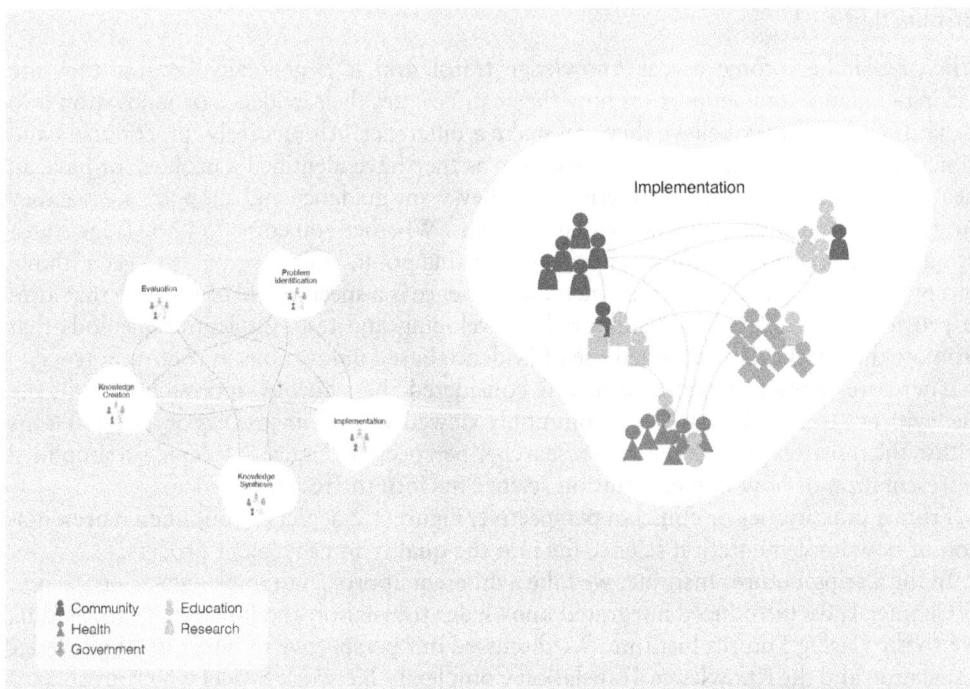

Figure 2.3 The Caring Futures Institute view of implementation science within integrated knowledge translation.
Source: https://doi.org/10.25451/flinders.29192621.v1

Futures Institute involved asking our research teams, in collaboration with our partners, to approach research in different ways and adopt new ways of working. We realised this was an ambitious ask and we did not want to deter our teams from integrated knowledge translation. Therefore, we wanted to utilise the existing strengths of our research teams and build on the approaches they were already using. We identified the opportunity to build on their skillset in applied research and implementation science, and to introduce an integrated knowledge translation lens to achieve this.

Figure 2.3 depicts our view of how implementation science is a research process that fits into the broader integrated knowledge translation process. We do not view implementation science as fitting into a linear process or being an isolated step in the process. Rather, utilising implementation science methodology is one research process that needs to be utilised alongside the research processes identified within the knowledge translation complexity network model (Kitson et al., 2018): problem identification, knowledge creation, knowledge synthesis, and evaluation.

Therefore, in this chapter we will provide a concise overview of implementation science. We will aim to share and explore how we have built on the skillset of our teams who have experience in applied research and implementation science and how we have worked with them in order to shift their thinking and practice from linear approaches to a more integrated approach.

What is implementation science?

It is important to establish an understanding of what implementation science is, how it fits within knowledge translation, and why it is important.

To implement evidence into health and social care is unpredictable, slow, and haphazard and can take several years, or may never happen at all. Foundational research has documented that it can take up to 17–20 years to get evidence into practice and fewer than 50% of clinical innovations make it into practice at all (Bauer & Kirchner, 2020; Morris et al., 2011). A significant amount of time and resources are invested into the production of high quality research evidence that could be of benefit to patients, providers, and society, cost effective, and could better use limited resources (Gagliardi et al., 2017; Straus, Tetroe, et al., 2009, Straus, Tetzlaff, et al., 2009; Wensing & Grol, 2019). But, there remains a consistent underuse, overuse, or misuse of research evidence in policy and practice and the delivery of care is not always in line with the best available evidence (Bauer & Kirchner, 2020).

The field of implementation science was specifically created to address the divide between evidence and practice and optimise the process of getting evidence into practice. Implementation science has been defined in several ways that are consistent with the definition put forward in the inaugural issue of the journal, Implementation Science: "… the scientific study of methods to promote the systematic uptake of research findings and other evidence-based practice into routine practice and, hence, to improve the quality and effectiveness of health services." (Eccles & Mittman, 2006, p.1). Hence the goal of implementation science is to maximise the health impact of a clinical innovation by identifying the factors that affect its uptake into routine use and by developing, testing, and refining strategies that account for those factors in successfully translating knowledge into practice (Bauer & Kirchner, 2020).

To support rigorous, systematic, and successful implementation, the field of implementation science has three key phases of implementation. These are: 1) pre-implementation planning, 2) conducting implementation with theories, models, and frameworks, and 3) evaluation (Handley et al., 2016). Below we provide an overview of each phase, and the activities involved within them.

Pre-implementation planning

Pre-implementation planning is the phase prior to conducting implementation (Handley et al., 2016). Pre-implementation planning requires you to think through and develop an approach for the who, what, when, where, why, and how of your implementation project.

Who involves identifying who you need to work with and who the key people are and engaging with them early to ensure you have a shared understanding of what the project is going to be. **What** involves you identifying what piece of evidence you are implementing into practice. **When** involves you identifying when the project will commence and the duration of your implementation period (e.g., 6 months, 12 months, 18 months, etc.). **Where** firstly involves you identifying if this project is being conducted in one site, multiple sites in one organisation, or multiple sites across multiple organisations. Identifying the sites will then lead to you needing to generate an understanding of the context of these sites and how the varying contexts of different sites may influence your implementation process. This may include a formalised context assessment that can aid in selecting implementation strategies to be used in the implementation process. Arguably, the most important thing to think through is your **why**. **Why** involves understanding why you are implementing evidence into practice and ensuring that everyone involved understands and agrees on this. People involved may have different perspectives on what the problem is and what needs to be addressed to overcome this problem, therefore having different perspectives on the why, can impact on implementation success. Taking the time to understand why and ensuring you have not missed key perspectives, will greatly improve implementation outcomes. So, then the **how** involves you identifying the appropriate implementation framework that will guide the process and specifying the details of the process. Ultimately, the information you gain from the who, what, when, where, and why will aid in you identifying and selecting a how.

Finally, to support clarity of the plan and to ensure that all aspects have been appropriately considered, implementation logic models are critical. Logic models are graphic depictions of what is going to be done, how it is going to happen, what is going to be impacted, and the intended outcomes. Logic models therefore provide a theory of action and a theory of change (Funnell & Rogers, 2011). An example includes the Implementation Research Logic Model which was developed to support the operationalisation of the complex process of implementation, this logic model can be seen in Figure 2.4.

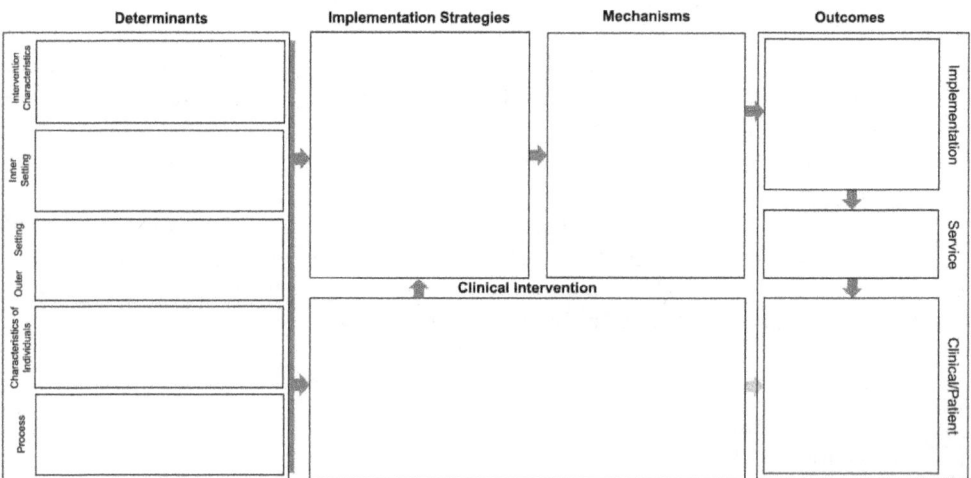

Figure 2.4 The Implementation Research Logic Model.
Source: Smith et al. (2020).

Conducting implementation: theories, models, and frameworks

The second phase is the 'doing' phase where you conduct implementation guided by implementation theories, models, and frameworks. Implementation science promotes a systematic approach and has thus dedicated years to studying which actions and processes aid in moving evidence into practice, why, and how. To harness this expertise, utilise implementation theories, models, and frameworks that have been developed, used, and tested. There are over 100 theories, models, and frameworks available (Birken et al., 2017), and they differ in their purpose due to the underpinning theories and the conceptual level in which they focus. They can offer guidance to 1) predict or guide the implementation process, 2) organise, understand, or explain factors that influence implementation, and 3) evaluate the implementation success (or failure) (Lynch et al., 2018; Nilsen, 2015; Presseau et al., 2022). They can be organised into five categories: process models, determinant frameworks, implementation theories, classic theories, and evaluation frameworks (Nilsen & Birken, 2020).

- **Process models** specify steps, stages, or phases in the process of implementing evidence into practice. The aim of process models is to describe or guide the process.
- **Determinant frameworks** specify domains or constructs which act as barriers or enablers that influence the implementation process or outcome. The aim is to understand, explain or predict influences on implementation outcomes.
- **Implementation theories** are theories which have been developed by implementation researchers. The aim is to provide an understanding or explanation of aspects of implementation.
- **Classic theories** are theories which have originated from fields external to implementation science. The aim is to apply these theories to provide an understanding or explanation of aspects of implementation.
- **Evaluation frameworks** specify outcomes that can be evaluated to determine implementation success.

Examples of commonly used theories, models and frameworks and which category they are, can be seen in Table 2.1.

Table 2.1 Types of commonly used theories, models, and frameworks

Theory, Model or Framework	Type of framework
Theory of Diffusion (Rogers, 2003)	Classic theory
Knowledge to Action (Graham et al., 2006)	Process model
Normalisation Process Theory (May & Finch, 2009)	Implementation theory
Theoretical Domains Framework (Cane et al., 2012; Michie et al., 2005)	Determinant framework
RE-AIM (Glasgow et al., 2006; Glasgow et al., 1999)	Evaluation framework
Consolidated Framework for Implementation Research (Damschroder et al., 2009)	Determinant framework
Integrated-Promoting Action on Research Implementation in Health Services framework (i-PARIHS; Harvey & Alison Kitson, 2016; Kitson et al., 1998)	Determinant framework

Evaluation

The third phase of implementation is evaluation. Implementation science is dedicated toward evaluating implementation interventions and strategies. Evaluation is critical for identifying if what you have done has worked. Your evaluation should focus on a few different components including: 1) understanding the process of implementation, 2) identifying barriers and enablers of change, and 3) outcomes. There are different approaches to evaluation to support these components, including:

- **Formative evaluation** ensures that a program or program activity is feasible, appropriate, and acceptable before it is implemented. It is usually conducted early on in a program to provide key information to implementers on how successful it is going to be, and to identify any barriers or enablers to implementation. This type of evaluation can be used to inform tailoring and adaptations along the way to enhance implementation success.
- **Process evaluation** focuses on understanding how a program or intervention was implemented, aiming to understand whether it was implemented as intended, that the intended outcomes were achieved, and the mechanisms of effect.
- **Outcome evaluation** measures whether the program impacted the target population by assessing outcomes that the program addresses.
- **Economic evaluation** examines the costs and consequences of implementing a program. One such evaluation is cost-benefit analysis, which comparatively assesses the costs of delivering a program with the outcomes of the program in monetary units. This allows you to identify, measure, value, and compare the costs and consequences of different programs. Another example is a cost-utility analysis in which costs of delivering a program are compared to a standardised unit of benefit that incorporates quality of life.

In addition to these broad evaluation approaches, dedicated implementation evaluation methods have been developed. Introduced by Curran et al. (2012) are effectiveness-implementation hybrid designs. In this seminal work, Curran et al. (2012) outline three trial designs, which are summarised in Table 2.2.

Implementation science and knowledge translation

We have provided a brief overview of implementation science and the phases of implementation. It is a specific and dedicated field to support the implementation of evidence into practice. Knowledge translation, by comparison, is a broader term referring to the process of generating, synthesising, and applying evidence within complex systems of relationships (Khalil, 2016). Implementation science and knowledge translation differ but are not mutually exclusive. This is evident through some implementation science theories, models, and frameworks also functioning as knowledge translation frameworks. For example, the Knowledge to Action framework is described by the developers as both an implementation and knowledge translation model (Rycroft-Malone & Bucknall, 2010). Similarly, the i-PARIHS framework (Harvey & Kitson, 2016) is an implementation-determinant framework, however, the facilitation construct allows for

Table 2.2 Hybrid trial designs

Hybrid Trial Design	Definition	Example of when you would use
Hybrid Type 1	Testing clinical effectiveness and gathering information on implementation	When you are implementing a brand-new innovation, your primary concern is with testing the clinical effectiveness. However, you want to learn about the implementation barriers and enablers to inform future implementation efforts.
Hybrid Type 2	Equally testing both clinical and implementation effectiveness	When you are implementing a complex intervention that bundles multiple clinically effective components and thus requires multi-faceted implementation strategies, you are equally concerned with testing clinical effectiveness and implementation effectiveness.
Hybrid Type 3	Testing implementation effectiveness and gathering information on clinical outcomes	When you are implementing an innovation that you know is clinically effective, but you want to implement into a new setting or at scale, your primary concern is with testing the implementation effectiveness. However, you want to collect clinical data to ensure your implementation approach did not impact the clinical effectiveness.

flexible application, lending its use across all phases of research. Within the Caring Futures Institute, we view implementation science as a rigorous research process that fits within the broader knowledge translation approach. Below we share our learnings and aim to demonstrate how we have supported our teams to view implementation science as part of integrated knowledge translation.

What we have learned

We have had many learnings through supporting our teams within the Caring Futures Institute to use implementation science and building their capacity and journey toward using implementation science within a broader integrated knowledge translation approach. In the previous section, we outlined the phases of implementation. However, what we aim to demonstrate in this section, is that whilst it is critical to have a logic model that outlines your working theory of change and theory of action, when undertaking knowledge translation, you cannot work through the phases of planning, doing, and evaluating neatly. The reality of implementation requires you to undertake many flexible cycles of planning, doing, and evaluation to see your theory of change and action come to fruition. This is why we position the rigor of implementation science as a critical tool within integrated knowledge translation.

Below we share some of our key learnings. We present these as the learnings that pertain to 1) doing implementation and 2) implementation through an integrated knowledge translation lens. We share case studies from our teams within the Caring Futures Institute to illustrate these learnings.

Implementation learnings

Planning is key

To successfully undertake an implementation project, pre-implementation planning is key. This is an important phase in the research project where you can set yourself up for success. However, this is usually the phase that is underestimated and overlooked, often because people are excited to get started and want to make a difference immediately. When writing a funding application or a project protocol generally the focus is too heavily weighted on the resources and time needed to 'do' the project. However, much more focus is required on the pre-implementation planning to allow time to understand the context and the people involved, and tailor the implementation approach.

Every piece of research and every project require detailed but adaptable planning. This notion of planning is not a new or novel concept. Research projects do not spontaneously come into being. However, planning for an implementation project requires specific preparatory tasks that may not be as emphasized in other types of research. For example, an implementation project is undertaken in close collaboration with clinical or practice partners. If you are a researcher and want to move evidence into practice, you will need to work in partnership with a practice site (or multiple sites). If you are a clinician and want to move evidence into your practice, working in partnership with a researcher (or multiple researchers) can help systematise your approach. Building these relationships and partnerships takes time.

This process of pre-implementation planning can be an informal process of developing relationships with your **who** and working with them to select the **what** and the **when** and they will help you understand the context of the **where** and the **why**, all of which will lead to the selection of your **how**. It can also be a systematic examination of the **who, what, when, where, why, and how,** that contributes to the science of implementation and is published as research.

A pre-implementation research project can be seen in the case study in Box 2.1. This team wrapped a rigorous research process around their pre-implementation planning to understand clinician and service-related barriers.

Case study 1, in Box 2.1, illustrates the value of taking a structured, implementation science-informed approach when uptake of evidence proves more complicated than anticipated. As the team discovered, early, well-intentioned efforts based on introducing guidelines and collaboration faltered when they underestimated contextual factors like workforce turnover and staff confidence. They then shifted focus to systematically unpacking the barriers and enablers, demonstrating the importance of implementation planning in navigating complexity, especially for early-career researchers learning to balance best available evidence with on-the-ground realities.

Box 2.1 *Case study 1* **Pre-implementation planning**

The acute recovery phase of traumatic brain injury involves a period of behavioural changes, commonly referred to as "challenging behaviours" (Marshman et al., 2013; Ponsford et al., 2021). Evidence-informed care for patients with acute traumatic brain injury experiencing challenging behaviours should encompass a multi-disciplinary, comprehensive approach with regular assessment of behaviour change; non-pharmacological management interventions; followed by pharmacological treatments if required (Bayley et al., 2016; Flanagan et al., 2009; Luauté et al., 2016). However, implementation of evidence-informed traumatic brain injury care is limited by variability in care practices, lack of rigorous research, and gaps in clinicians' knowledge and skills (Callender et al., 2017).

Recognising the importance of improving patient care, we dived into action and collaborated with clinicians working at two acute hospital settings to develop and implement a traumatic brain injury behaviour management approach for consistent identification of challenging behaviours, and a guide to management strategies (Block et al., 2022). Although the uptake of the traumatic brain injury behaviour management approach was initially high, this was not sustained after the evaluation period. It was evident there were multiple factors that influenced why the implemented approach was not sustained, including the rotational hospital workforce, staffing attitudes, limited skills, and knowledge. We reflected that we had not considered or thought through these factors prior to implementation, leading us to realise that implementation of evidence-informed care in this area of practice would require more than a guideline for consistency and occasional education sessions. We needed to comprehensively understand the barriers to implementing innovations for acute traumatic brain injury behaviour management; but also what factors could help inform better care.

We then set upon a program of research to focus on comprehensive preimplementation planning to identify factors relating to the evidence and guidelines, organisational, system and individual contextual factors, underpinned by the i-PARIHS framework (Harvey & Kitson, 2016). The innovation was examined through reviews of evidence (Block et al., 2021) and clinical practice guidelines (Block, Paul, et al., 2023). The recipients were the staff, patients, and families. Staff and service-related barriers and enablers were explored through focus groups with staff experienced in working with patients with traumatic brain injury (Block, Bellon, et al., 2023). We also needed to understand the perspectives of families on traumatic brain injury behaviour management in the acute setting, to explore the multifaceted individual, ward based, organisational barriers, therefore, we also conducted interviews with family members (Block et al., 2024). These studies highlighted the intricate difficulties in identifying and managing challenging behaviours; balancing safety, risk, patient-centred care; with a transient and rotational acute workforce; limited skills and experience of clinicians working in complex hospital environments that are overstimulating that trigger challenging behaviours, and the need for education and support to families. Further exploration of the context was conducted with a survey highlighting acute staffs' uncertainty in their knowledge and confidence in providing care to patients, and an audit of current practice demonstrating variability in care.

By understanding these barriers, enablers and contextual factors, we could then select the appropriate implementation strategies (Kirchner et al., 2020; Tucker et al., 2021) that could be targeted and tailored to promote successful and sustained implementation of evidence-informed practice and improvements for traumatic brain injury behaviour management relevant to the acute hospital context.

Along the way, we learnt that implementation of complex interventions in complex contexts requires thorough planning at multiple levels guided by an implementation framework to systematically assess and organize all relevant factors.

Author: Heather Block
Acknowledgements: Sarah Hunter, Stacey George, Michelle Bellon
Funded by the Lifetime Support Authority of South Australia

Selecting implementation theories, models, and frameworks

It is critical to select an appropriate 'how'. Many projects that implement evidence into practice may select an implementation strategy, such as education or training. However, there are many potential strategies to choose from. To help choose a strategy (or a combination of strategies) that is most appropriate for the particular evidence that you are looking to put into practice, especially given the specific contexts of your implementation sites, it is recommended that you select an implementation theory, model, or framework that is going to underpin what you do.

We have learnt that there is no such thing as the 'best' theory, model, or framework. Rather, selection of the 'right' approach is based on selecting the 'right' one for your project. To make the most of a theory, model, or framework, it is important to have a clear rationale and understanding for selecting it. An example of how teams can select a theory, model, or framework can be seen in the case study in Box 2.2. This case study highlights the importance of selecting an approach that aligns to the characteristics of the project. As described earlier in the chapter, there are many different implementation theories, models, and frameworks, and they vary in their purpose and guidance that they offer. To appropriately select a theory, model, or framework for your project, it can be useful to seek out support. Development and use of tools to help identify theories, models, or frameworks most relevant to specific implementation efforts are actively underway. For example, the Dissemination and Implementation Models in Health website hosts an interactive webtool to help you select and use implementation theories, models, and frameworks: https://dissemination-implementation.org/tool/. There are also various articles that have been published to support selection of theories, models, and frameworks, for example Birken et al. (2017), Lynch et al. (2018), and Moullin et al. (2020).

Case study 2, in Box 2.2, shows how thoughtful selection of theories, models, and frameworks can strengthen the design and equity of an implementation strategy. Faced with no single theory, model, or framework that addressed both structural and digital equity considerations, the team combined CFIR and the Digital Health Equity Framework to complexity of continuous glucose monitoring implementation in a large health system. Their approach demonstrates the value of a deliberate tailoring, especially implementing innovations with both technical demands and equity implications.

Box 2.2 *Case study* 2 Selecting a theory, model, or framework

To prevent undesirable health outcomes associated with diabetes, blood glucose levels must be maintained within a narrow target range. However, less than 60% of adults with diabetes successfully manage their glucose levels to be within the target range (Wang et al., 2021). Patients with type 2 diabetes mellitus (T2D), 1.2 million of whom are military veterans receiving United States Department of Veterans Affairs health care (Mahtta et al., 2020), are increasingly recommended to use continuous glucose monitoring (ElSayed et al., 2023; Fonseca et al., 2016; Klonoff et al., 2011), which is a notable innovation for glucose management. According to professional society guidelines for continuous glucose monitoring use, patients must learn both technical aspects about the device and how to interpret and respond to the data, and clinicians must learn to determine patients' eligibility as well as train and counsel them based on the data (Fonseca et al., 2016).

Concrete and integrated strategies to implement these important patient- and clinician-driven processes are currently lacking, which is concerning given that a substantially larger number of Veterans Affairs patients with T2D are eligible for continuous glucose monitoring since 2023. Implementation without clear and appropriate strategies, especially without strategies that account for social determinants of health relevant to racial and ethnic disparities, may critically impede equitable uptake and effective use of continuous glucose monitoring by eligible patients. Thus, our goal was to support the uptake, effectiveness, and health equity surrounding Veterans Affairs continuous glucose monitoring implementation by developing, piloting, and evaluating through mixed methods a continuous glucose monitoring implementation strategy bundle.

In seeking a conceptual framework to guide our study, we prioritized several characteristics that we wanted the framework to have. We wanted a framework that A) has specific operational definitions for its constructs and subconstructs, B) explicitly accounts for individual- to system-level factors that impact implementation, C) is associated with pre-developed tools and examples of their usage that we can adapt for our purposes, D) represents unique considerations surrounding implementation of technology-based (e.g., digital) innovations such as continuous glucose monitoring, and E) incorporates concepts related to health equity.

We consulted both the Theory, Model, and Framework Comparison and Selection Tool (T-CaST) (https://impsci.tracs.unc.edu/tcast/) and the Dissemination & Implementation Models Webtool (https://dissemination-implementation.org/) and found that no one framework alone could meet all our criteria. The Consolidated Framework for Implementation Research (CFIR) (Damschroder et al., 2009) met Criteria A-C and the Digital Health Equity Framework (DHEF) (Crawford & Serhal, 2020) met Criteria D-E. We thus decided to use a combination of the two – i.e., a DHEF-enhanced CFIR – as our guiding conceptual framework.

In bringing the two frameworks together, we determined the CFIR constructs for which we draw on DHEF to make explicit the construct's focus for our use. For example, we specified CFIR's "Policies and Laws" construct under its "Outer Setting" domain using DHEF's "National Digital Health Policy" and "Digital Health Governance" constructs under its "Health System as Digital Determinant of Health" domain. Another example under these same respective domains is that we specified CFIR's "financing" construct using DHEF's "digital health funding" construct.

By using both CFIR and DHEF, we were able to take advantage of each framework's strengths. For example, CFIR encompasses a large collection of factors associated with innovation implementation that we can consider (such as a patient's motivation to use an innovation), while DHEF makes it possible for us to specify those factors to be more directly relevant to continuous glucose monitoring as a digital innovation (such as a patient's motivation to use continuous glucose monitoring depending on how valuable they perceive continuous glucose monitoring to be).

Author: Bo Kim
Acknowledgements: Varsha Vimalananda, MD, MPH

Evaluation

The final key learning is to think of the end goal or the **so what** at the beginning. You need to decide early on what success will look like and how you are going to evaluate whether you have been successful. Evaluation plans for implementation projects can focus primarily on whether the **thing** was implemented and sustained, more than on whether the implemented thing worked. It is therefore important to build into your project plan, measures and data collection that will allow you to answer if your implementation was successful.

There are some key considerations that often only become front of mind at the **post-implementation phase**. However, it is important to recognise that everything we have discussed in this chapter are things that need to be considered in the **pre-implementation phase**. Hopefully you think of, and plan for, these things prior to the post-implementation phase. However, a key thing that you will want to know in the post-implementation phase is – were we successful? Evaluation is critical for determining if you have successfully implemented. It is important to be clear on the distinction between evaluation of the evidence and evaluation of the implementation process. Evaluation of the evidence draws on traditional effectiveness evaluation processes. This is where the focus is on testing whether the evidence or the **thing** works. Evaluation of the implementation process, however, is on evaluating whether the evidence was implemented as intended. This is where the focus is on measuring whether people are using the evidence or doing the **thing**. Proctor identified a taxonomy of implementation outcomes that can be evaluated, and these include acceptability, adoption, appropriateness, feasibility, fidelity, implementation cost, penetration, and sustainability (Proctor et al., 2011). Leveraging the field of implementation science will aid in developing a strong study design to ensure that you are clear on what you will measure as your indicators of success, the implementation theory, model, or framework that will best suit your project, the data you collect, and the resources and skills you require to undertake the evaluation.

Implementation learnings from an integrated knowledge translation perspective

Flexibility

In reality, implementation requires a lot of flexibility. It is important to be aware and accept that things will not go to plan. Despite the emphasis within implementation science on the importance of pre-implementation planning, conducting implementation in the real-world, means that many contextual and recipient factors will influence your project, and they will often be completely out of your control. This is why we believe viewing and approaching implementation through an integrated knowledge translation lens will provide you with the support and reassurance to navigate complexity and the flexibility required. An example of how this can look in practice is in the case study in Box 2.3.

Box 2.3 *Case study 3* Conducting implementation

Our experience of conducting implementation is a great example of something that may appear simple, actually, being incredibly difficult to implement due to the multi-level barriers that are at play.

Our project was a partnership between a university, a hospital, and a state-wide dental service and focused on implementing clinical guideline recommendations for oral healthcare for older adults in one geriatric evaluation and management ward in an acute hospital (Lewis et al., 2022; Murray et al., 2024; Murray et al., 2022). This project was a pilot Hybrid Type 2 (Curran et al., 2012) trial where we collected both clinical effectiveness and implementation outcomes.

Older adults are at high risk of poor oral health status, with caries, periodontal disease, and tooth loss prevalent in this cohort (Gil-Montoya et al., 2015). Poor oral health, in turn, carries an increased risk of systemic infection and malnutrition and therefore impacts older people's overall health (Scannapieco & Shay, 2014), psychological health, quality of life and wellbeing (Ohi et al., 2022). Many common oral health problems in older people can be prevented or managed by providing evidence-based oral healthcare and timely dental referral (Council of Australian Governments Health Council, 2016; Janssens et al., 2016; Lewis et al., 2016). A pivotal timepoint to instigate such intervention may be when an older adult is hospitalized, particularly when admitted to a specialist geriatric unit.

Unfortunately, the potential for oral healthcare intervention in healthcare institutions is often not realized; oral healthcare is described as one of the most missed aspects of fundamental care in hospital (Bail & Grealish, 2016; Kalisch et al., 2009).

Improving oral healthcare for older people in the acute care setting requires a multifaceted, interprofessional strategy underpinned by implementation science and knowledge translation principles (Hunter et al., 2020). Therefore, this project used the integrated-Promoting Action on Research Implementation in Health Services (i-PARIHS) framework (Harvey & Kitson, 2015) to inform implementation of an oral healthcare intervention in one acute geriatric unit.

i-PARIHS was used to assess the context and recipients at multiple timepoints and informed a multi-level facilitation approach. The multi-level facilitation approach navigated individuals and teams through the complex change processes involved, both at the local ward level and system wide level, and the contextual challenges encountered. Facilitation included two internal novice facilitators (one nurse and one speech pathologist), four external experienced facilitators (based at the university and dental service) and an external expert facilitator (based at the university). This facilitation team were supported by a project reference group that included various staff at the hospital in leadership roles.

The facilitation approach allowed for an examination of baseline oral healthcare practice, identification of gaps against clinical guideline recommendations, and the development of multi-disciplinary team strategies to implement and sustain evidence-based practice. The facilitation approach also allowed the project team to build hospital workforce capacity to undertake future implementation projects, inclusive of undertaking context assessments and tailoring evidence and implementation strategies.

Overall, we were able to successfully foster collaboration between clinical teams, hospital management and researchers to identify the gaps in current oral healthcare practice and improve awareness and attitudes of staff. However, while a suite of multilevel and multidisciplinary implementation strategies was designed to improve and sustain adherence to evidence-based oral healthcare, we were not able to show a change in clinical practice in terms of multidisciplinary oral healthcare improvements for individual patients within the timeframes of the project. This finding is consistent with other studies, which similarly concluded that, although oral healthcare may seem deceptively simple in terms of fundamental care provision, hospital staff often struggle to provide consistent and effective daily oral healthcare (Baker & Quinn, 2018; Kitson et al., 2014; Munro & Baker, 2018; National Health Service, 2019).

The biggest barrier to success within this project related to the active implementation period coinciding with the height of the COVID-19 pandemic where the organisation needed to pivot to address the state-wide emergency. In particular, staff at the forefront of care needed to upskill immediately about airborne disease and personal protective equipment and procedures. This context made it particularly difficult to prioritise and focus on oral healthcare. To adjust to the pressure placed on staff during this time, we pivoted from trying to bring our clinical partners along in the bigger picture co-design approach and instead focused on small actions that would make a noticeable difference to patients and support staff engagement and enthusiasm.

Upon reflection, despite the challenges and modifications, we do not view this project as a 'failure' but rather a huge success. Despite not seeing any immediate clinical improvement the iterative and facilitated approach taken in this project was viewed as a success and is now being rolled out across the entire health network. Further, the best practice guidelines we used in the project have now been adopted as a recommendation for all acute hospitals by the National Safety and Quality Commission of Australia.

Author: Joanne Murray
Acknowledgements: Adrienne Lewis, Sarah Hunter, Tiffany Conroy, Alison Kitson, Zita Splawinski, Debbie Courage, Amanda Challen-Jordan, Heather Block

Case study 3, in Box 2.3, shows how seemingly straightforward aspects of care like oral healthcare can lead to big implementation challenges when embedded in complex healthcare settings. The project shows how facilitation using the i-PARIHS framework supported a shift in awareness, relationship-building, and system-level engagement, even in the face of significant disruptions during the COVID-19 pandemic. Although immediate clinical improvements were not realised, the broader system-level impacts demonstrate that success in knowledge translation can take many forms often extending beyond the original project timeline.

You will need to have a plan for how you will manage modifications or tailoring your strategies to the local or wider context. Unlike traditional clinical trials or randomised controlled trials where the focus is on reducing bias and ensuring conditions are uniform, implementation projects are flexible and responsive to the real-world conditions, as the goal is to get the evidence embedded into the messiness of the real-world. If you think it is likely there will be changing or evolving factors that may influence how you deliver the intervention, it is important to have a process for identifying, monitoring, and documenting any adaptations or tailoring. Additionally, having flexible approaches to implementation allows for an equitable approach and can result in more equitable outcomes. This is where the selection of an appropriate implementation framework will support you. Some frameworks have embedded flexibility, such as the i-PARIHS framework that has facilitation as the meta-implementation strategy allowing for continual tailoring and iterative cycles of planning, doing, evaluating. This is evident in Case Study 3. Other implementation frameworks provide specific guidance and support for tailoring and adaptions. One example is the Framework for Reporting Adaptations and Modifications to Evidence-Based Interventions (FRAME) (Wiltsey Stirman et al., 2019), and there also exists its analogue FRAME-IS (Miller et al., 2021) for reporting modifications made to implementation strategies.

Partnerships

Partnerships are key for successful implementation. In the context of academia, the following African proverb applies: "if you want to go fast, go alone. If you want to go far, go together". To move evidence beyond academia and into clinical and social practice requires building partnerships with those who we are wanting to use the evidence. It is important, prior to implementation, to engage in a process of mapping who the individuals or groups of individuals are that have an interest in, can affect, be affected by, or perceive themselves to be affected by, the evidence you are wanting to implement into practice (Elwy et al., 2022). Specifically, it is important to engage with the recipients of your implementation efforts. Recipients are those whose actions an implementation effort aims to change – e.g., clinic staff for an implementation project aimed at improving staff's hand hygiene practices in a clinic (Harvey & Kitson, 2015). Before you commence any efforts to implement your evidence, you first need to understand the perspectives of various individuals and recipients. Through understanding their perspectives and experiences, you may achieve more implementation success by learning new information that could influence your implementation approach, understanding additional barriers or enablers that you can account for in implementation strategies that you use, and identifying some key decision makers or champions who can support you in your implementation process.

Identifying who needs to be involved early is crucial, not only as their perspectives and experiences can help in developing your implementation plan, but you also will have a greater understanding of the various individuals, groups, and organisations that will be involved in your project. It is easy to underestimate how much time you need to achieve and maintain these relationships and partnerships; you will need to dedicate time and resources to manage these, and this needs to be built into the project plan. This may be via setting up advisory groups, reference groups, or funding a dedicated project manager. There is no one correct way, and you will need a plan for whichever way you choose. More detail on working in partnership is provided in Chapter 3, however, adopting or framing your implementation project within a broader integrated knowledge translation approach will provide the necessary time and space required to dedicated to building relationships and working in partnership – the relational aspect of doing implementation.

'Success' and sustainability

Often when the 'active' implementation period has ended, the resources and efforts that have supported the implementation process are no longer being provided to the site where implementation occurred. This is a really critical time. Ideally, when planning your project, you have considered how the evidence or program will be sustained in practice following implementation. However, this is something that is often overlooked and is quite confronting when you get to this point. Removing resources and supports from a practice setting can cause rifts in the relationships or leave the practice feeling unsupported or no longer relevant. Embedding strategies for maintenance and sustainability are crucial.

One way to achieve this is through drawing on existing quality improvement processes and routine data collection. Drawing on local systems and processes as part of your implementation approach, as opposed to bringing in resource intensive approaches, will allow for continuous monitoring and evaluation of the program after the project is complete. Another way is through documentation. Clearly documenting the implementation process will enable the local site to maintain knowledge about what the implementation entailed and draw on that knowledge to sustain the program. Having complex, multifaceted strategies that are 'gatekept' offsite at a university and are not clearly documented and shared with the site, will guarantee the program will not be sustained after the project.

Capacity building and local ownership as guiding principles within an implementation project will lead to greater maintenance and sustainability. This links back to the importance of partnerships and viewing implementation through an integrated knowledge translation approach. Viewing the goal as broader than implementation, broader than getting evidence into practice, will drive sustainability. A broader focus on building capacity in the local staff to engage in the evidence-based practice being implemented and to be the drivers of the implementation project, will equip them with the skills to not only continue with the success of the immediate project, but have the skills to undertake future implementation projects. Local ownership of the project not only impacts sustainability but is also directly related to acceptability of the implementation effort. Rather than feeling like evidence is being 'pushed' onto them, local staff will value and be a part of the process, and thus will be more engaged in implementing the evidence into their practice.

Additionally, having a strong focus on partnership and plan for next steps or what happens when the active implementation period ends, not only supports sustainability of successful implementation, but negates the issue faced by many when implementation supposedly 'fails'. Sometimes, not implementing the evidence into practice is a good thing, as perhaps your partnership and flexible approach allowed for you to understand the context and recipients in greater detail, and you identified that the problem or 'gap' is more nuanced and requires a different evidence-based solution or perhaps requires new evidence to be developed. Through an implementation framing, this is not success. Through an integrated knowledge translation lens, this is success. If we frame our implementation efforts through integrated knowledge translation, we can position implementation failures as success as you have achieved what you set out to do – identify gaps in practice, work towards identifying, and implementing evidence-based solutions. What is important is that there is a shared understanding of what actually happened and how it can shape future actions.

Chapter summary

In this chapter we have introduced implementation science and discussed how implementation science can function within a broader integrated knowledge translation approach. The key learnings from an integrated knowledge translation perspective are shown in Figure 2.5. Implementing evidence into practice is complex and often does not follow clear steps or a linear process. The contexts we are trying to work within are much more complex than we can often appreciate, and the recipients of the evidence often have competing priorities and diverse experiences. To end this chapter, we want you to reflect on the significance and importance of the relational aspects of implementation. Successful implementation often comes from working in close partnership with others, exploring problems, generating solutions and implementing those solutions together. This is where we begin to shift toward embracing more dynamic and non-linear ways of researching within complex social systems. In Chapter 3, we will introduce ways we can

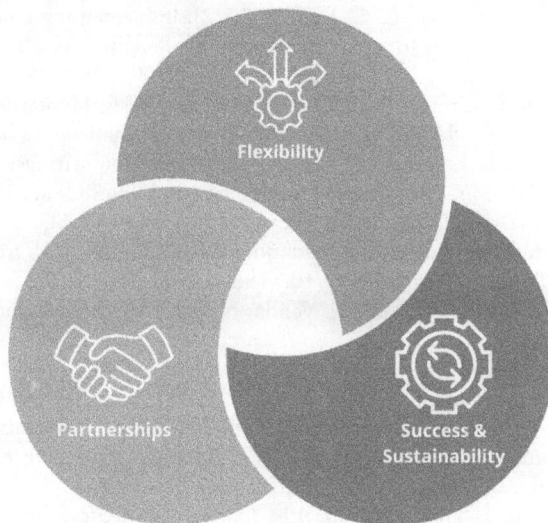

Figure 2.5 Integrated implementation key learnings.
Source: https://doi.org/10.25451/flinders.29192630.v1

work in partnership with people in different stages of the research journey to work in more integrated ways to enhance our knowledge translation success.

References

Bail, K., & Grealish, L. (2016). 'Failure to Maintain': A theoretical proposition for a new quality indicator of nurse care rationing for complex older people in hospital. *International Journal of Nursing Studies, 63*, 146–161. https://doi.org/10.1016/j.ijnurstu.2016.08.001

Baker, D., & Quinn, B. (2018). Hospital acquired Pneumonia Prevention Initiative-2: Incidence of nonventilator hospital-acquired pneumonia in the United States. *American Journal of Infection Control, 46*(1), 2–7. https://doi.org/10.1016/j.ajic.2017.08.036

Bauer, M. S., & Kirchner, J. (2020). Implementation science: What is it and why should I care? *Psychiatry Research, 283*, 112376–112376. https://doi.org/10.1016/j.psychres.2019.04.025

Bayley, M., Swaine, B., Lamontagne, M., Marshall, M., Allaire, A. S., Kua, A., & Marier-Deschenes, P. (2016). *INESSS-ONF Clinical Practice Guideline for the Rehabilitation of Adults with Moderate to Severe Traumatic Brain Injury*. Ontario Neurotrauma Foundation. https://braininjuryguidelines.org/modtosevere/

Birken, S. A., Powell, B. J., Shea, C. M., Haines, E. R., Alexis Kirk, M., Leeman, J., Rohweder, C., Damschroder, L., & Presseau, J. (2017). Criteria for selecting implementation science theories and frameworks: Results from an international survey. *Implementation Science: IS, 12*(1), 124–124. https://doi.org/10.1186/s13012-017-0656-y

Block, H., Bellon, M., Hunter, S. C., & George, S. (2023). Barriers and enablers to managing challenging behaviours after traumatic brain injury in the acute hospital setting: A qualitative study. *BMC Health Services Research, 23*(1), 1266. https://doi.org/10.1186/s12913-023-10279-z

Block, H., George, S., Hunter, S. C., & Bellon, M. (2024). Family experiences of the management of challenging behaviours after traumatic brain injury in the acute hospital setting. *Disability and Rehabilitation*, 1–10. https://doi.org/10.1080/09638288.2023.2280081

Block, H., George, S., Milanese, S., Dizon, J., Bowen-Salter, H., & Jenkinson, F. (2021). Evidence for the management of challenging behaviours in patients with acute traumatic brain injury or post-traumatic amnesia: An umbrella review. *Brain Impairment, 22*(1), 1–19. https://doi.org/10.1017/BrImp.2020.5

Block, H., Hunter, S. C., Bellon, M., & George, S. (2022). Implementing a behavior management approach in the hospital setting for individuals with challenging behaviors during acute traumatic brain injury. *Brain Injury*, 1–11. https://doi.org/10.1080/02699052.2022.2110941

Block, H., Paul, M., Muir-Cochrane, E., Bellon, M., George, S., & Hunter, S. C. (2023). Clinical practice guideline recommendations for the management of challenging behaviours after traumatic brain injury in acute hospital and inpatient rehabilitation settings: A systematic review. *Disability and Rehabilitation*, 1–11. https://doi.org/10.1080/09638288.2023.2169769

Callender, L., Brown, R., Driver, S., Dahdah, M., Collinsworth, A., & Shafi, S. (2017). Process for developing rehabilitation practice recommendations for individuals with traumatic brain injury. *BMC Neurology, 17*(1), 54. https://doi.org/10.1186/s12883-017-0828-z

Cane, J., O'Connor, D., & Michie, S. (2012). Validation of the theoretical domains framework for use in behaviour change and implementation research. *Implementation Science: IS, 7*(1), 37–37. https://doi.org/10.1186/1748-5908-7-37

Council of Australian Governments Health Council Health Council. (2016). *Healthy Mouths, Healthy Lives: Australia's National Oral Health Plan 2015-2024*. www.health.gov.au/resources/publications/healthy-mouths-healthy-lives-australias-national-oral-health-plan-2015-2024

Crawford, A., & Serhal, E. (2020). Digital health equity and COVID-19: The innovation curve cannot reinforce the social gradient of health. *Journal of Medical Internet Research, 22*(6), e19361–e19361. https://doi.org/10.2196/19361

Curran, G. M. (2020). Implementation science made too simple: A teaching tool. *Implementation Science Communications, 1*(1), 27–27. https://doi.org/10.1186/s43058-020-00001-z

Curran, G. M., Bauer, M., Mittman, B., Pyne, J. M., & Stetler, C. (2012). Effectiveness-implementation hybrid designs: Combining elements of clinical effectiveness and implementation research to enhance public health impact. *Medical Care, 50*(3), 217–226. https://doi.org/10.1097/MLR.0b013e3182408812

Damschroder, L. J., Aron, D. C., Keith, R. E., Kirsh, S. R., Alexander, J. A., & Lowery, J. C. (2009). Fostering implementation of health services research findings into practice: A consolidated framework for advancing implementation science. *Implementation Science: IS, 4*(1), 50–50. https://doi.org/10.1186/1748-5908-4-50

Eccles, M. P., & Mittman, B. S. (2006). Welcome to implementation science. *Implementation Science: IS, 1*(1), 1–1. https://doi.org/10.1186/1748-5908-1-1

ElSayed, N. A., Aleppo, G., Aroda, V. R., Bannuru, R. R., Brown, F. M., Bruemmer, D., Collins, B. S., Hilliard, M. E., Isaacs, D., Johnson, E. L., Kahan, S., Khunti, K., Leon, J., Lyons, S. K., Perry, M. L., Prahalad, P., Pratley, R. E., Seley, J. J., Stanton, R. C., ... on behalf of the American Diabetes, A. (2023). 7. Diabetes technology: Standards of care in diabetes-2023. *Diabetes Care, 46*(Suppl 1), S111–s127. https://doi.org/10.2337/dc23-S007

Elwy, A. R., Maguire, E. M., Kim, B., & West, G. S. (2022). Involving stakeholders as communication partners in research dissemination efforts. *Journal of General Internal Medicine: JGIM, 37*(Suppl 1), 123–127. https://doi.org/10.1007/s11606-021-07127-3

Flanagan, S. R., Elovic, E. P., & Sandel, E. (2009). Managing agitation associated with traumatic brain injury: Behavioral versus pharmacologic interventions? *The Journal of Physical Medicine and Rehabilitation, 1*(1), 76–80. https://doi.org/10.1016/j.pmrj.2008.10.013

Fonseca, V. A., Grunberger, G., Anhalt, H., Bailey, T. S., Blevins, T., Garg, S. K., Handelsman, Y., Hirsch, I. B., Orzeck, E. A., Roberts, V. L., & Tamborlane, W. (2016). Continuous glucose monitoring: A consensus conference of the American association of clinical endocrinologists and American College of endocrinology. *Endocrine Practice, 22*(8), 1008–1021. https://doi.org/10.4158/EP161392.CS

Funnell, S. C., & Rogers, P. J. (2011). *Purposeful program theory. Effective use of theories of change and logic models.* Jossey-Bass.

Gagliardi, A. R., Kothari, A., & Graham, I. D. (2017). Research agenda for integrated knowledge translation (IKT) in healthcare: What we know and do not yet know. *Journal of Epidemiology and Community Health (1979), 71*(2), 105–106. https://doi.org/10.1136/jech-2016-207743

Gil-Montoya, J. A., de Mello, A. L. F., Barrios, R., Gonzalez-Moles, M. A., & Bravo, M. (2015). Oral health in the elderly patient and its impact on general well-being: A nonsystematic review. *Clinical Interventions in Aging, 10*, 461–467. https://doi.org/10.2147/CIA.S54630

Glasgow, R. E., Klesges, L. M., Dzewaltowski, D. A., Estabrooks, P. A., & Vogt, T. M. (2006). Evaluating the impact of health promotion programs: Using the RE-AIM framework to form summary measures for decision making involving complex issues. *Health Education Research, 21*(5), 688–694. https://doi.org/10.1093/her/cyl081

Glasgow, R. E., Vogt, T. M., & Boles, S. M. (1999). Evaluating the public health impact of health promotion interventions: The RE-AIM framework. *American Journal of Public Health (1971), 89*(9), 1322–1327. https://doi.org/10.2105/AJPH.89.9.1322

Graham, I. D., Logan, J., Harrison, M. B., Straus, S. E., Tetroe, J., Caswell, W., & Robinson, N. (2006). Lost in knowledge translation: Time for a map? *The Journal of Continuing Education in the Health Professions, 26*(1), 13–24. https://doi.org/10.1002/chp.47

Handley, M. A., Gorukanti, A., & Cattamanchi, A. (2016). Strategies for implementing implementation science: A methodological overview. *Emergency Medicine Journal, 33*(9), 660–664. https://doi.org/10.1136/emermed-2015-205461

Harvey, G., & Kitson, A. L. (2015). *Implementing evidence-based practice in healthcare: A facilitation guide.* Routledge. https://doi.org/10.4324/9780203557334

Harvey, G., & Kitson, A. (2016). PARIHS revisited: From heuristic to integrated framework for the successful implementation of knowledge into practice. *Implementation Science: IS, 11*(1), 33–33. https://doi.org/10.1186/s13012-016-0398-2

Hunter, S. C., Kim, B., Mudge, A., Hall, L., Young, A., McRae, P., & Kitson, A. L. (2020). Experiences of using the i-PARIHS framework: A co-designed case study of four multi-site implementation projects. *BMC Health Services Research*, 20(1), 573–573. https://doi.org/10.1186/s12 913-020-05354-8

Janssens, B., De Visschere, L., van der Putten, G.-J., de Lugt-Lustig, K., Schols, J. M. G. A., & Vanobbergen, J. (2016). Effect of an oral healthcare protocol in nursing homes on care staffs' knowledge and attitude towards oral health care: A cluster-randomised controlled trial. *Gerodontology*, 33(2), 275–286. https://doi.org/10.1111/ger.12164

Kalisch, B. J., Landstrom, G., & Williams, R. A. (2009). Missed nursing care: Errors of omission. *Nursing Outlook*, 57(1), 3–9. https://doi.org/10.1016/j.outlook.2008.05.007

Khalil, H. (2016). Knowledge translation and implementation science: What is the difference? *International Journal of Evidence-Based Healthcare*, 14(2), 39–40. https://doi.org/10.1097/XEB.0000000000000086

Kirchner, J. E., Smith, J. L., Powell, B. J., Waltz, T. J., & Proctor, E. K. (2020). Getting a clinical innovation into practice: An introduction to implementation strategies. *Psychiatry Research*, 283, 112467. https://doi.org/10.1016/j.psychres.2019.06.042

Kitson, A., Brook, A., Harvey, G., Jordan, Z., Marshall, R., O'Shea, R., & Wilson, D. (2018). Using complexity and network concepts to inform healthcare knowledge translation. *International Journal of Health Policy and Management*, 7(3), 231–243. https://doi.org/10.15171/ijhpm.2017.79

Kitson, A., Harvey, G., & McCormack, B. (1998). Enabling the implementation of evidence based practice: A conceptual framework. *Quality in Health Care*, 7(3), 149–158. https://doi.org/10.1136/qshc.7.3.149

Kitson, A., Muntlin Athlin, Å., & Conroy, T. (2014). Anything but basic: Nursing's challenge in meeting patients' fundamental care needs. *Journal of Nursing Scholarship*, 46(5), 331–339. https://doi.org/10.1111/jnu.12081

Klonoff, D. C., Buckingham, B., Christiansen, J. S., Montori, V. M., Tamborlane, W. V., Vigersky, R. A., & Wolpert, H. (2011). Continuous glucose monitoring: An Endocrine Society Clinical Practice Guideline. *The Journal of Clinical Endocrinology and Metabolism*, 96(10), 2968–2979. https://doi.org/10.1210/jc.2010-2756

Lewis, A., Kitson, A., & Harvey, G. (2016). Improving oral health for older people in the home care setting: An exploratory implementation study. *Australasian Journal on Ageing*, 35(4), 273–280. https://doi.org/10.1111/ajag.12326

Lewis, A., Murray, J., Hunter, S. C., Conroy, T., Kitson, A., Splawinski, Z., Courage, D., Challen-Jordan, A., & Block, H. (2022). *REDUCE (tRanslating knowlEDge for fUndamental CareD): Missed oral healthcare: It takes a team (Whittaker Smiles): Project Report*. Adelaide, Australia: Flinders University.

Luauté, J., Plantier, D., Wiart, L., & Tell, L. (2016). Care management of the agitation or aggressiveness crisis in patients with TBI. Systematic review of the literature and practice recommendations. *Annals of Physical and Rehabilitation Medicine*, 59(1), 58–67. https://doi.org/10.1016/j.rehab.2015.11.001

Lynch, E. A., Mudge, A., Knowles, S., Kitson, A. L., Hunter, S. C., & Harvey, G. (2018). "There is nothing so practical as a good theory": A pragmatic guide for selecting theoretical approaches for implementation projects. *BMC Health Services Research*, 18(1), 857–857. https://doi.org/10.1186/s12913-018-3671-z

Mahtta, D., Ahmed, S. T., Shah, N. R., Ramsey, D. J., Akeroyd, J. M., Nasir, K., Hamzeh, I. R., Elgendy, I. Y., Waldo, S. W., Al-Mallah, M. H., Jneid, H., Ballantyne, C. M., Petersen, L. A., & Virani, S. S. (2020). Facility-level variation in cardiac stress test use among patients with diabetes: Findings from the Veterans Affairs National Database. *Diabetes Care*, 43(5), E58–E60. https://doi.org/10.2337/dc19-2160

Marshman, L. A., Jakabek, D., Hennessy, M., Quirk, F., & Guazzo, E. P. (2013). Post-traumatic amnesia. *Journal of Clinical Neuroscience*, 20(11), 1475–1481. https://doi.org/10.1016/j.jocn.2012.11.022

May, C., & Finch, T. (2009). Implementing, embedding, and integrating practices: An outline of normalization process theory. *Sociology (Oxford)*, 43(3), 535–554. https://doi.org/10.1177/0038038509103208

Michie, S., Johnston, M., Abraham, C., Lawton, R., Parker, D., & Walker, A. (2005). Making psychological theory useful for implementing evidence based practice: A consensus approach. *Quality & Safety in Health Care*, 14(1), 26–33. https://doi.org/10.1136/qshc.2004.011155

Miller, C. J., Barnett, M. L., Baumann, A. A., Gutner, C. A., & Wiltsey-Stirman, S. (2021). The FRAME-IS: A framework for documenting modifications to implementation strategies in healthcare. *Implementation Science: IS*, 16(1), 36–36. https://doi.org/10.1186/s13012-021-01105-3

Morris, Z. S., Wooding, S., & Grant, J. (2011). The answer is 17 years, what is the question: Understanding time lags in translational research. *Journal of the Royal Society of Medicine*, 104(12), 510–520. https://doi.org/10.1258/jrsm.2011.110180

Moullin, J. C., Dickson, K. S., Stadnick, N. A., Albers, B., Nilsen, P., Broder-Fingert, S., Mukasa, B., & Aarons, G. A. (2020). Ten recommendations for using implementation frameworks in research and practice. *Implementation Science Communications*, 1(1), 42–42. https://doi.org/10.1186/s43058-020-00023-7

Munro, S., & Baker, D. (2018). Reducing missed oral care opportunities to prevent non-ventilator associated hospital acquired pneumonia at the Department of Veterans Affairs. *Applied Nursing Research*, 44, 48–53. https://doi.org/10.1016/j.apnr.2018.09.004

Murray, J., Hunter, S. C., Conroy, T., Kitson, A. L., Splawinski, Z., Block, H., & Lewis, A. (2024). REDUCE missed oral healthcare: The outcomes of and learnings from an implementation project in an acute geriatric unit. *Research in Nursing & Health*, 47(5), 551–562. https://doi.org/https://doi.org/10.1002/nur.22408

Murray, J., Hunter, S. C., Splawinski, Z., & Conroy, T. (2022). Lessons learned from the preimplementation phase of an oral health care project. *JDR Clinical & Translational Research*, 8(3), 299–301. https://doi.org/10.1177/23800844221083966

National Health Service. (2019). *Mouth Care Matters programme.* http://mouthcarematters.hee.nhs.uk/index.html

Nilsen, P. (2015). Making sense of implementation theories, models, and frameworks. *Implementation Science*, 10(1), 53–53. https://doi.org/10.1186/s13012-015-0242-0

Nilsen, P., & Birken, S. A. (2020). *Handbook on implementation science.* Edward Elgar Publishing.

Ohi, T., Murakami, T., Komiyama, T., Miyoshi, Y., Endo, K., Hiratsuka, T., Satoh, M., Asayama, K., Inoue, R., Kikuya, M., Metoki, H., Hozawa, A., Imai, Y., Watanabe, M., Ohkubo, T., & Hattori, Y. (2022). Oral health-related quality of life is associated with the prevalence and development of depressive symptoms in older Japanese individuals: The Ohasama Study. *Gerodontology*, 39(2), 204–212. https://doi.org/10.1111/ger.12557

Ponsford, J., Carrier, S., Hicks, A., & McKay, A. (2021). Assessment and management of patients in the acute stages of recovery after traumatic brain injury in adults: A worldwide survey. *Journal of Neurotrauma*, 38(8), 1060–1067. https://doi.org/10.1089/neu.2020.7299

Presseau, J., Kasperavicius, D., Rodrigues, I. B., Braimoh, J., Chambers, A., Etherington, C., Giangregorio, L., Gibbs, J. C., Giguere, A., Graham, I. D., Hankivsky, O., Hoens, A. M., Holroyd-Leduc, J., Kelly, C., Moore, J. E., Ponzano, M., Sharma, M., Sibley, K. M., & Straus, S. (2022). Selecting implementation models, theories, and frameworks in which to integrate intersectional approaches. *BMC Medical Research Methodology*, 22(1), 1–212. https://doi.org/10.1186/s12874-022-01682-x

Proctor, E., Silmere, H., Raghavan, R., Hovmand, P., Aarons, G., Bunger, A., Griffey, R., & Hensley, M. (2011). Outcomes for implementation research: Conceptual distinctions, measurement challenges, and research agenda. *Administation and Policy in Mental Health*, 38(2), 65–76. https://doi.org/10.1007/s10488-010-0319-7

Rogers, E. M. (2003). *Diffusion of innovations* (5th ed.). Free Press.

Rycroft-Malone, J., & Bucknall, T. (2010). *Models and Frameworks for Implementing Evidence-Based Practice: Linking Evidence to Action*. Wiley. https://books.google.com.au/books?id=EpDbQSI1390C

Scannapieco, F. A., & Shay, K. (2014). Oral health disparities in older adults: Oral bacteria, inflammation, and aspiration pneumonia. *Dental Clinics*, 58(4), 771–782. https://doi.org/10.1016/j.cden.2014.06.005

Straus, S. E., Tetroe, J., & Graham, I. (2009). Defining knowledge translation. *Canadian Medical Association journal (CMAJ)*, 181(3–4), 165–168. https://doi.org/10.1503/cmaj.081229

Straus, S. E., Tetzlaff, J., Tricco, A. C., Moher, D., Brouwers, M. C., Stacey, D., O'Connor, A. M., McKibbon, K. A., & Lokker, C. (2009). Knowledge Creation. In S. E. Straus, J. Tetroe, & I. D. Graham (Eds.), *Knowledge Translation in Health Care*. Blackwell Publishing Ltd. https://doi.org/10.1002/9781444311747.ch2

Tucker, S., McNett, M., Mazurek Melnyk, B., Hanrahan, K., Hunter, S. C., Kim, B., Cullen, L., & Kitson, A. (2021). Implementation science: Application of evidence-based practice models to improve healthcare quality. *Worldviews on Evidence-Based Nursing*, 18, 76–84. https://doi.org/https://doi.org/10.1111/wvn.12495

Wang, L., Li, X., Wang, Z., Bancks, M. P., Carnethon, M. R., Greenland, P., Feng, Y.-Q., Wang, H., & Zhong, V. W. (2021). Trends in prevalence of diabetes and control of risk factors in diabetes among US adults, 1999–2018. *JAMA: The Journal of the American Medical Association*, 326(8), 704–716. https://doi.org/10.1001/jama.2021.9883

Wensing, M., & Grol, R. (2019). Knowledge translation in health: How implementation science could contribute more. *BMC Medicine*, 17(1), 88–88. https://doi.org/10.1186/s12916-019-1322-9

Wiltsey Stirman, S., Baumann, A. A., & Miller, C. J. (2019). The FRAME: An expanded framework for reporting adaptations and modifications to evidence-based interventions. *Implementation Science*, 14(1), 58. https://doi.org/10.1186/s13012-019-0898-y

3 Working in partnership

Sarah Hunter, Michael Lawless and Alison Kitson

Introduction

Researchers, practitioners, and clinicians often come to knowledge translation because they have a research- or practice-related goal in mind. Critical to achieving these goals is working in partnership with various people. In Chapter 1, we introduced integrated knowledge translation and the Knowledge Translation Complexity Network Model. Integrated knowledge translation is an approach that guides how we, at the Caring Futures Institute, undertake research. We built on this in Chapter 2 by focusing specifically on the implementation research process within the Knowledge Translation Complexity Network Model, which can be seen in Figure 3.1, as it is often where people begin when they come to knowledge translation.

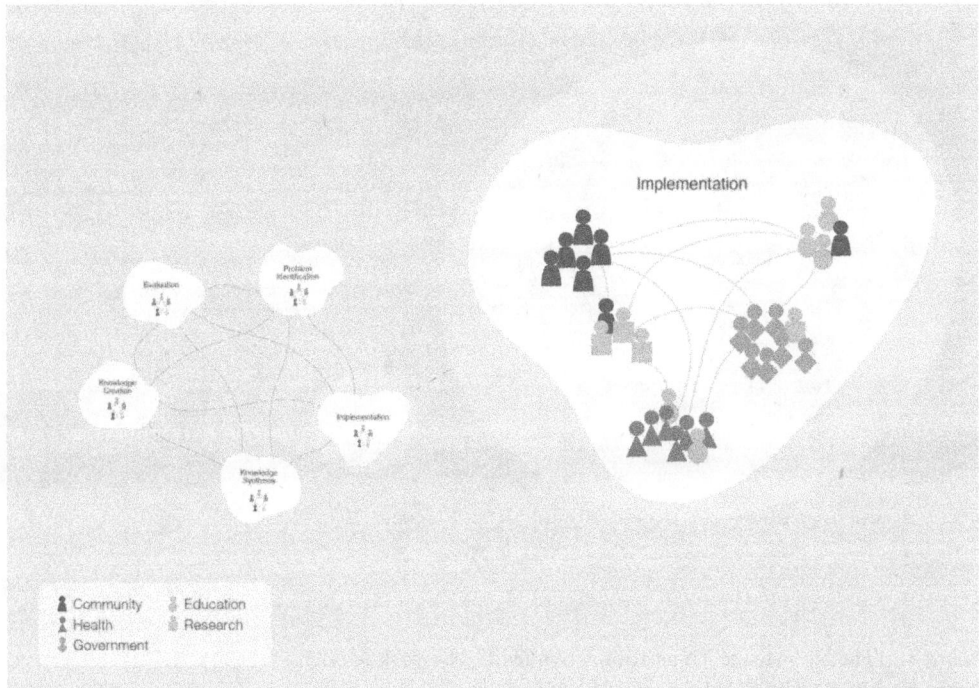

Figure 3.1 Implementation within the Knowledge Translation Complexity Network Model.
Source: https://doi.org/10.25451/flinders.29192642.v1

DOI: 10.4324/9781003245995-4

We demonstrated how we began our journey toward embracing integrated knowledge translation by building on our research teams' experiences of implementation science and shifting toward undertaking implementation through a broader integrated knowledge translation approach. That is, by viewing it as one of the research processes, as seen in Figure 3.2. This shift toward viewing implementation as a research process within integrated knowledge translation requires embracing complexity and flexibility. Critical to working in this way is working in partnership.

Once our teams had experience using and applying implementation science in an integrated way, we knew there was a growing interest in conducting different types of research in practice settings and working closely with various partners. Therefore, the next step in our journey was to explore how to work in partnership across the different research processes. Therefore, in this chapter, we are zooming out and not focusing on a particular research process (such as implementation or knowledge synthesis or problem identification). We will instead focus on the people in and across these processes that make knowledge creation, and knowledge use more likely to happen. Considering Figure 3.2, this chapter explores how we work in partnership with various people within the different research processes and start to introduce how to partner and work across the different research processes.

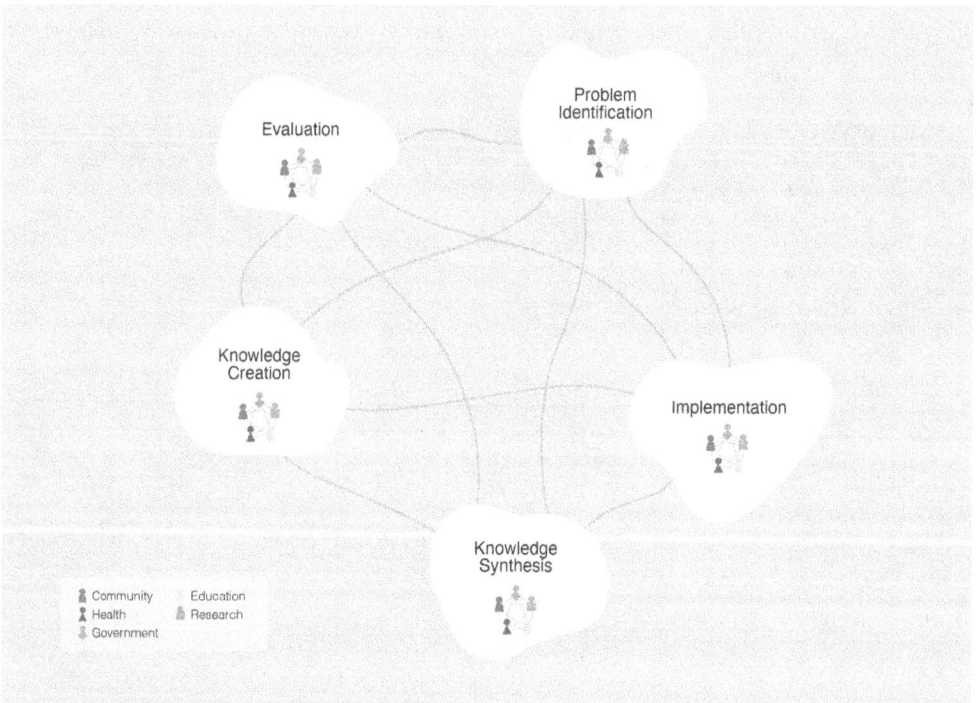

Figure 3.2 The Knowledge Translation Complexity Network Model.
Source: https://doi.org/10.25451/flinders.29192585.v1

What do we mean when we say working in partnership?

When we say it is important to work in partnership, what do we mean, and who are we referring to? 'Stakeholder' is a widely used term to describe any person, group, or organisation, with an interest in, or who are likely to be impacted by, the outcomes of research (Deverka et al., 2012). This can include, but is not limited to, patients, family members of patients, the general public, health care providers, executives and leadership in health or social care settings, public servants and policy decision makers, community groups, or organisations.

There are many different terms used to describe stakeholders within the knowledge translation literature and other fields of research and practice, such as communication and management science. These terms include stakeholders, end-users, consumers, decision makers, recipients, partners, and next users (Figure 3.3). There are contemporary discussions that critique the term stakeholder, and call for alternative terminology that is appropriate for the project (Reed et al., 2024). Instead of suggestions for a single, accepted term, there are recommendations to focus on the people and places themselves (Reed et al., 2024). Given there is no universally accepted term, we believe it is best to agree on the most appropriate term to use that is suitable for the context in which you are working. Throughout this chapter, we will refer to individuals or groups broadly, or specifically, when we are referring to a specific group.

The main takeaway is it is important to identify those who are affected by, or can affect, your research. If you are wanting to engage in knowledge translation, you need to ensure the people affected by research are aware of, and use, the evidence as well as ensuring research is informed and shaped by the experiences and needs of the people affected by it (Kitson et al., 2013).

Why partner?

The first question you may have is, why? Why do we need to work with various people?

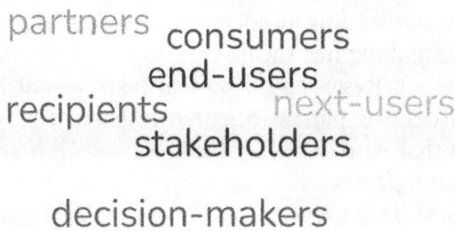

partners consumers
end-users
recipients next-users
stakeholders

decision-makers

Figure 3.3 Different terms used to describe partners.
Source: https://doi.org/10.25451/flinders.29192648.v1

Basic research teaches researchers to be objective or disengaged observers of 'reality'. Therefore, many of us are not taught the skills to conduct research in partnership. However, this notion of researching from a distance is becoming outdated, particularly in applied research. There is now an established recognition of the importance of conducting research that embeds principles and values aligned with collaborative approaches – where research is conducted 'with or by members of the public rather than to, about, or for them' (National Institute for Health and Care Research, 2021, paragraph 5). This is very much aligned with the movement **nothing about us without us** (Charlton, 1998; Chu et al., 2016).

No one single person or group holds all the knowledge or experience to answer complex problems faced in society. Whilst researchers may hold the research expertise to provide a process for generating evidence, collaboration is required across various groups spanning multiple individuals, organisations, industries, and sectors to generate and translate knowledge into meaningful outcomes.

Thus, appropriate, and meaningful engagement of various and diverse people has been highlighted as a key mechanism to improve the relevance, efficiency, and impact of research (Banner et al., 2019). Chapter 2 mentioned how evidence does not easily get into practice and so researchers cannot, and should not, work in isolation.

This approach to conducting research is not unique to knowledge translation approaches and is rather part of a wider cultural and political shift in research. This is clear through many of the major national research strategies, frameworks, and funding bodies outlining the need for engagement in research. For example:

- **United Kingdom:** The National Institute of Health and Care Research developed the "INVOLVE Framework" (National Institute for Health and Care Research, 2023) in 1996 to support active public involvement in the National Health Service, public health, and social care research. This framework outlines the requirement of the public voice across the entire research process and provides the values, principles, and standards for public involvement. In 2020, the National Institute for Health and Care Research launched a new Centre for Engagement and Dissemination (National Institute for Health and Care Research, 2020) which builds on the INVOLVE framework and is dedicated to strengthening the collaborative culture of engaging the public across the health and care system.
- **United States:** The Patient-Centred Outcomes Research Institute (Patient-Centred Outcomes Research Institute, 2023) is the leading funder of health research in the United States that empowers patients in making healthcare decisions.
- **Canada:** The Canadian Institutes of Health Research (Canadian Institutes of Health Research, 2023) has developed a strategy for patient-oriented research focused on transforming the role of patients from that of passive recipients of research and evidence to proactive partners in the research process.
- **Australia:** The Australian Government Department of Health and Aged Care (2023) funded by the Medical Research Future Fund developed the Emerging Priorities and Consumer-Driven Research initiative. This initiative involves providing $613 million over 2022–2033 to support consumers and researchers to work together.

Even if you cannot see the immediate value, it is an established expectation and requirement from research institutions and funders that consumers and others are involved in research (Archibald et al., 2023).

Methods for working in partnership

There are different methods, approaches, or strategies for identifying who you should partner with and how to partner or work together. The first step is often identifying who to partner with. 'Stakeholder mapping', or 'stakeholder analysis', is a method for identifying individuals, groups, or organisations, understanding their relationships to each other, and their unique motivators that may support or oppose your research (Bernstein et al., 2020; Brugha & Varvasovszky, 2000).

A widely used matrix for mapping is the Mendelow Matrix, originally conceptualised by Mendelow (1991) but revised and adapted by many over the decades to map groups based on their relative power and perceived interest. Figure 3.4 is one version of the Mendelow Matrix. This matrix helps to visualise the various individuals or groups that may relate to your research and how they may have varying power or interest in what you are doing and the resulting way that may be best to engage with them. This approach to mapping your reality/context is an aid in the planning stage. There is no 'one size fits all' approach to engaging or working with others and is something that is context- and project-dependent.

Meet their needs: These are individuals or groups who have high power, but low interest, it is important to put enough effort to keep them satisfied, but not so much that they become bored with your message.

Keep informed: These are individuals or groups who have low power, and low interest, it is important to keep them informed but not engage them too much.

Key player: These are individuals or groups who have high power, and high interest, these are your key partners. These are the people who you need to have engaged and keep their needs and interests front of mind.

Show consideration: These are individuals or groups who have low power, but high interest, are important to have involved and show consideration for their perspective and interest.

Once you know who you are partnering with it is important to identify or define what working together looks like. Figure 3.5 illustrates some common partnership

		Low	High
Power	High	Meet their needs	Key player
	Low	Keep informed	Show consideration

Level of interest

Figure 3.4 Mendelow's Matrix.

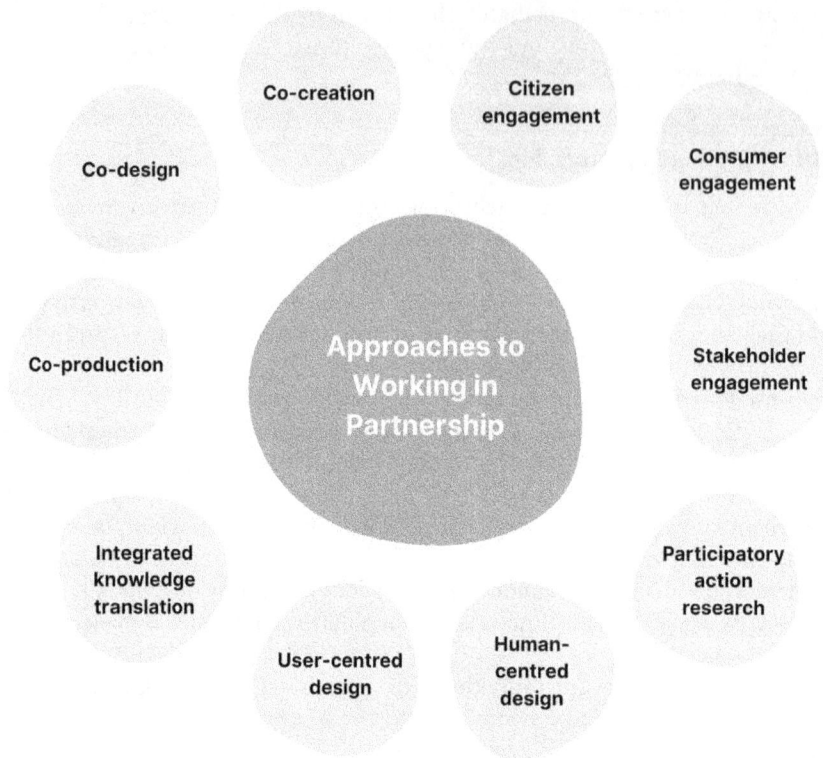

Figure 3.5 Common knowledge translation approaches to working in partnership.
Source: https://doi.org/10.25451/flinders.29192657.v1

approaches and their key characteristics, which we explore in the examples throughout this book.

- **Stakeholder engagement:** Interactions between researchers (knowledge producers) and knowledge users that may vary in intensity, complexity, and level of engagement depending on the nature of the research, the findings, as well as the needs of the particular knowledge user (Straus et al., 2009). Stakeholder engagement in knowledge translation increases the likelihood that research is relevant, understandable, and applicable to the needs of all stakeholders (Cargo & Mercer, 2008).
- **Consumer engagement:** The process by which consumers' knowledge and experience is shared in a collaborative dialogue with program developers, practitioners, researchers, and policymakers (Sanders & Kirby, 2012). Consumer engagement in knowledge translation ensures research is relevant, understandable, and actionable by those directly affected by it.
- **Citizen engagement:** The process of active two-way interaction between individuals or groups from the public and researchers, policymakers or practitioners that involves citizens in generating, sharing, and using knowledge to inform decision making. Citizen engagement in knowledge translation helps ensure that research findings are relevant, accessible, and applicable to the needs and priorities of citizens, ultimately enhancing the impact and effectiveness of evidence-informed policies and practices (Canadian Institutes for Health Research, 2012).

- **Patient and public involvement:** The phrase 'with' or 'by' the public, rather than 'to', 'about', or 'for' the public is a widely used phrase or concept to describe patient and public involvement in research (Boote et al., 2011; National Institute for Health and Care Research, 2021). Patient and public involvement in knowledge translation underscores the importance of engaging the public as active partners in the research process rather than treating them as research subjects or beneficiaries (Staley, 2015).
- **Co-design, co-production, and co-creation:** These co-approaches in the context of knowledge translation focuses on a collaborative process of developing and implementing research projects, interventions, or policies in which researchers work closely with stakeholders and consumers to co-create solutions to real world problems (Cowdell et al., 2022). Co-approaches in the context of knowledge translation prioritises iterative processes and empowering stakeholders.
- **Participatory action research:** A systematic inquiry with the collaboration of those affected by the issue being studied for the purposes of taking action or promoting change (Greene et al., 1995). Participatory action research in the context of knowledge translation aims to generate actionable knowledge through a cyclical process of reflection, action, and learning.
- **User-centred design (also called human-centred design):** An iterative method of involving prospective users in repeated cycles of development intended to optimise the user experience of a system, service, or product (Garrett, 2011). User-centred design in the context of knowledge translation involves understanding the perspectives, experiences, and context of those who will use or benefit from the knowledge being translated and ensuring it is tailored to their specific needs and circumstances.
- **Integrated Knowledge Translation:** An approach developed by the Canadian Institutes of Health Research that outlines that 'knowledge users' should be engaged throughout the research process and results in research and evidence that are more likely to be relevant and used by 'knowledge users' (Canadian Institutes of Health Research, 2015).

It is important to select the method that is most suitable for you and your partners, as well the research or work you are undertaking together. Despite the various terms and methods, generally, engaging individuals or groups in research ranges on a spectrum from involving, engaging, collaborating, consulting, participating to empowering, and partnering (International Association for Public Participation, 2018). The International Association for Public Participation developed this spectrum, and it provides useful support in determining the scope of the working relationship, see Table 3.1.

Table 3.1 International Association for Public Participation Spectrum

Activity	Definition
Inform	To keep partners informed with balanced and objective information to assist them in understanding the project and provide opportunities for feedback and input
Consult	To obtain partner feedback or input to influence the project direction and ensure partners are listened to and their concerns or interests are considered.
Involve	To work directly with partners throughout the project to ensure their concerns or interests directly affect and influence the project.
Collaborate	To partner throughout the project and their advice and input is incorporated into the project.
Empower	To ensure partners make the final decision within the project and their decisions are implemented.

Source: International Association for Public Participation (2018).

To support with selecting the right approach for you and your partners, we developed our own visual process to develop a plan. This can be seen in Table 3.2.

1) First, you start by trying to identify who:
   Audience: Here you can map out a list of all individuals, groups, or organisations that may have an interest in, affect, or be affected by your research.
2) Second, you identify their 'what':
   Power/interest: Here you use Mendelow's Matrix to map their perceived power or interest.
   Key interests and issues: Here you articulate what their interest in, or issue with, your project may be.
3) Third, you take this knowledge of the who and the what to articulate how you will work with them:
   Communication vehicle: Here you identify how you will communicate with each of your individuals, groups, or organisations. For example, if they are key to what you are doing, you may plan to meet with them via a direct meeting. Even though you have used Mendelow's Matrix, it's important to recognise this tool is best for mapping needs and interests, as a starting point. It's critical to work with the people to identify their preferences for communication. For example, those that may be mapped into the 'show consideration' box may in fact be a 'key player' as they have the time and interest to be engaged in your project. It is critical then, once you have identified the 'who' and 'what' to commence working with people to develop the 'how' and 'why' together.
   Frequency: Here you identify how regularly you will communicate with each of your stakeholders. For example, if they are key to what we are doing, you may have regular meetings monthly or quarterly. Whereas other stakeholders may want to be engaged less frequently.
4) Finally, we think it is crucial to articulate, in partnership with your stakeholders, the why:
   Justification: Here you need to identify why you are engaging each individual, group, or organisation. Individuals, groups, and organisations are busy and have competing demands and priorities. If you are to engage them in a research project, you need to be clear on why you are engaging them and what you are asking them to do. What is the purpose or goal of the engagement, are you asking them to contribute, are you trying to let them know about what you are doing because you think it may affect them? It

Table 3.2 Caring Futures Institute Partner Planning Tool

Audience	Power/Interest	Key interests and issues	Communication medium	Frequency	Justification
Insert	Insert	Insert	Insert	Insert	Insert
"Who?"	"What?"		"How?"		"Why?"

is critical this is discussed and clarified with them as this will ensure the engagement is meaningful and authentic for both parties and this will support in developing a clear plan and understanding of how to work together.

In addition to traditional, linear approaches to planning partnerships, we encourage you to think of your collaborations as part of a broader network. Visual tools like network diagrams (Glegg et al., 2019) can support knowledge translation processes by mapping out roles and relationships, clarifying who is contributing to what, and clarifying how different people and groups interact (Figure 3.6). These diagrams can also show more efficient pathways for knowledge sharing, making the process more explicit and systematic. By showing weak links or isolated individuals and groups, network diagrams can help address social and relational barriers to knowledge translation. Likewise, they can help identify key players with strong relationships across various groups who can speed up the sharing and adoption of knowledge. Understanding networks and using visualisations highlights the interconnected, systemic nature of knowledge translation, shifting the focus from isolated projects to collaborative, dynamic problem solving. In the example below, we have developed a hypothetical network diagram to visualise various roles, relationships, and collaborations.

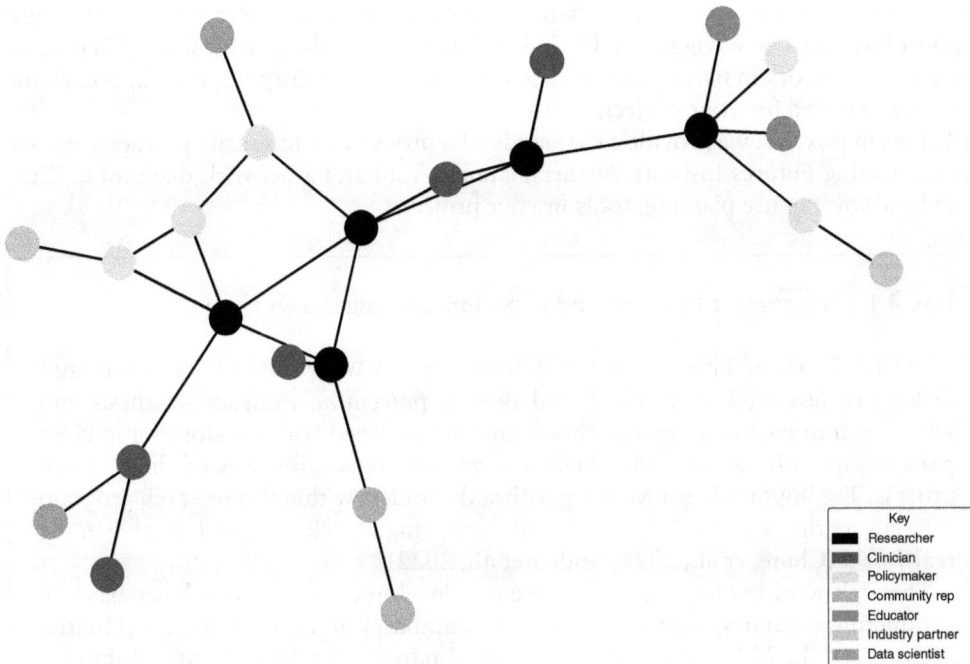

Key	
■	Researcher
■	Clinician
▦	Policymaker
▦	Community rep
▦	Educator
▦	Industry partner
▦	Data scientist

Figure 3.6 Example of a network diagram.
Source: https://doi.org/10.25451/flinders.29192663.v1

What we learned

We have had many learnings through supporting our teams within the Caring Futures Institute to work in partnership across various types of research. These experiences have helped shape our journey towards an integrated knowledge translation approach to conducting research. Broadly, we have learnt that connections, interactions, and partnerships are at the heart of, and what drives, the knowledge translation process (Kitson et al., 2013). Understanding the various priorities, experiences, and perspectives of others allows us to understand the 'problem' we are trying to address and supports us in generating relevant and meaningful evidence. Further, this partnership increases the likelihood that our evidence will be used in practice, as we have developed it in a way that it can be adopted, adapted, and tailored to suit diverse needs.

Below we share some of our key learnings. We present these as the learnings that pertain to 1) working in partnership within a discrete project, and 2) working in partnership in an integrated knowledge translation way. We share case studies from our teams within the Caring Futures Institute to illustrate these learnings.

Partnership learnings

Developing a plan

Before you reach out and engage, there are some practical considerations to plan and support how you can navigate, build, and maintain productive partnerships. There is no correct way to work in partnership, rather, it is key to select the appropriate approach for your partners and for your project.

Below, in Box 3.1, we provide a case study of a project that has many partners, and we use the Caring Futures Institute Partner Planning Tool and a network diagram to illustrate how you can use planning tools in your project:

Box 3.1 *Case study 1* **Planning and importance of engagement**

TOPCHILD is an international collaboration (www.topchildcollaboration.org/) seeking to fast-track early childhood obesity prevention evidence synthesis and adoption into routine practice. This cannot be achieved without working in close partnership with various individuals and groups across all stages of the research process. The importance of working with stakeholders within this research program is to ensure the evidence base developed is meaningful, relevant, and useable in the real world (Chung et al., 2024; Seidler et al., 2022).

Through working in partnership, we are developing a living evidence base by conducting regular systematic searches of databases and trial registries (Hunter, Webster, et al., 2022), combining individual participant data (Hunter, Johnson, et al., 2022) and coding of intervention content (Johnson et al., 2022) to understand which intervention components work for which populations. A simplified illustration of this partnership is shown in the network diagram below (Figure 3.7).

Our goal was ambitious in that we did not want to conduct a review of average intervention effects from published literature, but rather, to generate a meaningful and useful living evidence base of individual participant outcomes and intervention components, that can incorporate new evidence from planned and ongoing research (Seidler et al., 2019). We wanted the evidence base to be accessible, practical, and tailorable for those who need this evidence in their everyday decision making and routine practice.

To achieve this, the people we partner with include other research teams, policy makers, practitioners, and families of young children. Given the individuals and groups we work with cover a breadth of needs and experiences we chose to work with people aligned to the inform and consult end of the engagement spectrum (International Association for Public Participation, 2018).

In the early stages of the project, we engaged four stakeholder representatives, two policy makers, one nurse, and one parent, to act as advisors and provide a sounding board to ensure the practical needs were included in project planning. We engaged four representatives to ensure that our funding could provide financial reimbursement over the life of the project. These individuals continued to engage and advise on the project throughout the formation of the collaboration, through to interpreting the findings four years later. Other research teams engaged were the trial representatives for the interventions included in the living evidence base. Trial representatives shared their trial dataset and intervention materials and had input into the protocol development, engaged in annual interactive collaborator meetings (including results interpretation), and received regular newsletters.

Author: Brittany Johnson
Acknowledgements: Rebecca Golley, Anna Lene Seidler, Kylie Hunter

Case study 1, in Box 3.1, shows the importance of embedding stakeholder engagement from the start, particularly when developing large-scale, dynamic research infrastructure like a living evidence base. The TOPCHILD collaboration demonstrates how sustained partnerships, even at the 'inform and consult' end of the spectrum, can help ensure that evidence synthesis remains relevant and accessible to practice. It also reflects how thoughtful engagement planning, including considerations around reimbursement, roles, and continuity, can build trust and ensure partners' voices shape both process and outcomes over the life of a project.

Table 3.3 is given as an example to help you think through and map your key stakeholders across different areas of your project. We have applied the Caring Futures Institute Partner Planning Tool to Case Study 4. Under each heading, we have included brief illustrative details to show how the tool can be used to plan stakeholder engagement effectively. This example is not exhaustive – it's intended to demonstrate how you might begin developing your own stakeholder engagement plan in a practical and structured way.

Table 3.3 Case Study 4 and the Caring Futures Institute Partner Planning Tool

Audience	Power/Interest	Key interests and issues	Communication medium	Frequency	Justification
Policy makers	High Power/High Interest	Need high-quality evidence that is timely, relevant, and usable for policymaking	Advisory meetings, written briefs, newsletters	Quarterly or aligned with project milestones	Their input ensures the evidence generated is fit-for-policy-use; key avenue for eventual policy translation
Health professionals (e.g., nurses)	Medium Power/High Interest	Practicality and feasibility of interventions in routine care; clear, implementable findings	Advisory meetings, workshops	Every six months or as needed	Their practical perspective ensures the tool is useful in health service settings
Consumers/parents	Low Power/High Interest	Ensuring the evidence is relevant, understandable and reflects lived experience	Workshops, plain language summaries	Every six months or project-specific check-ins	Keeps the project grounded in practical concerns and ensures relevance for families
Trial representatives (other research teams)	Medium to High Power/High Interest	Data sharing, protocol fidelity, accurate interpretation, contribution recognition	Email, newsletters, annual collaborator meetings	Ongoing with periodic in-depth engagement	Key for building and maintaining the living evidence base and ensuring scientific accuracy and collaboration
Broader research community	Low Power/Medium Interest	Updates on project progress, opportunities for collaboration, sharing publication	Website, newsletters, social media	Biannual	Dissemination builds visibility and invites future collaboration or use of evidence base
"Who?"	"What?"		"How?"		"Why?"

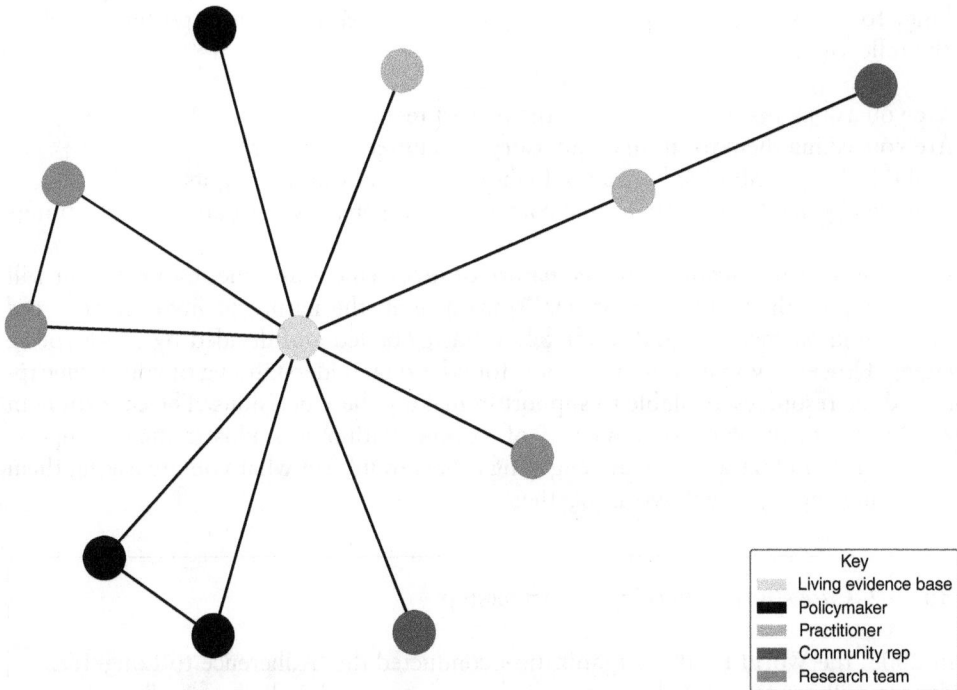

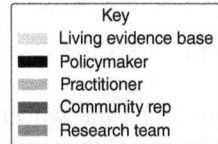

Figure 3.7 Simplified network diagram based on Case Study 1.
Source: https://doi.org/10.25451/flinders.29192669.v1

How to partner with others?

We have shared our learnings of how to identify who to partner with and how to develop a plan for engagement. It is important to think about how you are going to partner with others in your own project. Working on your own project with your own colleagues and team often means you share a common understanding, language, and similar skills, expertise, and experience. While this familiarity can make collaboration feel easier, it can also lead to prioritising efficiency over impact. Sticking to those who think and work like us blocks diverse perspectives and innovative solutions, reducing the potential for broader, more meaningful change. Working in partnership with various different individuals and groups often flips this, with relationships and trust being prioritised over efficiency. Working in partnership means the richness in experience and perspective also brings diversity in language and skill. Therefore, it may be a messy and iterative experience, and you may come up against challenges along the way. To maximise the chances of a positive experience with meaningful outcomes, you need to know how you will work together. Therefore, we want to share some of our key learnings and the below can support you in navigating your engagement.

A crucial thing to consider before you dive headfirst into reaching out to people and making plans and promises around how they can be involved is what resources you will need. It is important to be clear in your own mind on what your expectations are, what their roles and responsibilities may be and how this might change over the lifetime of the project, and how you can support and resource this.

It is therefore important to reflect on that type of involvement or relationship you are seeking. To determine what type of involvement you are seeking it is important to reflect on the following:

- Are you asking people to be part of the project team?
- Are you asking them to sit on an advisory committee or similar?
- Will they be contributing by way of high-level feedback and thoughts?
- Will they be involved in intellectual contributions such as writing and critical editing?

These all have implications for the nature of involvement and the resources you will need to support their involvement. Decisions around the nature of involvement need to be made in partnership, and ultimately needs to be led and decided by those you're engaging. However, you need to have some foundational understanding of your own capacity and the resources available to support in making these decisions. The case study in Box 3.2 provides an example of one way of working with others, illustrating the importance of understanding why you are engaging others to inform what you are asking them to do to guide how you will work together.

Box 3.2   *Case study* 2 Working in partnership

In 2003, the World Health Organization conducted the 'Adherence to Long-Term Therapies Project', a global initiative aiming to improve global rates of adherence to therapies, including physical activity programs, in people with chronic conditions (World Health Organization, 2003). The report concluded that increasing the effectiveness of adherence to interventions may have a far greater impact on the health of the population than any improvement in specific medical treatments. To enhance adherence and empower clinicians, it was recommended that 'adherence counselling toolkits' should be developed.

Using co-design methodology (Nguyen et al., 2020), this project aimed to develop a toolkit for clinicians who work with survivors of stroke, aiming to promote adherence to physical activity or exercise recommendations based on the key features outlined in the World Health Organization report. Evidence shows that many survivors of stroke have reduced adherence and do not meet physical activity guideline recommendations (Fini et al., 2021).

The aim of this toolkit was to help clinicians; therefore, we saw it as critical to include them in the process. We realised that if we developed the toolkit without considering the usability and acceptability it would be a waste of our time and resources. We also saw it as critical to engage survivors of stroke in the process. We really wanted to understand their individual barriers to adherence and hear their ideas about the toolkit, its use, design, and contents.

Before commencing the project, the researchers engaged clinicians from the local affiliated health service. To secure funding to support this work, we worked collaboratively with two clinicians and a person with lived experience, discussed the ideas, developed the research team, and submitted a grant application.

Upon receiving the grant, we secured the resources required to work together and formally commenced the project. We conducted focus groups with two groups,

1) clinicians and 2) survivors of stroke and family members, to understand what they would want from a toolkit. Through these focus groups we were able to develop a preliminary idea about the needs of key stakeholders. The clinician researchers led the clinician focus groups, and the lived experience researcher led the survivor of stroke and family member focus groups. This was important to ensure there was effective co-design within the focus groups.

All participants were then invited to join an 'expert working group' to support the research team in the process of working with a design company to develop the toolkit. Essential, desirable, and non-desirable features were explored. Working through cycles of feedback and toolkit updates, this ensured that the stakeholders had ongoing input in the design and development of the toolkit.

The toolkit has now been developed in a paper-based and online version. This project has used co-design at every stage; hence the toolkit has been designed by and for stakeholders. User testing has been conducted in the health service at the local level (Curran et al., 2012) and the toolkit is currently being evaluated for feasibility in a hybrid type 1 (Curran et al., 2012) implementation effectiveness study.

Author: Tamina Levy
Acknowledgements: Elizabeth Lynch, Lucy Lewis, Kelly Huxley, Saran Chamberlain

Case study 5, in Box 3.2, provides an example of how co-design can be embedded throughout a project from initial grant development through to designing and evaluating tools. By involving clinicians and survivors of stroke at different stages, the project demonstrates stakeholder-led innovation, ensuring the end product is both usable and relevant. It also demonstrates how co-design can improve implementation readiness by anticipating real-world barriers, enabling more tailored and acceptable strategies.

Partnership learnings from an integrated knowledge translation perspective

Managing diversity

Engaging partners to work on a discrete project requires the goals and objectives to be specific. However, when we start to broaden the engagement of partners beyond a specific project and move toward partnering within and across various projects, this creates opportunity for diverse perspectives and involvement, which can create tension. It is not uncommon for external partners, particularly community members, to feel uncomfortable or even silenced in meetings that are led by academic researchers (Bowen & Martens, 2005). Therefore, there is an ethical and practical imperative to ensure you appropriately select who you are engaging and have a process for managing varied and diverse perspectives. For example, you need to ensure that your engagement does not reinforce social inequalities by only including those who already have strong voices or are already embedded within academic culture. It is important to remain mindful that representation of large groups of people is not possible, and one person cannot speak on behalf of a community (Murtagh et al., 2017). Likewise, it is important to be mindful that when bringing together people with diverse perspectives, the goal cannot always be consensus as this may create tensions and ultimately privilege certain perspectives (Murtagh et al., 2017; Tieu et al., 2023).

You therefore need strategies in place for managing these tensions. You cannot pull together a diverse range of people and request their perspectives, which may be contradictory, and not have a plan for appropriately managing and respecting these varied views. There are many ways to do this but having a clear governance process is one such way. Through establishing your governance process, you can clearly outline how perspectives will be collected, navigated, and considered in the research. We have learnt that governance strategies such as meeting agendas, developing terms of reference, external facilitators or meeting chairs, and opportunities for both verbal and written contributions, are examples of strategies that can be used to manage diverse perspectives and any tensions or conflicts that might emerge.

It is also important to have processes, tools, or techniques to build rapport and foster trust. For people to make a meaningful contribution it is important to build trust, develop a strong foundation of safety for sharing ideas, identify common priorities and work in a truly collaborative way (Jansson et al., 2010). This can take time and is often not achieved within one project. Trust and rapport may need to be developed and built upon across many projects. Strategies such as establishing formalised partnerships between organisations and utilising knowledge brokers (i.e., people or groups that help move knowledge from those who create the knowledge to those that use the knowledge) are useful in managing these dynamics and building this longer-term trusting partnerships (Jansson et al., 2010). For example, within the Caring Futures Institute, we are co-located with the Flinders Medical Centre, a large metropolitan public hospital where much of our health and medical research is conducted. Therefore, we often engage patients, family members, and service providers in our research (such as the case study in Table 3.5). The ongoing partnership between the two organisations, allows us to have clear governance and ways of working together which facilitates trust, rapport, and a shared understanding. Another example, within the Caring Futures Institute, is that we have research academics who are employed in joint positions with health services and government departments, to function as knowledge brokers and as implementation science partners. These staff members work in collaboration with the site to develop and implement research into policy and practice. They also focus on building the research capacity and capability of our health, education, and social care workforce. This strategic approach, exemplified by Case Study 3, highlights how close collaboration and a clear plan can facilitate working in partnership.

Box 3.3 *Case study 3* **Working in partnership**

Outpatient waiting times for specialist review are a challenge in public health. Long wait times negatively impact: quality of life, patient outcomes, and health system efficiencies (Lynch et al., 2018). At the commencement of this project, the state health department identified priority areas for reform including the redesign of models of outpatient care. Non-urgent neurosurgical specialist wait time at the project site was ranked the second longest in the state, with 708 patients on the waiting list, with median waiting times of 26.4 months (>2 years) and a maximum waiting time of 122.6 months (>10 years). Due to the scale of this problem and the urgent need to implement redesigned models of care, a project team was formed including clinicians at the project site, allied health researchers, and a health economist.

Stage 1: A stakeholder group was formed with representation from the project team, allied health leadership, neurosurgeons, nursing, and administration. This stakeholder group met regularly over the 12 months of the project.

The project used the Knowledge to Action Framework (Graham et al., 2006) where knowledge creation was featured in stages 2 to 4.

Stage 2: A prospective observational study of people on the waiting list involved:

Surveys (n= 200 sent, n= 30 responses) described symptoms/effects on quality of life and out-of-hospital health care and identified that majority had worsening symptoms and low quality of life.

Semi-structured interviews (n=12) indicated that waitlisted patients were negatively impacted, feeling frustrated and demoralised, "the not knowing is really bad".

Stage 3: A retrospective observational study of hospital utilisation. It was identified that for a cohort of 183 patients, costs for Emergency Department presentations and inpatient admissions were $30,495. This equates to $116,000 per year with approximately 700 people on waitlist.

Stage 4: An evidence review of models of care for managing neurosurgical waiting lists. It was identified that supporting physiotherapy led assessment/triage of non-urgent spinal patients is safe, cost-effective, correlated with surgeon assessments, higher levels of patient and referrer satisfaction.

The project team led the knowledge synthesis with the results from Stages 2- 4 to develop feasible evidence-based solutions. The Knowledge to Action Framework (Graham et al., 2006) action cycle was then enacted through two workshops:

Stage 5: A first workshop was held where the knowledge synthesis was shared with the stakeholder group. Additional stakeholders were invited to this workshop including primary care practitioners and consumers. Stakeholders selected and suggested adaptations to the feasible evidence-based solutions.

Stage 6: Options that were selected in the first workshop were developed and refined to reflect the local context, including resources required to implement different models and expected effects on the waiting list, healthcare resources and patient outcomes.

Stage 7: A second workshop was held where the stakeholder group were presented with developed model of care options, which were described in terms of cost, benefits, and implementation. As a group, the final model selected which was an advanced practice physiotherapist assessment and management strategy recommendations.

This seven-stage co-design project guided by the Knowledge to Action Framework was successful in bringing together the diverse perspectives of key stakeholders to identify and tailor a new model of care. The engagement of the diverse stakeholders was critical to develop a solution that considered the local context to aid in implementation.

Since completing this project, a business case was submitted to the hospital executive to improve care for patients who are on the neurosurgical wait list. From this, a Senior Physiotherapist position was approved for 1 year to lead this new model of care. This role will be evaluated in terms of patient satisfaction, referrer/stakeholder satisfaction, cost effectiveness and impact on wait lists.

Author: Stacey George
Acknowledgements: Jane Bickford, Jon Karnon, Ema Knight, and Duncan Lodge

Case study 3, in Box 3.3, demonstrates the systematic application of the Knowledge-to-Action framework to redesign outpatient neurosurgical care. A particular strength is its structured stakeholder engagement across different phases of the project. The approach illustrates how an integrated knowledge translation approach can inform practical solutions by combining multiple data sources with end-user input. By involving stakeholders early and often, this project not only co-designed a contextually relevant model but also secured organisational buy-in and resourcing for implementation.

Evaluating 'success'

Completing or delivering a project is not a sufficient outcome to say that a partnership or engagement was successful. How success is defined or understood can vary across different partners. Therefore, it is critical to identify what your partners view as measures of success. For them, traditional outputs like academic publications or conference presentations may be of low priority. Instead, developing a resource or product they can use, business cases, or policy briefs, may be what matters most. The goals or outcomes that may be considered success for your partners, may not be achievable within a discrete project. This again, is where taking an integrated knowledge translation approach can support ongoing partnership and support delivering success for all partners involved.

Consider the following questions when determining what successful engagement is:

- Who has benefited from the project?
- Has the project had impact for all involved?
- Does everyone involved feel like they achieved what they expected?
- Is everyone happy with the end result?
- Were there any unexpected challenges or outcomes and does everyone feel like these were managed appropriately?
- Is there still interest to continue working together?

It is also important to acknowledge and celebrate successes and achievements to ensure partners feel valued and as though their contribution made a significant impact. Similarly, it is important for both researchers and partners to understand how their involvement fits into the bigger picture and how they are making a distinct valuable contribution. If you and your partners are unable to understand or articulate this, you are at risk of engaging people in a tokenistic way, which may cause more damage to relationships and reputations, than if no engagement were to occur (Romsland et al., 2019).

Chapter summary

We have introduced working in partnership, shared our learnings of working with others, and highlighted how an integrated knowledge translation approach to partnership supports sustained and diverse engagement within and across projects. Our key learnings in this chapter revolved around developing a plan for engagement, managing diversity, and evaluating what 'success' looks like in partnerships (Figure 3.8).

In Chapter 4, we will explore integrated knowledge translation in more detail and begin to explore how you can move your engagement with partners from a method to a mindset.

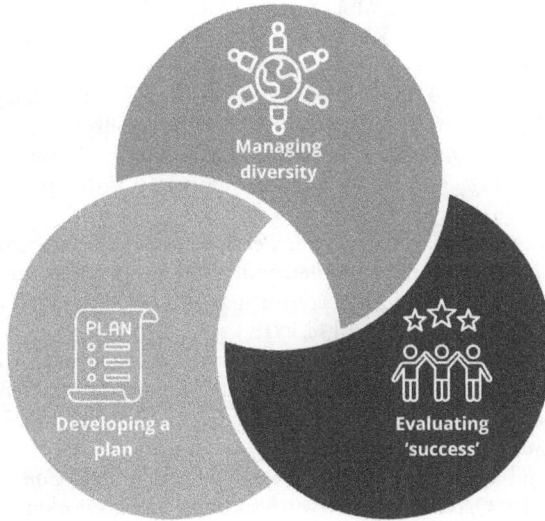

Figure 3.8 Partnership key learnings.
Source: https://doi.org/10.25451/flinders.29192681.v1

References

Archibald, M., Lawless, M. T., de Plaza, M. A. P., & Kitson, A. L. (2023). How transdisciplinary research teams learn to do knowledge translation (KT), and how KT in turn impacts transdisciplinary research: A realist evaluation and longitudinal case study. *Health Research Policy and Systems*, 21(1), 20–20. https://doi.org/10.1186/s12961-023-00967-x

Banner, D., Bains, M., Carroll, S., Kandola, D. K., Rolfe, D. E., Wong, C., & Graham, I. D. (2019). Patient and public engagement in integrated knowledge translation research: Are we there yet? *Research Involvement and Engagement*, 5(1), 8–8. https://doi.org/10.1186/s40900-019-0139-1

Bernstein, S. L., Weiss, J., & Curry, L. (2020). Visualizing implementation: Contextual and organizational support mapping of stakeholders (COSMOS). *Implementation Science Communications*, 1(1), 48–48. https://doi.org/10.1186/s43058-020-00030-8

Boote, J., Baird, W., & Sutton, A. (2011). Public involvement in the systematic review process in health and social care: A narrative review of case examples. *Health policy (Amsterdam)*, 102(2), 105–116. https://doi.org/10.1016/j.healthpol.2011.05.002

Bowen, S. J., & Martens, P. (2005). Demystifying knowledge translation: Learning from the community. *Journal of Health Services Research & Policy*, 10(4), 203–211. https://doi.org/10.1258/135581905774414213

Brugha, R., & Varvasovszky, Z. (2000). Stakeholder analysis: A review. *Health Policy and Planning*, 15(3), 239–246. https://doi.org/10.1093/heapol/15.3.239

Canadian Institutes for Health Research. (2012). *CIHR's Framework for Citizen Engagement*. Retrieved 23 May from www.cihr-irsc.gc.ca/e/41270.html.

Canadian Institutes of Health Research. (2015). *Guide to knowledge translation planning at CIHR: Integrated and end-of-grant approaches*. https://cihr-irsc.gc.ca/e/45321.html

Canadian Institutes of Health Research. (2023). *Strategy for patient-oriented research*. Canadian Institutes of Health Research. www.cihr-irsc.gc.ca/e/41204.html

Cargo, M., & Mercer, S. L. (2008). The value and challenges of participatory research: Strengthening its practice. *Annual Review of Public Health*, 29(1), 325–350. https://doi.org/10.1146/annurev.publhealth.29.091307.083824

Charlton, J. I. (1998). *Nothing about us without us: Disability oppression and empowerment.* University of California Press. https://doi.org/10.1525/9780520925441

Chu, L. F., Utengen, A., Kadry, B., Kucharski, S. E., Campos, H., Crockett, J., Dawson, N., & Clauson, K. A. (2016). "Nothing about us without us"-patient partnership in medical conferences. *BMJ (Online), 354,* i3883–i3883. https://doi.org/10.1136/bmj.i3883

Chung, A., Kuswara, K., Johnson, B., Seidler, A. L., Hall, A., & Brown, V. (2024). Collaborating with end-users in evidence synthesis: Case studies for prevention in the first 2000 days. *Public Health Research & Practice, 34*(1 DOI – http://dx.doi.org/10.17061/phrp3412410), e3412410. http://dx.doi.org/10.17061/phrp3412410

Cowdell, F., Dyson, J., Sykes, M., Dam, R., & Pendleton, R. (2022). How and how well have older people been engaged in healthcare intervention design, development or delivery using co-methodologies: A scoping review with narrative summary. *Health & Social Care Community, 30*(2), 776–798. https://doi.org/10.1111/hsc.13199

Curran, G. M., Bauer, M., Mittman, B., Pyne, J. M., & Stetler, C. (2012). Effectiveness-implementation hybrid designs: Combining elements of clinical effectiveness and implementation research to enhance public health impact. *Medical Care, 50*(3), 217–226. https://doi.org/10.1097/MLR.0b013e3182408812

Department of Health and Aged Care. (2023). *Emerging Priorities and Consumer-Driven Research Initiative.* Retrieved 25 October from www.health.gov.au/our-work/mrff-emerging-priorities-and-consumer-driven-research-initiative

Deverka, P. A., Lavallee, D. C., Desai, P. J., Esmail, L. C., Ramsey, S. D., Veenstra, D. L., & Tunis, S. R. (2012). Stakeholder participation in comparative effectiveness research: Defining a framework for effective engagement. *Journal of Comparative Effectiveness Research, 1*(2), 181–194. https://doi.org/10.2217/cer.12.7

Fini, N. A., Bernhardt, J., Churilov, L., Clark, R., & Holland, A. E. (2021). Adherence to physical activity and cardiovascular recommendations during the 2 years after stroke rehabilitation discharge. *Annals of Physical and Rehabilitation Medicine, 64*(2), 101455. https://doi.org/10.1016/j.rehab.2020.03.018

Garrett, J. J. (2011). *The elements of user experience, 2nd edition.* New Riders Publishing.

Glegg, S. M. N., Jenkins, E., & Kothari, A. (2019). How the study of networks informs knowledge translation and implementation: A scoping review. *Implementation Science: IS, 14*(1), 34–34. https://doi.org/10.1186/s13012-019-0879-1

Graham, I. D., Logan, J., Harrison, M. B., Straus, S. E., Tetroe, J., Caswell, W., & Robinson, N. (2006). Lost in knowledge translation: Time for a map? *The Journal of Continuing Education in the Health Professions, 26*(1), 13–24. https://doi.org/10.1002/chp.47

Greene, L. W., George, M. A., Daniel, M., Frankish, C. J., Herbert, C., Bowie, W. R., & O'Neill, M. (1995). Study of participatory research in health promotion. *Royal Society of Canada, 45*(50).

Hunter, K. E., Johnson, B. J., Askie, L., Golley, R. K., Baur, L. A., Taylor, R. W., Wolfenden, L., Wood, C. T., Mihrshahi, S., Hayes, A. J., Rissel, C., Robledo, K. P., O'Connor, D. A., Espinoza, D., Staub, L. P., Barba, A., Libesman, S., Smith, W. A., Sue-See, M., ... Widen, E. (2022). Transforming Obesity Prevention for CHILDren (TOPCHILD) Collaboration: Protocol for a systematic review with individual participant data meta-analysis of behavioural interventions for the prevention of early childhood obesity. *BMJ Open, 12*(1), e048166–e048166. https://doi.org/10.1136/bmjopen-2020-048166

Hunter, K. E., Webster, A. C., Page, M. J., Willson, M., McDonald, S., Berber, S., Skeers, P., Tan-Koay, A. G., Parkhill, A., & Seidler, A. L. (2022). Searching clinical trials registers: Guide for systematic reviewers. *BMJ (Online), 377,* e068791–e068791. https://doi.org/10.1136/bmj-2021-068791

International Association for Public Participation. (2018). IAP2 Spectrum of Public Participation. www.iap2.org/page/pillars

Jansson, S. M., Benoit, C., Casey, L., Phillips, R., & Burns, D. (2010). In for the long Haul: Knowledge translation between academic and nonprofit organizations. *Qualitative Health Research, 20*(1), 131–143. https://doi.org/10.1177/1049732309349808

Johnson, B. J., Hunter, K. E., Golley, R. K., Chadwick, P., Barba, A., Aberoumand, M., Libesman, S., Askie, L., Taylor, R. W., Robledo, K. P., Mihrshahi, S., O'Connor, D. A., Hayes, A. J., Wolfenden, L., Wood, C. T., Baur, L. A., Rissel, C., Staub, L. P., Taki, S., . . . Transforming Obesity Prevention for, C. C. (2022). Unpacking the behavioural components and delivery features of early childhood obesity prevention interventions in the TOPCHILD Collaboration: A systematic review and intervention coding protocol. *BMJ open*, *12*(1), 1–9. https://doi.org/10.17863/CAM.80702; https://link.springer.com/article/10.1186/s12966-025-01708-9

Kitson, A., Powell, K., Hoon, E., Newbury, J., Wilson, A., & Beilby, J. (2013). Knowledge translation within a population health study: How do you do it? *Implementation Science: IS, 8*(1), 54–54. https://doi.org/10.1186/1748-5908-8-54

Lynch, E. A., Mudge, A., Knowles, S., Kitson, A. L., Hunter, S. C., & Harvey, G. (2018). "There is nothing so practical as a good theory": A pragmatic guide for selecting theoretical approaches for implementation projects. *BMC Health Services Research*, *18*(1), 857–857. https://doi.org/10.1186/s12913-018-3671-z

Mendelow, A. L. (1991). Environmental Scanning: The Impact of the Stakeholder Concept. Second International Conference on Information Systems, Cambridge, MA.

Murtagh, M. J., Minion, J. T., Turner, A., Wilson, R. C., Blell, M., Ochieng, C., Murtagh, B., Roberts, S., Butters, O. W., & Burton, P. R. (2017). The ECOUTER methodology for stakeholder engagement in translational research. *BMC Medical Ethics*, *18*(1), 24–24. https://doi.org/10.1186/s12910-017-0167-z

National Institute for Health and Care Research. (2020). *NIHR launches new Centre for Engagement and Dissemination*. Retrieved 25 October from www.nihr.ac.uk/news/nihr-launches-new-centre-for-engagement-and-dissemination/24576

National Institute for Health and Care Research. (2021). *Briefing notes for researchers*. Retrieved 25 October from www.nihr.ac.uk/documents/briefing-notes-for-researchers-public-involvement-in-nhs-health-and-social-care-research/27371

National Institute for Health and Care Research. (2023). *NIHR INVOLVE*. Retrieved 25 October from www.invo.org.uk/

Nguyen, T., Graham, I. D., Mrklas, K. J., Bowen, S., Cargo, M., Estabrooks, C. A., Kothari, A., Lavis, J., MacAulay, A. C., MacLeod, M., Phipps, D., Ramsden, V. R., Renfrew, M. J., Salsberg, J., & Wallerstein, N. (2020). How does integrated knowledge translation (IKT) compare to other collaborative research approaches to generating and translating knowledge? Learning from experts in the field. *Health Research Policy and Systems*, *18*(1), 35–35. https://doi.org/10.1186/s12961-020-0539-6

Patient-Centred Outcomes Research Institute. (2023). *Patient-Centred Outcomes Research Institute*. Retrieved 25 October from www.pcori.org/

Reed, M. S., Merkle, B. G., Cook, E. J., Hafferty, C., Hejnowicz, A. P., Holliman, R., Marder, I. D., Pool, U., Raymond, C. M., Wallen, K. E., Whyte, D., Ballesteros, M., Bhanbhro, S., Borota, S., Brennan, M. L., Carmen, E., Conway, E. A., Everett, R., Armstrong-Gibbs, F., ... Stroobant, M. (2024). Reimagining the language of engagement in a post-stakeholder world. *Sustainability Science*, *19*(4), 1481–1490. https://doi.org/10.1007/s11625-024-01496-4

Romsland, G. I., Milosavljevic, K. L., & Andreassen, T. A. (2019). Facilitating non-tokenistic user involvement in research. *Research Involvement and Engagement*, *5*(1), 18–18. https://doi.org/10.1186/s40900-019-0153-3

Sanders, M. R., & Kirby, J. N. (2012). Consumer engagement and the development, evaluation, and dissemination of evidence-based parenting programs. *Behavior Therapy*, *43*(2), 236–250. https://doi.org/10.1016/j.beth.2011.01.005

Seidler, A. L., Hunter, K. E., Cheyne, S., Ghersi, D., Berlin, J. A., & Askie, L. (2019). A guide to prospective meta-analysis. *BMJ (Online)*, *367*, l5342–l5342. https://doi.org/10.1136/bmj.l5342

Seidler, A. L., Johnson, B. J., Golley, R. K., & Hunter, K. E. (2022). The complex quest of preventing obesity in early childhood: Describing challenges and solutions through collaboration and innovation. *Frontiers in Endocrinology (Lausanne)*, *12*, 803545–803545. https://doi.org/10.3389/fendo.2021.803545

Staley, K. (2015). 'Is it worth doing?' Measuring the impact of patient and public involvement in research. *Research Involvement and Engagement, 1*(1), 6. https://doi.org/10.1186/s40 900-015-0008-5

Straus, S. E., Tetroe, J., & Graham, I. (2009). Defining knowledge translation. *Canadian Medical Association Journal (CMAJ), 181*(3–4), 165–168. https://doi.org/10.1503/cmaj.081229

Tieu, M., Lawless, M., Hunter, S. C., Pinero de Plaza, M. A., Darko, F., Mudd, A., Yadav, L., & Kitson, A. (2023). Wicked problems in a post-truth political economy: A dilemma for knowledge translation. *Humanities & Social Sciences Communications, 10*(1), 280–280. https://doi.org/10.1057/s41599-023-01789-6

World Health Organization. (2003). Adherence to long-term therapies: Evidence for action. Geneva: World Health Organization.

4 Integrated knowledge translation meets complexity science

Alison Kitson, Michael Lawless and Sarah Hunter

Introduction

Knowledge translation is now widely acknowledged and increasingly expected in applied health and social care research. This growing emphasis reflects a broader movement towards ensuring that publicly funded research is used more effectively, efficiently, and promptly in policy and practice. Over time, there has been a shift in the way we think and talk about knowledge translation approaches, moving from linear, rational process descriptions, to acknowledging the interconnectedness of behavioural, social, and system-level factors. Getting the conditions right to ensure that evidence-informed interventions, tools, or strategies are recognised and used appropriately in policy and practice is as much about behavioural, social, and organisational factors as it is about the logical, rational ways of thinking about knowledge production and use.

We have reached a stage where the focus on evidence or new knowledge implementation has expanded to consider the whole knowledge translation process. This includes dissemination, synthesis, problem identification, knowledge generation and refining, as well as implementation and evaluation. Integrated knowledge translation approaches are gaining momentum as they help to tell the whole story (the rational, behavioural, and social) and explain why things didn't work as much as why they did work. This means that knowledge translation researchers need to be familiar with a range of methodological approaches, while developing key relational and management skills. These approaches can help us understand and work across multiple levels of influence: individual and inter-personal behaviours, motivations, and relationships (micro level); social and organisa-tional structures, power dynamics, hierarchies, and routines (meso level); and broader system influences such as policy, regulation, and political environments (macro level).

In this chapter we will summarise some common integrated knowledge translation theories, models, and frameworks that you are likely to come across. We are not pro-viding you with an exhaustive list but giving you an idea of what the main elements are (these elements are summarised in Chapter 8). We will then briefly explain how integrated knowledge translation and complexity science came together. This will be followed by a more detailed description of the Knowledge Translation Complexity Network Model. This is the working model that we use to help us understand and work with knowledge translation in the Caring Futures Institute.

In introducing you to the Knowledge Translation Complexity Network Model, which essentially is where 'integrated knowledge translation meets complexity science', we will outline why we think this approach offers more insight into understanding the messy world of getting new knowledge into policy and practice. We will describe each of the

DOI: 10.4324/9781003245995-5

processes of the model. In Chapter 5, you will find case studies that illustrate knowledge translation in action. If you prefer, you can skip ahead and read these first before exploring the theoretical underpinnings in this chapter. Seeing how these concepts play out in real-world research might help the frameworks and constructs we discuss in this chapter feel more concrete and intuitive. These case studies also highlight that integrated knowledge translation is an evolving process, often shaped by trial and error. None of our teams deliberately started out using the Knowledge Translation Complexity Network Model to shape their knowledge translation methods. What we present in these chapters is more of a reflective journey, describing how teams made sense of what worked, what didn't, and why and how they could improve outcomes by understanding what was happening within the micro-, meso-, and macro-levels of the systems they were working.

Integrated knowledge translation: a recap

As introduced in Chapter 1, the most widely used definition of integrated knowledge translation comes from the Canadian Institutes of Health Research:

> "An approach to doing research that involves applying the principles of knowledge translation (synthesis, dissemination, exchange, and ethically sound application of knowledge) to the **entire research process**."
> (Canadian Institutes of Health Research, 2015;
> Kothari et al., 2017) (emphasis added)

Despite the Canadian Institutes of Health Research defining integrated knowledge translation as collaborative and iterative, traditional, linear (or 'pipeline') models seem to be the default approach (see Chapter 1). These models generally assume that 'knowledge producers' (e.g., researchers) and 'knowledge users' (e.g., clinicians, policymakers, patients, communities) are separate communities and that knowledge translation mostly follows a predictable and orderly set of steps. As we have seen, though, this perspective tends to ignore or downplay the dynamic and unpredictable movement and transformation of knowledge within complex social systems. In Chapter 1, we discussed how applied research approaches, the Canadian Institutes of Health Research's influential definition of integrated Knowledge Translation and the Medical Research Council's Complex Intervention guidance (Campbell et al., 2000; Craig et al., 2006; Craig et al., 2008; Skivington et al., 2021) all embrace the basic idea that 'bridging' the research-practice gap means that we need context-sensitive, collaborative, and adaptive approaches (Braithwaite et al., 2018; Greenhalgh et al., 2017; Kitson et al., 2018).

What sets integrated knowledge translation apart from what has been termed 'end-of-grant' knowledge translation is that it marks a fundamental shift from researcher-led knowledge creation and dissemination to ongoing, purposeful engagement. Instead of treating research as a one-way process, integrated knowledge translation involves 'knowledge users' as equal partners across various research processes. This collaborative approach helps ensure that research is relevant, useable, and more likely to lead to meaningful societal benefits. Figure 4.1 illustrates the distinction between integrated and end-of-grant knowledge translation. While end-of-grant knowledge translation typically focuses on communicating findings after a study finishes, integrated knowledge translation spans the full spectrum of knowledge translation processes and can be embedded across all stages of research (Esmail et al., 2020; Strifler et al., 2018).

Integrated Versus End-of-Grant Knowledge Translation

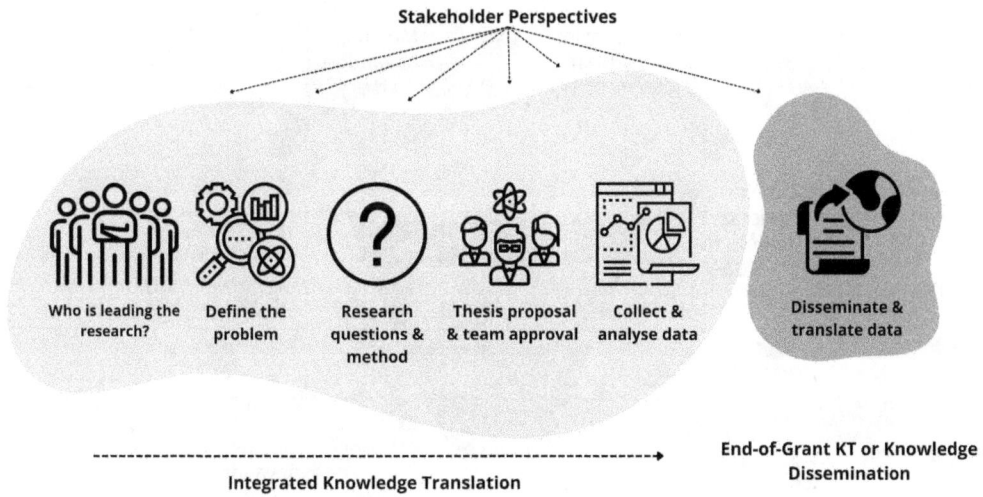

Figure 4.1 Integrated versus end-of-grant knowledge translation.
Source: https://doi.org/10.25451/flinders.29192690.v1

Integrated knowledge translation emphasises co-production, relationship-building, and shared decision-making, setting up conditions for research that are not only methodologically rigorous but also contextually relevant and geared towards action.

Integrated knowledge translation: theories, models, and frameworks

Integrated knowledge translation is put into practice using a range of theories, models, and frameworks. Although these theories, models, and frameworks often emphasise similar principles like working closely with the various people and groups who will use or be affected by the research from the very start of the project, they are grounded in different epistemologies and disciplinary traditions. For more in-depth discussion of the range of integrated and 'full spectrum' knowledge translation theories, models, and frameworks, we encourage readers to consult existing sources (e.g., Esmail et al., 2020; Nilsen & Birken, 2020). Here, we provide a brief overview of three examples that can be used to guide an integrated knowledge translation approach. Our aim is not to be exhaustive, but to offer a sense of their shared principles and how they might be applied in practice. Whichever theory, model, or framework your team selects, it's important to be clear about why it was chosen and how it fits the specific goals and context of your project. Below, we summarise each theory, model, or framework, and include the visual representations that have been used to communicate their key ideas.

Knowledge-to-Action Framework (Graham et al., 2006)

The Knowledge-to-Action framework (Figure 4.2) is a widely used approach that conceptualises the dynamic and iterative processes involved in moving research-based

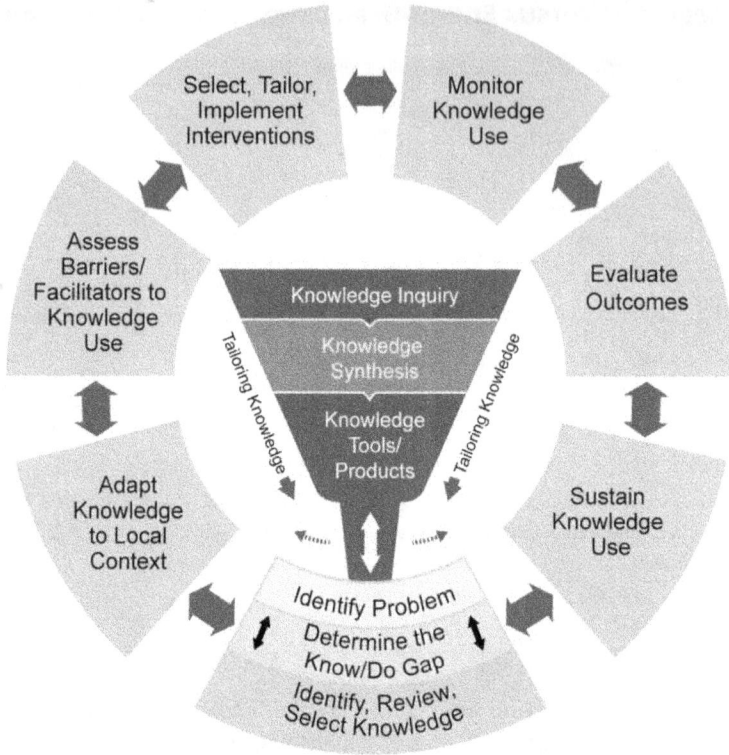

Figure 4.2 Knowledge-to-Action Framework.
Source: Graham et al. (2006).

knowledge into practice. The framework is composed of two key components: Knowledge Creation, represented by a funnel, illustrates the refinement of knowledge through the stages of inquiry, synthesis, and the development of tools and products; and the Action Cycle, which surrounds the funnel and describes a sequence of activities that support the application of knowledge, including adapting knowledge to the local context, assessing barriers and enablers, monitoring knowledge use, evaluating outcomes, and ensuring sustainability. The Knowledge-to-Action framework is appropriate when specific change is desired (e.g., implementing clinical guidelines). It outlines specific steps to generate, adapt, and apply knowledge in context-sensitive ways that integrate multiple partner perspectives.

Co-creating Knowledge Translation Framework (Kitson et al., 2013)

The Co-creating Knowledge Translation framework (Figure 4.3) aims to support collaboration between researchers and communities from the outset of the project. It was developed to support the co-creation, refinement, implementation, and evaluation of knowledge that is sensitive to local needs, values, and contextual factors. Knowledge for improving health service delivery and outcomes through interdisciplinary

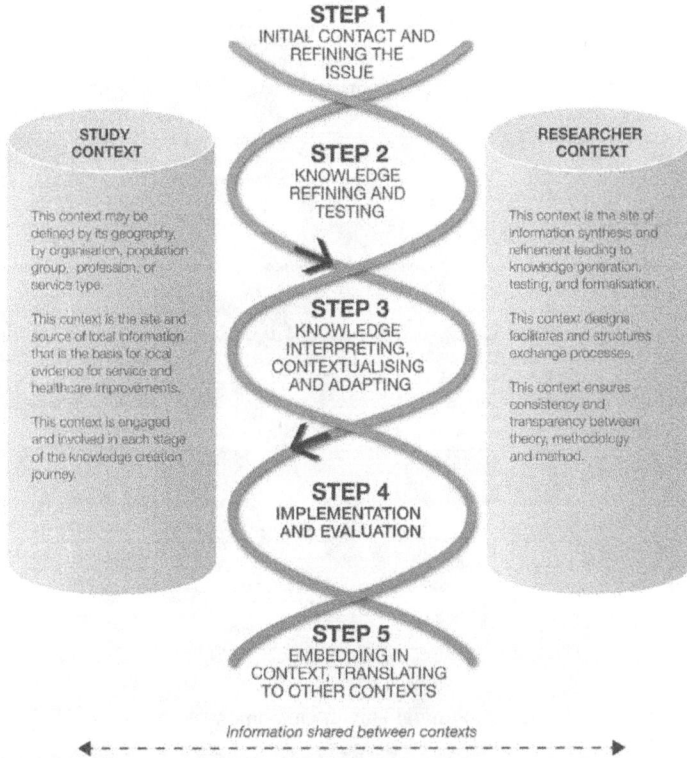

Figure 4.3 Co-creating Knowledge Translation Framework.
Source: Kitson et al. (2013).

collaboration. Influenced by participatory action research, the Co-creating Knowledge Translation framework recognises both explicit (e.g., research, manuals, protocols, clinical guidelines) and tacit knowledge forms and sources, (e.g., practice-based decision-making, patient and caregiver experiences), and promotes ongoing and multi-directional knowledge exchange. The framework is particularly well suited to community-based or population health studies where equitable partner engagement and local applicability are required.

CollaboraKTion Framework (Jenkins et al., 2016)

The CollaboraKTion framework (Figure 4.4) focuses on community-based knowledge translation through a theory-driven approach that incorporates insights from both knowledge translation and participatory action research. It outlines an iterative process consisting of five overarching activities, including contacting, and connecting, deepening understandings, adapting, and applying knowledge, supporting, and evaluating continued action, and transitioning and embedding knowledge. Each activity includes key process elements that serve as contextual considerations and outcomes within the community-based knowledge translation process.

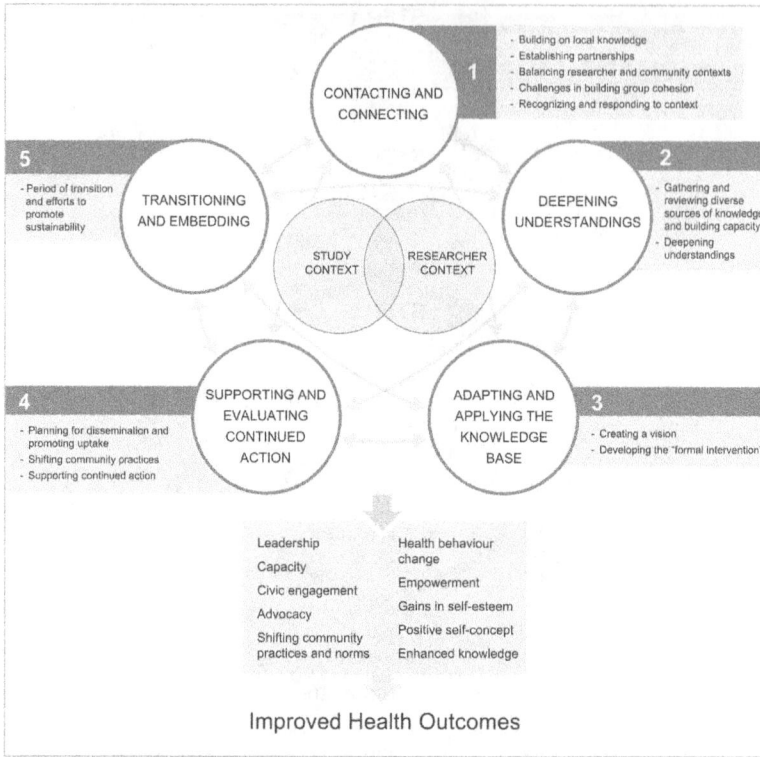

Figure 4.4 CollaboraKTion Framework.
Source: Jenkins et al. (2016).

Integrated knowledge translation involves paying attention to relationships and interactions. This requires trust-building, negotiation, and shared decision-making. These social processes are dynamic and hard to standardise and predict. This level of engagement makes it hard to create a standard research or implementation plan or protocol in a traditional sense. The challenge, then, is to have an idea of where you want to get to but be prepared for diversions and unexpected events on the journey. Documenting this and responding to it in a systematic, reflective way is part of the new skill set that knowledge translation researchers need to develop.

The most common conceptualisation of integrated knowledge translation emerged from sociological traditions and focuses on interpersonal and social aspects (Nguyen et al., 2020; Thomas et al., 2014). More recently in knowledge translation research there has been an acknowledgement of contextual and organisational factors (McCormack et al., 2002; Nilsen & Bernhardsson, 2019; Squires et al., 2022), which, in turn, have led to thinking about organisational and system complexity (May et al., 2016). We now move into a short summary of how complexity science teamed up with integrated knowledge translation in healthcare settings.

When complexity science meets integrated knowledge translation

The roots of complexity theory or science in healthcare can be traced back to the broader application of complexity science in various fields such as computer science, physics, sociology, and economics (Churruca et al., 2019). Complexity science is closely linked with the study of complex adaptive systems (among other influences), which are systems made up of diverse agents (individual components or entities, including human agents, organisations, and technologies) that continuously interact with each other and their environment, influencing each other's actions and responses. This perspective recognises that such systems exhibit behaviours that are more than the sum of their parts, often showing non-linear, unpredictable, and emergent properties.

The adoption of complexity science in healthcare research started to gain momentum in the early 2000s, with seminal papers (e.g., Plsek & Greenhalgh, 2001) making a compelling case for introducing complexity science thinking to medical research and practice. These initial contributions framed healthcare systems as complex, adaptive, and inherently unpredictable environments, emphasising the need for flexible and adaptive approaches to healthcare delivery and research.

Despite the early publications in the 2000s, there has not been a huge uptake in complexity science thinking in health services research. Knowledge translation researchers have tended to focus on 'context' as the substitute construct for complex adaptive systems and significant work has been undertaken to develop and refine measures of context (Damschroder et al., 2022; Harvey & Kitson, 2016; Pfadenhauer et al., 2017), measures of organisational readiness for change (Weiner, 2020), and measures of leadership effectiveness in systems (Aarons et al., 2014; Gifford et al., 2017). Whilst these are important contributions to our understanding of contextual factors and how to moderate their impact, they still tend to be deterministic and rigid in their application.

You could think that these context measures are grafted onto an integrated knowledge translation approach to help you understand the wider system or organisational factors that need to be considered. But if your knowledge translation research approach does not allow you to change or moderate your activity because of local contextual (system and organisational) variation, then you are not able to adapt to the complex systems you are studying. That means that while you may try and change individual behaviour using an approach like the Theoretical Domains Framework (Cane et al., 2012; Michie et al., 2005), you may not have the equivalent understanding of how you are going to shape some of the contextual factors (leadership, power, culture, resource, routines for example) that you will come up against. Or else, you assume that people who are changing their behaviour are also developing the skills and competencies to influence the wider system. This essentially is what complexity science is offering integrated knowledge translation approaches – the ability not only to adapt and respond to individual and interpersonal differences, but also to take account of system and organisational complexities and variations.

We have come across four theories, models, and frameworks that we believe connect integrated knowledge translation principles with complexity science thinking. We summarise these below

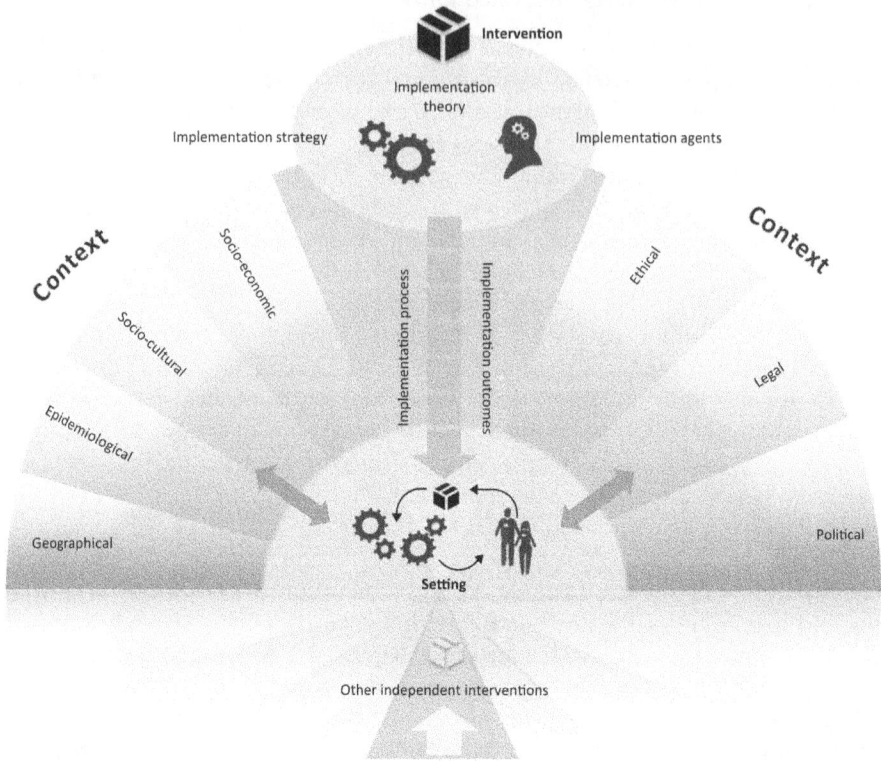

Figure 4.5 Context and Implementation of Complex Interventions Framework.
Source: Pfadenhauer et al. (2017).

Context and Implementation of Complex Interventions Framework (Pfadenhauer et al., 2017)

The Context and Implementation of Complex Interventions framework (Figure 4.5) integrates complexity theory into the evaluation and implementation of complex interventions by considering the context in which these interventions are implemented. It was developed to facilitate the structured and comprehensive conceptualisation and assessment of context and implementation of complex interventions.

Non-adoption, Abandonment, Scale-Up, Spread, and Sustainability (NASSS) Framework (Greenhalgh & Papoutsi, 2018)

The NASSS framework (Figure 4.6) is specifically designed to understand and address the challenges related to the adoption and scaling up of health technologies. It incorporates complexity theory by recognising that technology adoption in healthcare is influenced by multiple interacting domains: the illness, the technology, the value proposition, the

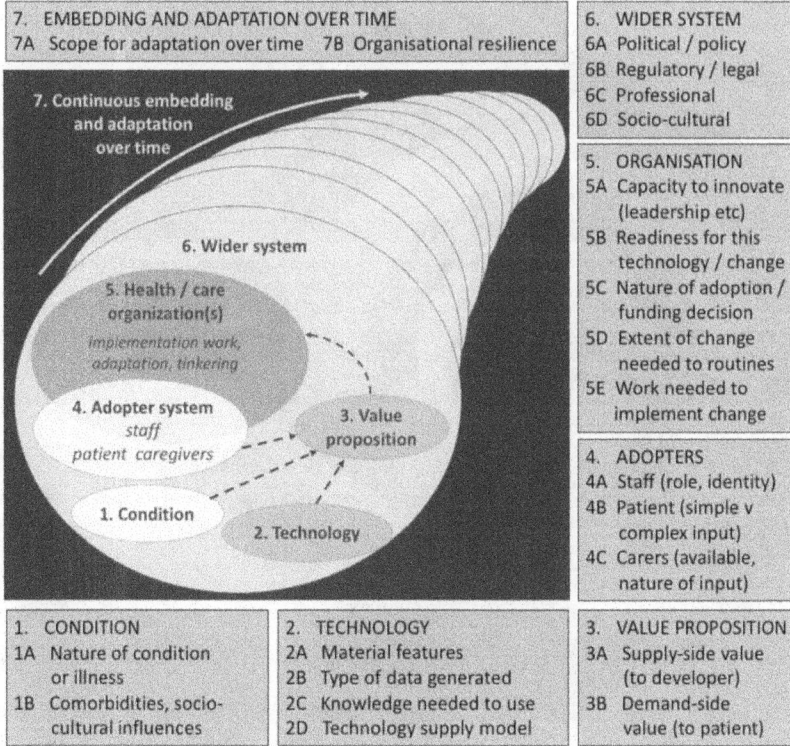

Figure 4.6 Non-adoption, Abandonment, Scale-Up, Spread, and Sustainability (NASSS) Framework.

Source: Greenhalgh & Papoutsi (2018).

adopter system (patients, healthcare staff, etc.), the healthcare organisation, the wider institutional and regulatory context, and the temporal aspects over time. The NASSS framework (see Figure 4.6) allows researchers to surface and explain the multiple forms and manifestations of complexity in technology-supported change projects.

Successful Healthcare Improvement from Translating Evidence (SHIFT-Evidence) Framework (Reed et al., 2018)

The SHIFT-Evidence framework (Figure 4.7) emphasises iterative and adaptive approaches to knowledge translation. It draws on complexity theory by recognising that healthcare systems are dynamic, and that evidence must be translated in a way that can adapt to changes within the system. The framework identifies three key principles: acting scientifically and pragmatically, embracing complexity, and engaging and empowering partners.

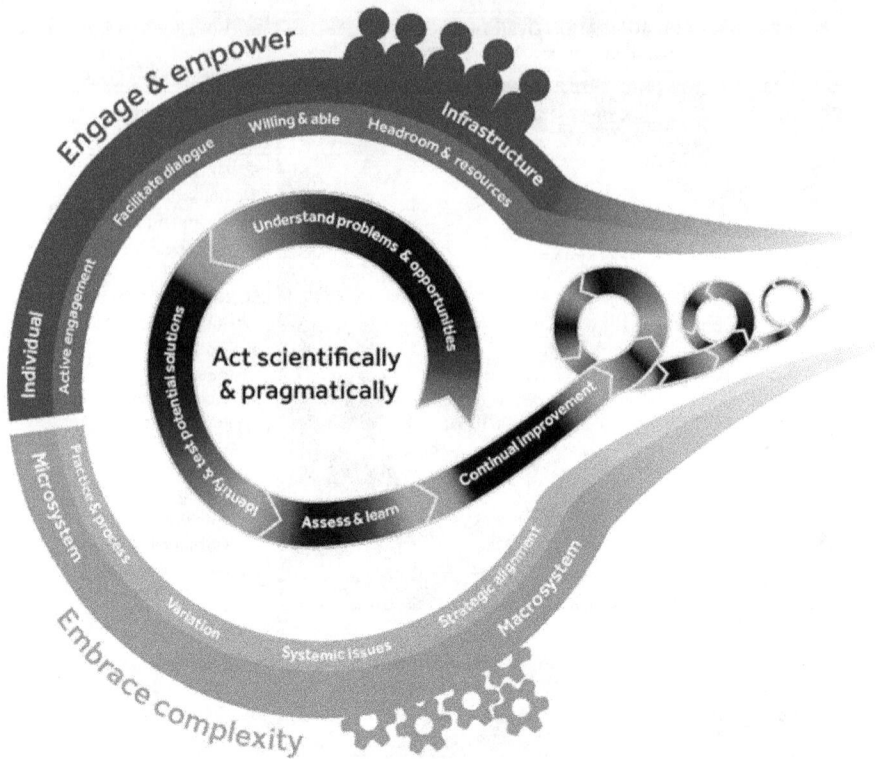

Figure 4.7 Successful Healthcare Improvement from Translating Evidence (SHIFT-Evidence) Framework.
Source: Reed et al. (2018).

Knowledge Translation Complexity Network Model (Kitson et al., 2018)

The Knowledge Translation Complexity Network Model (Figure 4.8) is based in complexity science and network concepts, offering a more integrated and dynamic approach to knowledge translation. It incorporates five key processes: problem identification, knowledge creation, knowledge synthesis, implementation, and evaluation. The Knowledge Translation Complexity Network Model views these processes as part of a dynamic and complex process, interacting within the structural components of the entire knowledge translation system.

It recognises that healthcare is a complex adaptive system characterised by non-linearity, interdependence, and emergent behaviour. The model emphasises that successful knowledge translation requires understanding and engaging with these complexities.

These theories, models, and frameworks integrate aspects of complexity science thinking into their conceptualisations to address the challenges of knowledge translation specifically in healthcare. They all recognise that healthcare systems are dynamic, adaptive, and influenced by multiple interacting factors, to varying degrees, but differ in their focus (e.g., adopting and scaling health technologies in the case of NASSS). Together, they illustrate the importance of considering multiple, interacting factors and

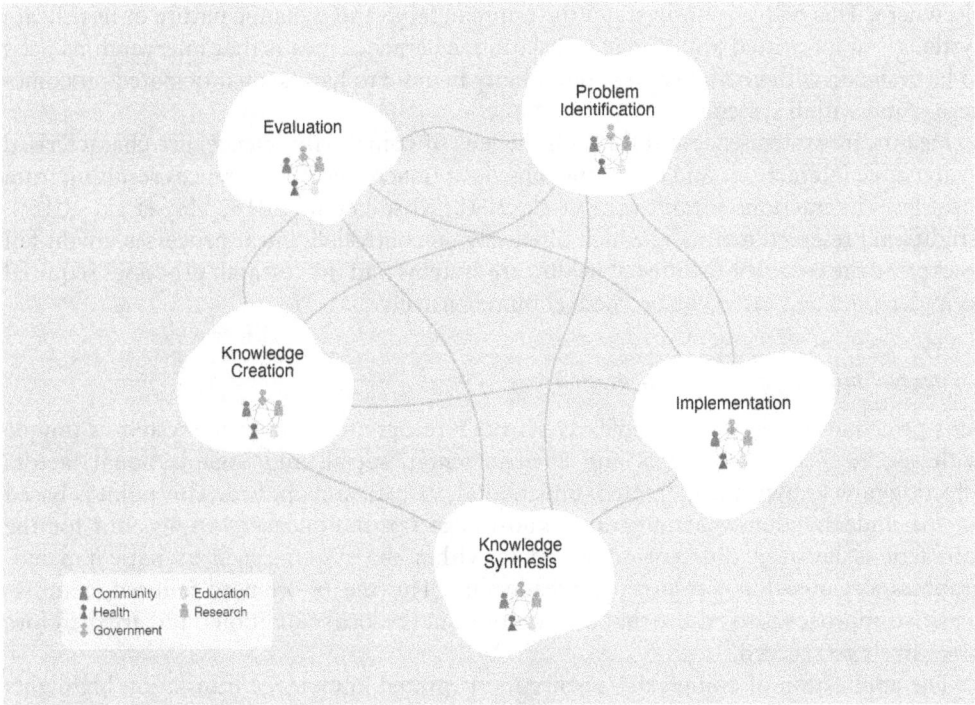

Figure 4.8 The Knowledge Translation Complexity Network Model.
Source: https://doi.org/10.25451/flinders.29192585.v1

the adaptability needed to effectively translate knowledge in complex healthcare systems. So, we can see that in practice successful knowledge translation means we can't rely on 'one-size-fits all' solutions but instead consider local contextual variations, adapt strategies to changing conditions, while making and monitoring connections with different partners at every stage.

While complexity science thinking rarely offers predictive explanations about what happens in systems, it does seek to generate working or guiding principles that people can use to explain what's happening in the systems being studied. These are sometimes referred to in the complexity science literature as guiding principles or 'rules of thumb'. These principles reflect key ideas in complexity science and are synthesised from some of the emerging frameworks and models. They include acknowledging non-linearity and emergence, tailoring and local adaptation to the context, transdisciplinary collaboration, and managing uncertainty and adaptive learning.

Guiding principles of complexity science

Acknowledging non-linearity and emergence

This principle is grounded in the central concept of non-linearity, which states that cause-and-effect relationships in complex systems are not straightforward. Instead, small changes in one part of the system can have disproportionate and unpredictable impacts elsewhere. This helps us understand the unpredictable and dynamic nature of healthcare systems – in integrated knowledge translation, emergence means that interventions need to be designed with flexibility and adaptability in mind to handle unanticipated outcomes across and within systems.

Healthcare systems, viewed through the lens of complexity science, are characterised by dynamic interactions and emergent behaviour (macro-level occurrences resulting from local-level interactions (Braithwaite et al., 2018; Kitson et al., 2018; May et al., 2016)). Traditional research methods, which often rely on controlled, linear processes, might fail to capture the complex realities of healthcare systems and the research processes required to understand and intervene on them comprehensively.

Contextual tailoring and local adaptation

This principle comes from complexity science's recognition that every system is unique with specific historical origins and environmental, social, and organisational factors affecting how knowledge is created, understood, valued, and applied. This point is based on the understanding that integrated knowledge translation needs to account for the interactions between different components within the system, such as patient demographics, organisational culture, and leadership. This means we need tailored, context-sensitive approaches to ensure that interventions fit the local conditions, and are therefore more likely to succeed.

The application of complexity science in integrated knowledge translation highlights the importance of contextual tailoring of interventions. Churruca et al., (Churruca et al., 2019) emphasise that understanding the local environment and its unique barriers and enablers is crucial for successful implementation.

Promoting transdisciplinary collaboration

Complexity emphasises the importance of diverse agents interacting within and across multiple systems. This means that generating and getting new knowledge into these systems requires collaboration across multiple disciplines and partners outside academia. This principle reflects the idea that in complex systems, no single person or group has all the answers. Collaboration with a diverse range of people and organisations helps us draw on collective knowledge and better respond to the multifaceted and evolving nature of healthcare systems.

Complexity science highlights the value of transdisciplinary collaboration in integrated knowledge translation. Braithwaite et al. (2018) argue that successful implementation requires collaboration across these different groups to understand the complex interplays within the system. We use the term transdisciplinary because it aligns with the basic tenets of integrated knowledge translation – collaboration, co-creation, and the integration of diverse perspectives, including those of non-academic partners such as community members, policymakers, and practitioners (Archibald et al., 2023). This kind of work requires flexible, integrative leadership that can unite multiple voices to co-create practical, meaningful solutions that go beyond the boundaries of any specific discipline (Belcher et al., 2015; Pineo et al., 2021).

Embracing uncertainty and adaptive learning

This principle stems from the non-deterministic nature of complex systems, where outcomes are often uncertain and evolve over time (Braithwaite et al., 2018). In these situations, we need an iterative approach to learning that allows interventions to be continuously adapted based on timely feedback. In integrated knowledge translation, this means building in adaptive learning mechanisms – tools or processes that support ongoing evaluation and refinements. Rather than following a fixed plan, teams learn as you go, adjusting strategies based on what is happening (Martin et al., 2020). This is especially useful in uncertain or fast-changing environments where being flexible and responsive is key to staying on track and making progress.

Given the inherent uncertainty and unpredictability of complex systems, integrated knowledge translation informed by complexity science prioritises adaptive learning. Instead of trying to eliminate uncertainty, this approach recognises it as part of the process and focuses on building resilience and capacity to respond to change. Reed et al. (2018), for example, highlight the use of iterative processes and continuous feedback mechanisms as critical elements of complexity-informed research, allowing for real-time adjustments and improvements based on ongoing learning. Table 4.1 summarises the main ideas emerging from each of these guiding principles or 'rules of thumb'.

What happens at the individual level in complexity science and how does it link to integrated knowledge translation?

The final piece of the jigsaw in connecting integrated knowledge translation with complexity science is how we have approached the individuals in the systems that make the

Table 4.1 Guiding principles of complexity science shaping integrated knowledge translation activity

Guiding principle	What it means in practice
Non-linearity and emergence	Cause and effect can be difficult to predict
	Small events or actions can have large and unanticipated impacts
	Systems are unpredictable – surprises are part of the process
Tailoring and local adaption	Every system is unique
	Teams need to understand how knowledge is created, valued, understood, and applied in the local context
	This naturally leads to local adaptations
Transdisciplinary collaboration	Many different people (individual agents) interact within systems
	Effective collaboration requires leadership, relationship-building, and influencing
	Teams need to work across disciplines, sectors, and systems
Managing uncertainty and adaptive learning	Uncertainty is expected – embrace a learning mindset
	Foster a culture of continuous improvement
	Use tools like audit, feedback, and real-time data to guide adaptation and learning

desired changes happen. In integrated knowledge translation these individuals have been described in various ways from stakeholders and recipients (see Chapter 3) (Canadian Institutes of Health Research, 2016; Kothari et al., 2017) to particular roles that shape and influence the adoption of new knowledge into policy and practice – most notably knowledge brokers (Bornbaum et al., 2015; Dobbins et al., 2019), boundary spanners (Evans & Scarbrough, 2014), opinion leaders (Grimshaw et al., 2012; Spyridonidis et al., 2015), local champions (Flynn et al., 2023), change agents (Kitson, 2009), local, experienced, expert, internal or external facilitators (Harvey & Kitson, 2015; Ritchie et al., 2020). In complexity science and fields like network science – which study complex networks such as technological, biological, and social systems – the roles driving change are often described as 'nodes' and 'hubs' (Kitson et al., 2018).

- **Nodes** represent the individual agents or entities within a system
- **Hubs** represent highly connected nodes that play a central role in facilitating communication and coordination
- **When** a critical mass of nodes and hubs come together to drive change, this forms a cluster – a small or emerging network (or sub-network) that, as it grows, begins to function as a larger network.

Figure 4.9 shows how nodes (individual agents) connect within and across two clusters (sub-networks) in a knowledge translation complexity network. We have found that terms like node, hub, and cluster are not widely understood in knowledge translation and health research. To bridge this gap, Table 4.2 provides a 'translation' of complexity science terms into more familiar knowledge translation language. However, throughout this book, we will continue using the terms as they appeared in our 2018

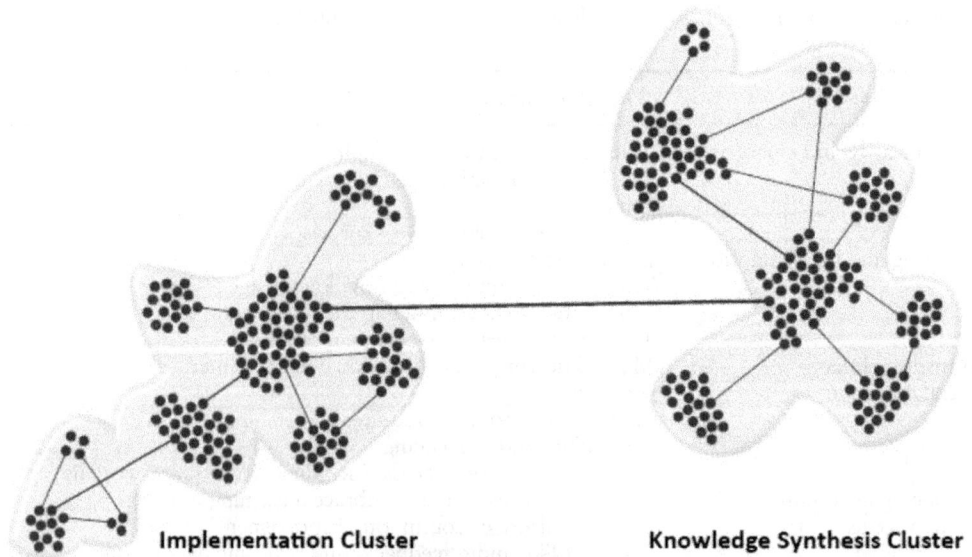

Implementation Cluster   **Knowledge Synthesis Cluster**

Figure 4.9 Representations of two clusters (sub-networks) within a knowledge translation complexity network.

Source: Kitson et al. (2018).

Table 4.2 Mapping complexity science terms to integrated knowledge translation concepts

Complexity science term	Integrated knowledge translation term (examples)	Role in system change
Node A single agent interacting with others	**Stakeholder,** recipient, consumer, partner	Recognises that individual agents within systems are essential participants in any activity; they are pivotal in driving broader system change
Hub A single agent with extensive interactions, acting as a champion within and between clusters	**Knowledge broker,** facilitator, boundary spanner, opinion leader, local champion	Acknowledges that certain agents within systems assume roles that mobilise and facilitate change. They employ leadership, negotiation, and facilitation skills to engage others in the change process
Cluster A sub-network comprising nodes and hubs working collectively towards shared goals	**Implementation team,** collaboration team, focus groups	Emphasises the importance of building a critical mass to reach a 'tipping point' where there is sufficient momentum (desire and ability) to implement desired changes. This involves having a clear plan, purpose, and willingness to test new ideas
Network A collection of nodes, hubs, and clusters and the connections between them	**Social networks,** communities of practice	Facilitates the dissemination or adoption of innovations or ideas from a small group of agents to a broader community. This can be intentionally supported through roles like external facilitators, boundary spanners, or knowledge brokers, and/or organically through individuals acting as champions or opinion leaders.

paper (Kitson et al., 2018), but with integrated knowledge translation equivalents, so that we remain consistent in our application of the Knowledge Translation Complexity Network Model.

Complexity science therefore helps to highlight principles around complex adaptive system behaviour and change that can guide and inform the development of integrated knowledge translation strategies. What happens is that characteristics of the system (non-linearity and emergence, local adaptation and tailoring, transdisciplinary collaboration, and adaptive learning and managing uncertainty) are connected to the principles of individual and interpersonal behaviour change describing the deliberate work of opinion leaders, teams, and networks who drive the responses of people in the system to respond and adopt new knowledge being presented to them. This means that we do indeed have the capacity to connect individual experiences with wider systems behaviours. The Knowledge Translation Complexity Network Model is the bridge between these two ways of understanding the world.

Working with the Knowledge Translation Complexity Network Model

At the Caring Futures Institute, we are using the Knowledge Translation Complexity Network Model to help us plan and carry out knowledge translation in an integrated, interactive, and dynamic way –although we're still very much on the journey. To recap, the Knowledge Translation Complexity Network Model outlines five key research processes: Problem Identification, Knowledge Creation, Knowledge Synthesis, Implementation and Evaluation (Table 4.3). Each process includes specific activities that are shaped by how researchers and partners interact at different system levels. These processes are interconnected and shaped by the nature of the problem the research team is addressing in collaboration with their partners. And those partners can come from many different systems – health, education, government, community – each with their own priorities, values, and ways of working.

Think of Knowledge Translation Complexity Network Model as a map. It helps you figure out:

- Where to start conversations
- Who you're working with
- What methods or tools might be useful
- How to build and maintain successful partnerships.

It also prompts you to think who the key agents in your system are (often called stakeholders, recipients, partners or end-users in knowledge translation), and how to work with them to introduce and embed change. These agents might include local champions, facilitators, or knowledge brokers (often described as nodes or hubs in network science), who help spread new ideas within and across systems, forming clusters and networks that support uptake and sustainability.

Table 4.3 Terminology used and working definitions of knowledge translation complexity network elements

Term	Definition
Knowledge Translation Complexity Network	The umbrella term that describes the components of the overall network that connect and interplay in order for knowledge translation to occur. Different individuals collaborate within a dynamic discursive space to ensure that appropriate information is being developed, refined, and mobilised throughout the network to the appropriate nodes, hubs, clusters and sectors.
Problem Identification	The process by which societal challenges, issues or problems are formulated, defined and constructed to proceed to systematic investigation.
Knowledge Creation	Describes what is traditionally termed basic, clinical, pre-clinical, epidemiological, health services, and population health research approaches to answering health related problems.
Knowledge Synthesis	The rigorous and systematic generation of evidence-based products (patents, materials, tools, programs, and guidelines) for application in policy and practice.
Implementation	The rigorous application of new knowledge into policy and practice in a theory informed and reflective way.
Evaluation	The explicit and systematic review of key processes of knowledge translation and broader objectives within and across a range of complex and interconnected sectors and networks.

Chapter summary

This chapter has explored how integrated knowledge translation and complexity science come together, mapping out some of the key moments in this journey. We explored the Knowledge Translation Complexity Network Model as the outcome of this fusion of ideas and worldviews. While the descriptions may have been dense at times, they provide a solid theoretical and conceptual base to help researchers and teams understand where these ideas have come from, how they align, and, most importantly, how they can be used in practice.

As an integrated knowledge translation researcher or practitioner, you will never be too far away from theory. The challenge – and the opportunity – is knowing *how* to put those theories into action. While integrated knowledge translation can feel messy and unpredictable, it's a shared journey, and our collective commitment to rigorous, high-quality research remains equally important.

In the next chapter (Chapter 5), we shift gears and offer a more hands-on perspective by providing a range of case studies and reflections. Additionally, in Chapter 8, we provide a practical guide designed to help translate the concepts from this chapter into thoughts, reflections, and actions. We hope that any integrated knowledge translation researcher, enthusiast, or curious clinician can use this resource support integrated, collaborative, and context-sensitive knowledge translation in their work.

References

Aarons, G. A., Ehrhart, M. G., & Farahnak, L. R. (2014). The implementation leadership scale (ILS): Development of a brief measure of unit level implementation leadership. *Implementation Science, 9*(1), 45. https://doi.org/10.1186/1748-5908-9-45

Archibald, M., Lawless, M. T., de Plaza, M. A. P., & Kitson, A. L. (2023). How transdisciplinary research teams learn to do knowledge translation (KT), and how KT in turn impacts transdisciplinary research: A realist evaluation and longitudinal case study. *Health Research Policy and Systems, 21*(1), 20–20. https://doi.org/10.1186/s12961-023-00967-x

Belcher, B. M., Rasmussen, K. E., Kemshaw, M. R., & Zornes, D. A. (2015). Defining and assessing research quality in a transdisciplinary context. *Research Evaluation, 25*(1), 1–17. https://doi.org/10.1093/reseval/rvv025

Bornbaum, C. C., Kornas, K., Peirson, L., & Rosella, L. C. (2015). Exploring the function and effectiveness of knowledge brokers as facilitators of knowledge translation in health-related settings: A systematic review and thematic analysis. *Implementation Science, 10*(1), 162. https://doi.org/10.1186/s13012-015-0351-9

Braithwaite, J., Churruca, K., Long, J. C., Ellis, L. A., & Herkes, J. (2018). When complexity science meets implementation science: A theoretical and empirical analysis of systems change. *BMC Medicine, 16*(1), 63–63. https://doi.org/10.1186/s12916-018-1057-z

Campbell, M., Fitzpatrick, R., Haines, A., Kinmonth, A. L., Sandercock, P., Spiegelhalter, D., & Tyrer, P. (2000). Framework for design and evaluation of complex interventions to improve health. *British Medical Journal, 321*(7262), 694–696. https://doi.org/10.1136/bmj.321.7262.694

Canadian Institutes of Health Research. (2015). *Guide to knowledge translation planning at CIHR: Integrated and end-of-grant approaches.* https://cihr-irsc.gc.ca/e/45321.html

Canadian Institutes of Health Research. (2016). *Knowledge translation at CIHR.* https://cihr-irsc.gc.ca/e/29418.html

Cane, J., O'Connor, D., & Michie, S. (2012). Validation of the theoretical domains framework for use in behaviour change and implementation research. *Implementation Science: IS, 7*(1), 37–37. https://doi.org/10.1186/1748-5908-7-37

Churruca, K., Pomare, C., Ellis, L. A., Long, J. C., & Braithwaite, J. (2019). The influence of complexity: A bibliometric analysis of complexity science in healthcare. *BMJ Open*, *9*(3), e027308. https://doi.org/10.1136/bmjopen-2018-027308

Craig, P., Dieppe, P., Macintyre, S., Michie, S., Nazareth, I., & Petticrew, M. (2006). *Developing and Evaluating Complex Interventions*. Medical Research Council.

Craig, P., Dieppe, P., Macintyre, S., Michie, S., Nazareth, I., Petticrew, M., & Medical Research Council, G. (2008). Developing and evaluating complex interventions: The new Medical Research Council guidance. *BMJ*, *337*, a1655. https://doi.org/10.1136/bmj.a1655

Damschroder, L. J., Reardon, C. M., Widerquist, M. A. O., & Lowery, J. (2022). The updated Consolidated Framework for Implementation Research based on user feedback. *Implementation Science: IS*, *17*(1), 1–75. https://doi.org/10.1186/s13012-022-01245-0

Dobbins, M., Greco, L., Yost, J., Traynor, R., Decorby-Watson, K., & Yousefi-Nooraie, R. (2019). A description of a tailored knowledge translation intervention delivered by knowledge brokers within public health departments in Canada. *Health Research Policy and Systems*, *17*(1), 63. https://doi.org/10.1186/s12961-019-0460-z

Esmail, R., Hanson, H. M., Holroyd-Leduc, J., Brown, S., Strifler, L., Straus, S. E., Niven, D. J., & Clement, F. M. (2020). A scoping review of full-spectrum knowledge translation theories, models, and frameworks. *Implementation Science: IS*, *15*(1), 11–11. https://doi.org/10.1186/s13012-020-0964-5

Evans, S., & Scarbrough, H. (2014). Supporting knowledge translation through Collaborative translational research initiatives: 'Bridging' versus 'blurring' BOUNDARY-spanning approaches in the UK CLAHRC initiative. *Social Science and Medicine*, *106*, 119–127. https://doi.org/10.1016/j.socscimed.2014.01.025

Flynn, R., Cassidy, C., Dobson, L., Al-Rassi, J., Langley, J., Swindle, J., Graham, I. D., & Scott, S. D. (2023). Knowledge translation strategies to support the sustainability of evidence-based interventions in healthcare: A scoping review. *Implementation Science*, *18*(1), 69. https://doi.org/10.1186/s13012-023-01320-0

Gifford, W., Graham, I. D., Ehrhart, M. G., Davies, B. L., & Aarons, G. A. (2017). Ottawa model of implementation leadership and implementation leadership scale: Mapping concepts for developing and evaluating theory-based leadership interventions. *Journal of Healthcare Leadership*, *9*, 15–23. https://doi.org/10.2147/jhl.S125558

Graham, I. D., Logan, J., Harrison, M. B., Straus, S. E., Tetroe, J., Caswell, W., & Robinson, N. (2006). Lost in knowledge translation: Time for a map? *The Journal of Continuing Education in the Health Professions*, *26*(1), 13–24. https://doi.org/10.1002/chp.47

Greenhalgh, T., & Papoutsi, C. (2018). Studying complexity in health services research: Desperately seeking an overdue paradigm shift. *BMC Medicine*, *16*(1), 95–95. https://doi.org/10.1186/s12916-018-1089-4

Greenhalgh, T., Pawson, R., Wong, G., Westhorp, G., Greenhalgh, J., & Manzano, A. (2017). *What Realists Mean by Context; or Why Nothing Works Everywhere or for Everyone*. National Institute for Health Research.

Grimshaw, J. M., Eccles, M. P., Lavis, J. N., Hill, S. J., & Squires, J. E. (2012). Knowledge translation of research findings. *Implementation Science: IS*, *7*(1), 50–50. https://doi.org/10.1186/1748-5908-7-50

Harvey, G., & Kitson, A. (2016). PARIHS revisited: From heuristic to integrated framework for the successful implementation of knowledge into practice. *Implementation Science: IS*, *11*(1), 33–33. https://doi.org/10.1186/s13012-016-0398-2

Harvey, G., & Kitson, A. L. (2015). *Implementing Evidence-based Practice in Healthcare: A Facilitation Guide*. Routledge. https://doi.org/10.4324/9780203557334

Jenkins, E. K., Kothari, A., Bungay, V., Johnson, J. L., & Oliffe, J. L. (2016). Strengthening population health interventions: Developing the CollaboraKTion Framework for Community-Based Knowledge Translation. *Health Research Policy and Systems*, *14*(1), 65–65. https://doi.org/10.1186/s12961-016-0138-8

Kitson, A. L. (2009). The need for systems change: reflections on knowledge translation and organizational change. *Journal of advanced nursing, 65*(1), 217–228.

Kitson, A., Brook, A., Harvey, G., Jordan, Z., Marshall, R., O'Shea, R., & Wilson, D. (2018). Using complexity and network concepts to inform healthcare knowledge translation. *International Journal of Health Policy and Management, 7*(3), 231–243. https://doi.org/10.15171/ijhpm.2017.79

Kitson, A., Powell, K., Hoon, E., Newbury, J., Wilson, A., & Beilby, J. (2013). Knowledge translation within a population health study: How do you do it? *Implementation Science: IS, 8*(1), 54–54. https://doi.org/10.1186/1748-5908-8-54

Kothari, A., McCutcheon, C., & Graham, I. D. (2017). Defining integrated knowledge translation and moving forward: A response to recent commentaries. *International Journal of Health Policy and Management, 6*(5), 299–300. https://doi.org/10.15171/ijhpm.2017.15

Martin, F., Chen, Y., Moore, R. L., & Westine, C. D. (2020). Systematic review of adaptive learning research designs, context, strategies, and technologies from 2009 to 2018. *Educational Technology Research and Development, 68*(4), 1903–1929. https://doi.org/10.1007/s11 423-020-09793-2

May, C. R., Johnson, M., & Finch, T. (2016). Implementation, context and complexity. *Implementation Science: IS, 11*(1), 141–141. https://doi.org/10.1186/s13012-016-0506-3

McCormack, B., Kitson, A., Harvey, G., Rycroft-Malone, J., Titchen, A., & Seers, K. (2002). Getting evidence into practice: The meaning of 'context'. *Journal of Advanced Nursing, 38*(1), 94–104. https://doi.org/10.1046/j.1365-2648.2002.02150.x

Michie, S., Johnston, M., Abraham, C., Lawton, R., Parker, D., & Walker, A. (2005). Making psychological theory useful for implementing evidence based practice: A consensus approach. *Quality & Safety in Health Care, 14*(1), 26–33. https://doi.org/10.1136/qshc.2004.011155

Nguyen, T., Graham, I. D., Mrklas, K. J., Bowen, S., Cargo, M., Estabrooks, C. A., Kothari, A., Lavis, J., MacAulay, A. C., MacLeod, M., Phipps, D., Ramsden, V. R., Renfrew, M. J., Salsberg, J., & Wallerstein, N. (2020). How does integrated knowledge translation (IKT) compare to other collaborative research approaches to generating and translating knowledge? Learning from experts in the field. *Health Research Policy and Systems, 18*(1), 35–35. https://doi.org/10.1186/s12961-020-0539-6

Nilsen, P., & Bernhardsson, S. (2019). Context matters in implementation science: A scoping review of determinant frameworks that describe contextual determinants for implementation outcomes. *BMC Health Services Research, 19*(1), 189. https://doi.org/10.1186/s12 913-019-4015-3

Nilsen, P., & Birken, S. A. (2020). *Handbook on Implementation Science.* Edward Elgar Publishing.

Pfadenhauer, L. M., Gerhardus, A., Mozygemba, K., Lysdahl, K. B., Booth, A., Hofmann, B., Wahlster, P., Polus, S., Burns, J., Brereton, L., & Rehfuess, E. (2017). Making sense of complexity in context and implementation: The Context and Implementation of Complex Interventions (CICI) framework. *Implementation Science: IS, 12*(1), 21–21. https://doi.org/10.1186/s13 012-017-0552-5

Pineo, H., Turnbull, E. R., Davies, M., Rowson, M., Hayward, A. C., Hart, G., Johnson, A. M., & Aldridge, R. W. (2021). A new transdisciplinary research model to investigate and improve the health of the public. *Health Promotion International, 36*(2), 481–492. https://doi.org/10.1093/heapro/daaa125

Plsek, P. E., & Greenhalgh, T. (2001). Complexity science: The challenge of complexity in health care. *BMJ, 323*(7313), 625–628. https://doi.org/10.1136/bmj.323.7313.625

Reed, J. E., Howe, C., Doyle, C., & Bell, D. (2018). Simple rules for evidence translation in complex systems: A qualitative study. *BMC Medicine, 16*(1), 92–92. https://doi.org/10.1186/s12 916-018-1076-9

Ritchie, M. J., Parker, L. E., & Kirchner, J. E. (2020). From novice to expert: A qualitative study of implementation facilitation skills. *Implementation Science Communications, 1*(1), 25. https://doi.org/10.1186/s43058-020-00006-8

Skivington, K., Matthews, L., Simpson, S. A., Craig, P., Baird, J., Blazeby, J. M., Boyd, K. A., Craig, N., French, D. P., McIntosh, E., Petticrew, M., Rycroft-Malone, J., White, M., & Moore, L. (2021). Framework for the development and evaluation of complex interventions: Gap analysis, workshop and consultation-informed update. *Health Technology Assessment*, 25(57). https://doi.org/10.3310/hta25570

Spyridonidis, D., Hendy, J., & Barlow, J. (2015). Leadership for knowledge translation: The case of CLAHRCs. *Qualitative Health Research*, 25(11), 1492–1505. https://doi.org/10.1177/10497 32315583268

Squires, J. E., Hutchinson, A. M., Coughlin, M., Bashir, K., Curran, J., Grimshaw, J. M., Dorrance, K., Aloisio, L., Brehaut, J., Francis, J. J., Ivers, N., Lavis, J., Michie, S., Hillmer, M., Noseworthy, T., Vine, J., & Graham, I. D. (2022). Stakeholder perspectives of attributes and features of context relevant to knowledge translation in health settings: A multi-country analysis. *International Journal of Health Policy and Management*, 11(8), 1373–1390. https://doi.org/10.34172/ ijhpm.2021.32

Strifler, L., Cardoso, R., McGowan, J., Cogo, E., Nincic, V., Khan, P. A., Scott, A., Ghassemi, M., MacDonald, H., Lai, Y., Treister, V., Tricco, A. C., & Straus, S. E. (2018). Scoping review identifies significant number of knowledge translation theories, models, and frameworks with limited use. *Journal of Clinical Epidemiology*, 100, 92–102. https://doi.org/10.1016/j.jclin epi.2018.04.008

Thomas, A., Menon, A., Boruff, J., Rodriguez, A. M., & Ahmed, S. (2014). Applications of social constructivist learning theories in knowledge translation for healthcare professionals: A scoping review. *Implementation Science: IS*, 9(1), 54–54. https://doi.org/10.1186/1748-5908-9-54

Weiner, B. J. (2020). A theory of organizational readiness for change. In P Nilsen & S. A. Birken (Eds.), *Handbook on Implementation Science* (pp. 215–232). Edward Elgar Publishing. https:// EconPapers.repec.org/RePEc:elg:eechap:18688_8

Section II

Navigating the journey

5 Integrated knowledge translation within the Caring Futures Institute

Sarah Hunter, Michael Lawless and Alison Kitson

Introduction

In the previous chapter, we provided a detailed description of how integrated knowledge translation approaches have developed. As we move into the second section of this book, we take a more practical approach by sharing how we at the Flinders University Caring Futures Institute have navigated our own integrated knowledge translation journey. In this chapter, we share seven short and diverse case studies from teams who currently or previously work across the Caring Futures Institute. A researcher from each team shares their experience of undertaking a project or a program of research and how they navigated the various knowledge translation processes and partners involved. Following each case study, we provide a visual representation of their story in context of the knowledge translation complexity network model, and we share our (the book editors) reflections of their case study. If any of the case studies particularly pique your interest, we have provided at the end of this chapter, a list of key references relating to these projects.

Through this chapter, we hope to illustrate that there is no 'correct' way to do integrated knowledge translation. There is no recipe, or one size fits all approach. Undertaking integrated knowledge translation looks different in each project as the journey is dependent on the dynamic nature of the relationships we establish with our research partners.

But first, we will recap the Knowledge Translation Complexity Network Model, as introduced in Chapters 1 and 4. The model integrates five key knowledge translation processes. These five processes are: Problem Identification, Knowledge Creation, Knowledge Synthesis, Implementation, and Evaluation. Figure 5.1 provides a visual representation of the model.

Case studies

We begin by sharing a case study from Professor Jeroen Hendriks which explores implementation of an evidence-based model of care to improve cardiac care. We then share a case study from Dr Brittany Johnson which explores knowledge synthesis to generate a living database for the prevention of early childhood obesity. Whilst these two case studies vary in their primary knowledge translation processes (implementation and knowledge synthesis, respectively), what we see is that both commenced as researcher led, and success only came about through engaging in the additional knowledge translation processes with engaged partners.

DOI: 10.4324/9781003245995-7

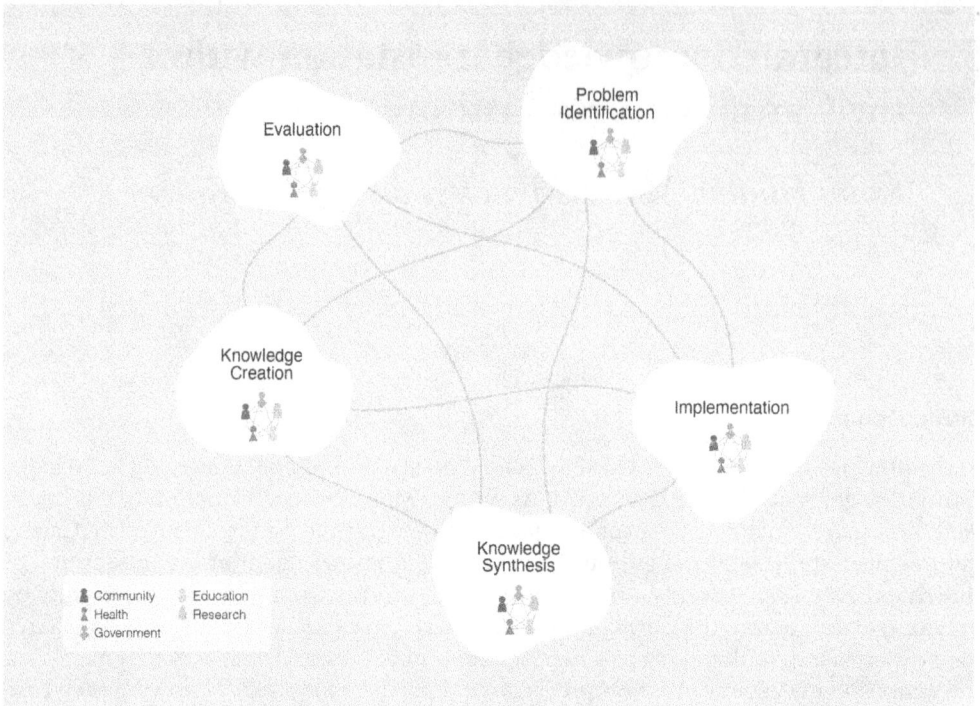

Figure 5.1 Knowledge Translation Complexity Network Model.
Source: https://doi.org/10.25451/flinders.29192585.v1

We then share a case study from Associate Professor Elizabeth Lynch, which explores co-designing implementation of clinical guideline recommendations to improve stroke rehabilitation in inpatient settings. This is followed by a case study Associate Professor Michelle Bellon which explores co-designing cancer care solutions with people with intellectual disabilities. These two case studies demonstrate research collaborations with community members and how this facilitates movement between the knowledge translation processes.

The case studies so far have demonstrated what we would consider relatively linear movement between the knowledge translation processes. The case studies we share next illustrate more complex movements, where there is movement between and across processes. We share a case study from Professor Jennifer Tieman which explores developing a home care app to support end-of-line care. We then share a case study from Dr Matthew Wallen which explores developing nurse-led shared care models in care survivorship care. We end on a case study from Professor Gill Harvey which explores tackling the problem of repeated hospital presentations for older people. In Gill's case study, we can see a program of research that was set up and guided by the knowledge translation complexity network model. We see not only movement across and between knowledge translation processes but also multiple projects or phases addressing a single knowledge translation process with varied engagement of partners.

A final note before sharing the case studies, is the visual representations of these case studies are designed to be illustrative. They are designed to aid in understanding the key elements and dynamics of the projects. However, please note that these visuals are not intended to be perfectly accurate depictions.

Box 5.1 *Case study 1* **Implementation of an evidence-based model of care to improve cardiac care**

Atrial fibrillation is the most prevalent cardiac arrhythmia. Patients with atrial fibrillation often have symptoms like palpitations, shortness of breath, and or chest pain, and there may be a lot of anxiety surrounding that. There are also multiple lifestyle risk factors that contribute to the development or worsening of atrial fibrillation. So, to imagine having only one healthcare professional addressing all these issues within one approximate 15-minute consult, that may be considered insufficient care, and we realised we need to redesign the care processes.

Based on previous research conducted in the Netherlands (Hendriks et al., 2012; Hendriks et al., 2010; Hendriks et al., 2019), we developed a novel model of care based on the concept of integrated care, the i-CARE-AF clinic. This clinic and model of care is underpinned by four fundamentals: 1) patient centred approach, 2) multidisciplinary team, 3) comprehensive treatment approach, and 4) use of technology to support this integrated approach.

Implementing this model of care required a whole redesign of current practice. Therefore, prior to being able to implement or trial our intervention, we had to dedicate a significant amount of time developing partnerships. We engaged and talked to people within the service, presenting our ideas to them over and over again, in different ways. This social aspect is important because once you get people on board, the next step is to work together and co-design the implementation process.

What worked for us, was using this social approach to gaining entrance into the service with the executives and leadership. We started with informing all key partners and then focused on the front runners, the early adopters, and started small. But, we had to keep talking, keep engaging and informing people, and we were iterative in our approach, going where there were successes and wins. Knowing that this facilitative approach is within implementation frameworks, allowed us to not feel like we were failing, as we were not deviating from a structured, set out plan.

Whilst what we have done is an implementation project, unlike many implementation projects that are structured much like a clinical trial with a discrete beginning and end, we were able to embed this model of care as routine care.

We took an integrated approach to conducting our research, whilst we followed implementation science, we also had this social pathway. Much of our focus was on working closely with our partners across multiple grants and projects to navigate how to resource this continuous piece of work. Through this we are working together to build the evidence around the i-CARE-AF clinic, implementing it into routine care, and showcasing its success and impact.

Author: Jeroen Hendriks
Acknowledgements: Team of the Centre for Heart Rhythm Disorders, University of Adelaide

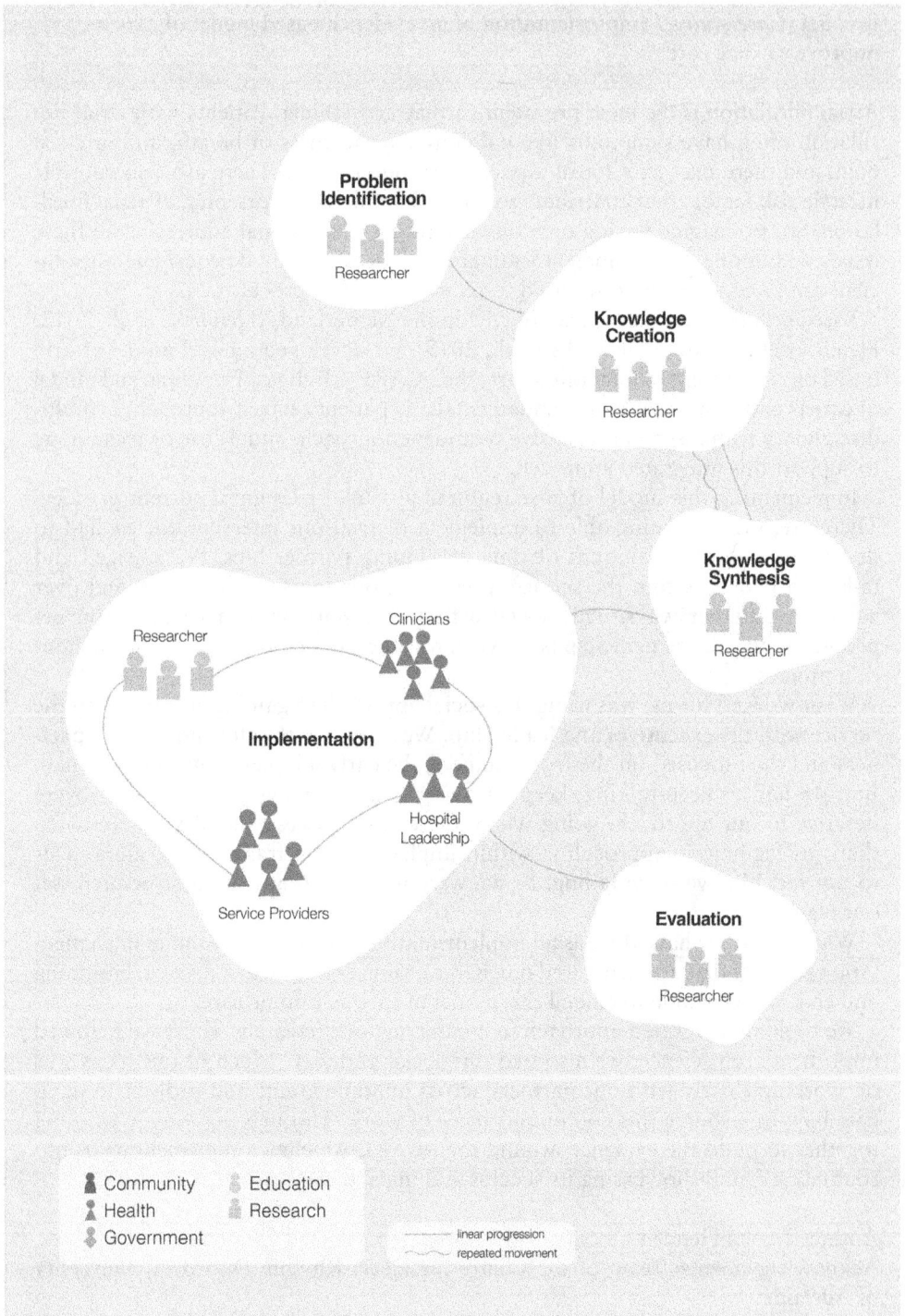

Figure 5.2 Case study 1 through the Knowledge Translation Complexity Network Model.
Source: https://doi.org/10.25451/flinders.29192714.v1

Case study 1 (Figure 5.2) demonstrates a focus on implementation of an evidence-based model of care. In this example, the problem identification, knowledge creation, and knowledge synthesis were researcher led. The wavy lines between knowledge creation and knowledge synthesis illustrate the continual movement often needed between synthesising existing evidence and generating new knowledge to develop a model of care. The implementation process being visually represented as the largest, reflects the amount of work and new relationships required to implement the new model of care. Jeroen's honest description of the unexpected challenges he and his team encountered during the implementation process is not uncommon and the description of the need for a 'social approach' illustrates the complexity of implementing without prior partnership. Ideally, had this team been aware of the methods of integrated knowledge translation sooner, they would have engaged partners in the development of the new model of care which would have aided in implementation.

Box 5.2 *Case study* 2 **Knowledge synthesis to generate a living database for the prevention of early childhood obesity**

In our experience of conducting a knowledge synthesis project where we worked with partners in varying ways in our TOPCHILD Collaboration (www.topchildco llaboration.org/) (introduced in Case Study 4, in Chapter 3), we realised the complexity of what we were trying to achieve. We recognised for people to use the evidence we are synthesising, there is a greater need for partner engagement, especially given the increasing focus on having partners drive research. As an early career researcher, I felt more confident taking on an integrated knowledge translation approach due to experience from the initial project, and the increasing focus and support on conducting this type of research within the Caring Futures Institute.

Our project deviates from the traditional and common approach of translating gold-standard systematic reviews of meta-analyses into healthcare via clinical practice guidelines as there are no clinical practice guidelines for the prevention of early childhood obesity (i.e. promotion of optimal diet, movement, and sleep behaviours). Therefore, we appreciate the need to engage and collaborate with partners to ultimately ensure implementation of the evidence into practice.

Overall, our TOPCHILD-Policy program is guided by the Knowledge to Action Framework (Graham et al., 2006). The initial TOPCHILD Collaboration project established a living evidence base of individual participant outcomes and intervention components (including target behaviours, delivery features, and behaviour change techniques), forming part of the Knowledge to Action Framework knowledge creation funnel.

Through the TOPCHILD Policy program, we are now simultaneously undertaking the Knowledge to Action Framework knowledge creation funnel and the Knowledge to Action Framework action cycle. We have formed a Consumer Advisory Panel consisting of 14 parents/caregivers, practitioners, policy makers, and boundary spanners, who guide the entire research process. We are working in collaboration with these partners to gain a deeper understanding of their needs and the problems they are facing. This is resulting in additional knowledge creation and synthesis to develop products and tools to be used by program planners/service managers to use and embed this evidence in policy and practice settings. As part of this process, we are working with our partners to develop our implementation and evaluation plan.

We are still in the early stages of the program; however, already I feel more comfortable with the integrated knowledge translation approach of collaborating regularly and meaningfully with partners and have seen the resulting benefits for the program. Working closely with partners to iteratively incorporate their ideas and perspectives also helps to reinforce the importance of the work and keep motivated throughout the research process roller-coaster.

Author: Brittany Johnson
Acknowledgements: Rebecca Golley, Anna Lene Seidler, Kylie Hunter, Sarah Hunter

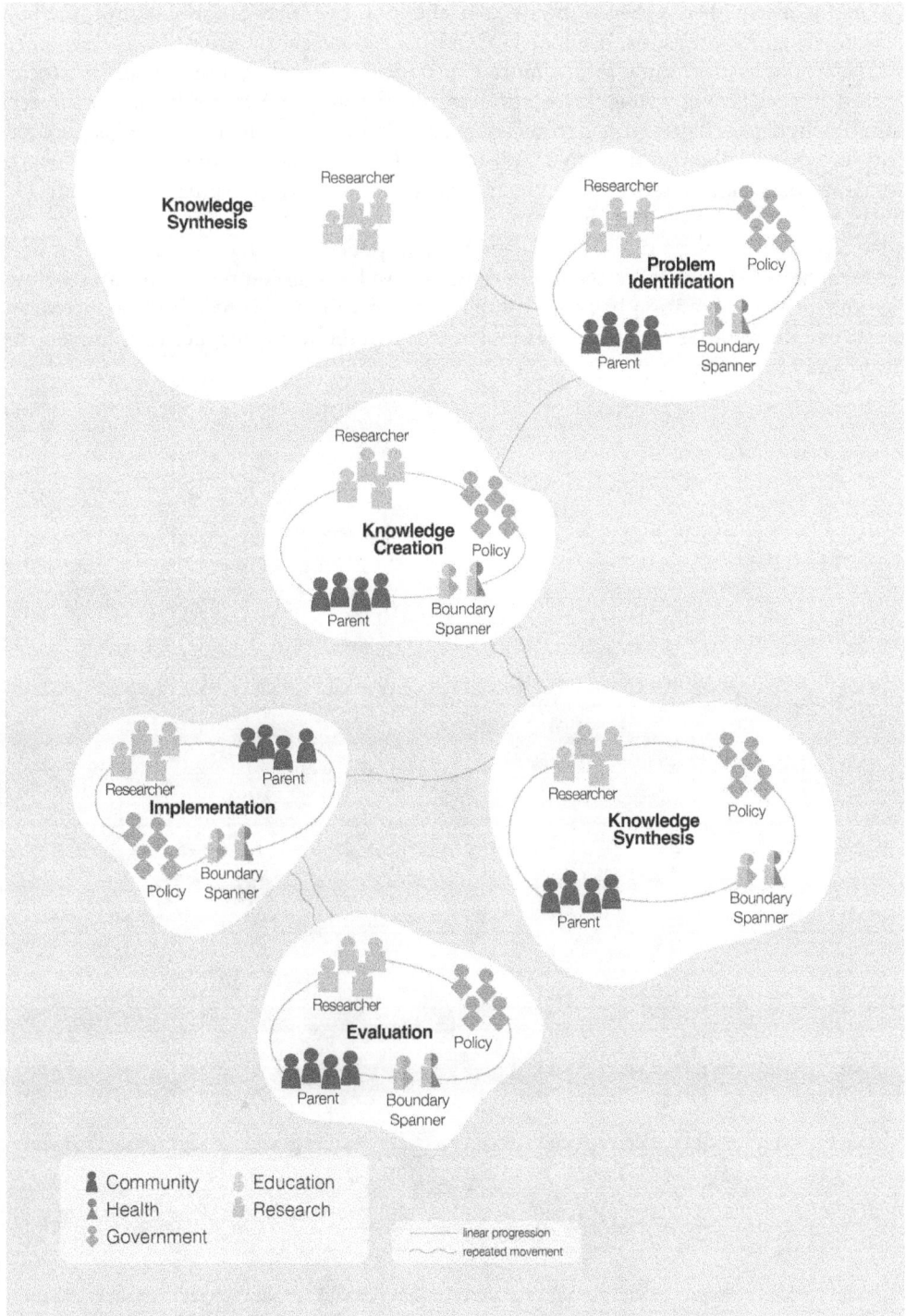

Figure 5.3 Case study 2 through the Knowledge Translation Complexity Network Model.
Source: https://doi.org/10.25451/flinders.29192726.v1

Case study 2 (Figure 5.3) demonstrates a focus on knowledge synthesis to generate a living database for the prevention of early childhood obesity. In this example, the initial knowledge synthesis, the original TOPCHILD Collaboration project, was researcher led. However, as Britt grew into a more experienced researcher, and the shifting focus toward integrated knowledge translation within the Caring Futures Institute, she felt more confident to work with partners throughout the research process. This enabled Britt to work collaboratively with a Consumer Advisory Panel to explore in more depth the issues being faced and to subsequently work together to move back and forth (as illustrated with the wavy line) between creating new knowledge and synthesising knowledge to create products to enable evidence use in policy and practice. Whilst Britt and her team have yet to move to the implementation and evaluation phase, we can see how the authentic collaboration has been established and will set this team up for success in navigating the iterative movement (as illustrated with the wavy line) between implementation and evaluation.

Box 5.3 *Case study 3* Co-designing implementation of clinical guideline recommendations to improve stroke rehabilitation in inpatient settings

Stroke rehabilitation is a critical phase for patients transitioning from hospital care back to community living. However, there are gaps between the stroke clinical guidelines, patient needs, and what is actually being delivered in inpatient rehabilitation settings. Many of the key recommendations from clinical guidelines were not being implemented effectively, despite strong evidence supporting their benefits. Patients and carers frequently reported dissatisfaction with certain aspects of their care, which highlighted the need for improvements. We published two systematic reviews examining patient and carer experiences in stroke rehabilitation, which underscored the misalignment between clinical practice and patient preferences. Additionally, national audit data revealed that key guideline recommendations were not being met consistently in practice. This evidence laid the foundation for a project aimed at addressing these gaps.

Our project aimed to implement four key strong recommendations from the stroke clinical guidelines that were directly aligned with what patients and carers wanted from their rehabilitation experience. Our approach was informed by experience-based co-design, and we brought together healthcare staff, patients, and carers to collaboratively design solutions that improve healthcare delivery. Our goal was to integrate the voices of people with lived experience of stroke and their carers into the process of translating evidence into practice.

At the heart of the project was the active engagement of partners. We brought together a diverse group of participants, including stroke survivors, carers, and healthcare professionals. This group co-designed the solutions to address the identified gaps in care. In the beginning, we made a "rookie error" of planning the project without having any people with lived experience on the initial team. However, we quickly corrected course, incorporating patients and carers as co-designers and co-researchers.

To maintain engagement throughout the project, we had monthly facilitated meetings with both staff and patients. These sessions provided opportunities for the healthcare team to receive direct feedback from patients and carers, fostering a sense of accountability among the clinicians. The meetings also enabled stakeholders to collaboratively monitor the progress of the project and adjust the implementation strategies as needed. Although efforts were made to recruit a diverse group of participants, including individuals from different cultural backgrounds and people with communication difficulties, the team faced challenges in achieving the desired level of diversity.

While the project did not succeed in fully implementing the guideline recommendations in the targeted inpatient setting, we did achieve significant process-based successes. One of the key successes was the high level of engagement from the core group of patients and carers who consistently participated in the meetings. Many participants even rearranged personal commitments to continue attending the monthly sessions, reflecting their strong commitment to the project.

For the healthcare staff, the process provided a form of professional "self-care". Amid the stress of their regular clinical duties, interacting with patients and carers through the project reminded them of the core purpose of their work—improving patient outcomes and experiences. This reconnection with the "why" behind their roles was deeply meaningful for the staff, even if the project did not result in significant measurable changes in practice.

As a team, we also reflected on the broader lessons learned from the project, particularly the feasibility of engaging people with lived experience to drive change in healthcare settings. This experience helped us refine our approach to co-design and partner engagement, emphasising the importance of practical considerations such as meeting participants' logistical needs and ensuring fair reimbursement for their time.

Author: Dr Elizabeth Lynch
Acknowledgements: Maria West, Dominique Cadilhac, Fawn Cooper, Gillian Harvey, lived experience advisors, health professional team involved

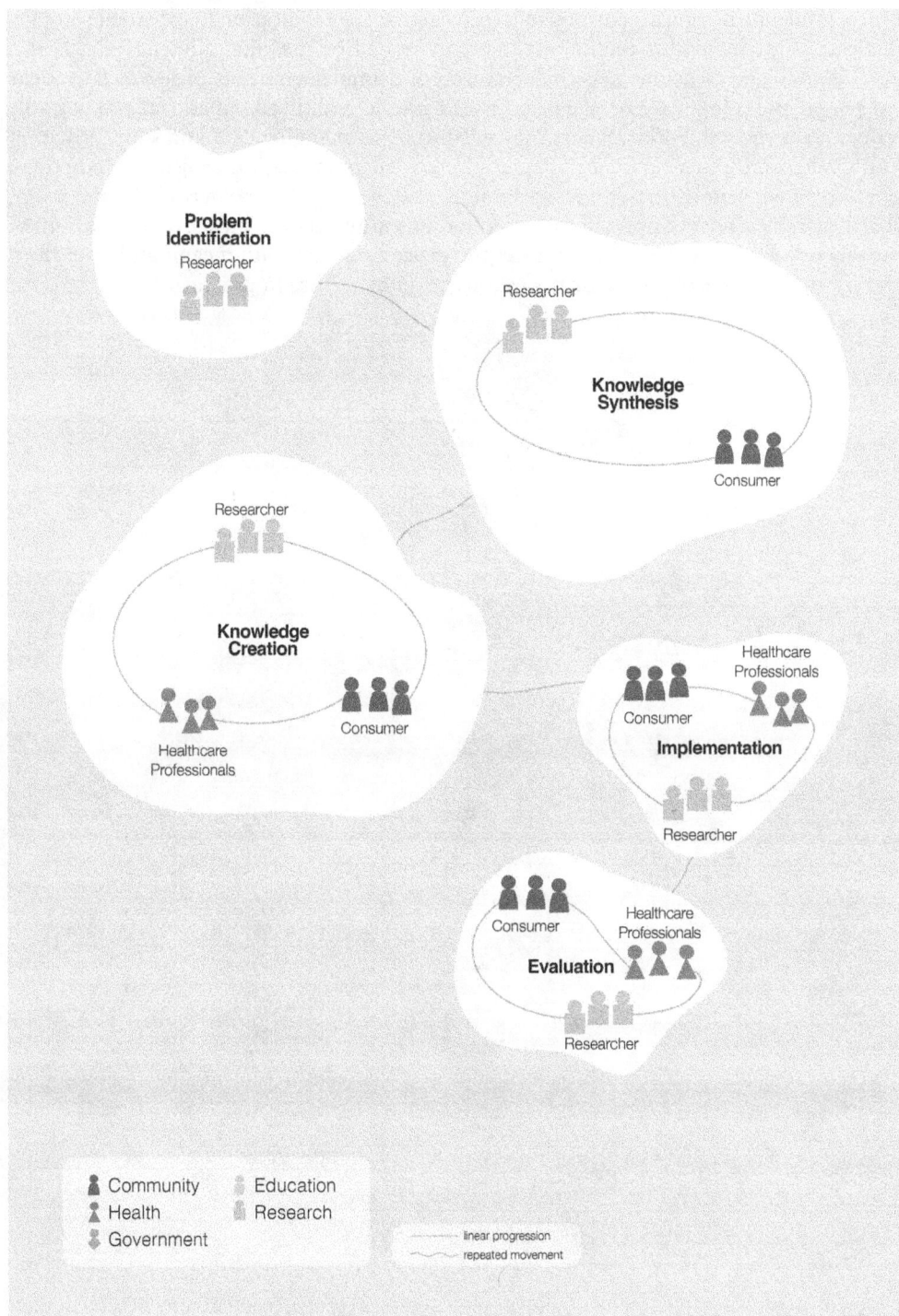

Figure 5.4 Case study 3 through the Knowledge Translation Complexity Network Model.
Source: https://doi.org/10.25451/flinders.29192738.v1

Case study 3 (Figure 5.4) demonstrates a focus on co-designing implementation of clinical guideline recommendations to improve stroke rehabilitation in inpatient settings. This case study highlights the impact that can be had by meaningfully engaging health professionals and consumers within research and implementation projects. It is clear that people providing care on the ground and people with lived experience are not able to operate as the influential leaders they wish to be in changing care and support within health systems. Partnering on an integrated knowledge translation project can empower people even when immediate changes are not achieved, which is powerful. For this team, what began as a novel approach to co-design has now become business as usual in the team's work. The next step is to connect the process success with meaningful impact on relevant outcome measures that can sustain the guideline use in practice.

Box 5.4 *Case study 4* Co-designing cancer care solutions with people with intellectual disabilities

People with intellectual disability often face significant barriers to good health care, including stigma, discrimination, and a lack of appropriate and accessible health care services. To examine and address this issue, a joint Research Lead position was established between Disability and Community Inclusion at Flinders University and the South Australian Intellectual Disability Health Service within Northern Adelaide Local Health Network.

The South Australian Intellectual Disability Health Service includes a multidisciplinary team of health professions spanning psychiatry, physical medicine, general practice, nursing, occupational therapy, speech pathology, pharmacy, social work and positive behaviour support. A central focus of the Research Lead role is to lead inclusive research practice and co-produce solutions together with people with intellectual disability and other stakeholders. We have developed a community researcher team with people with intellectual disability as co-researchers. This team is instrumental in guiding the entire research process, from identifying problems and priorities, to co-producing solutions and resources. Community researchers are key members of the team and contribute to all aspects of the research, including design, interviews, observations, analysis, and dissemination.

We are currently conducting a collaborative research project funded by the Medical Research Future Fund to co-produce cancer survivorship resources with and for people with intellectual disability. The initiative was prompted by gaps identified by Cancer Council South Australia and the South Australian Intellectual Disability Health Service, who observed that information after a cancer diagnosis was often not available in accessible formats, many people with intellectual disability were not empowered to be part of decision making about their own healthcare, and in some cases, were offered only palliative care when other options were available. This project aims to ensure that cancer survivorship resources are accessible, relevant, and inclusive of the needs and experiences of people with intellectual disability.

Although the project is still in its early stages, strong partnerships have laid the groundwork for long-term impact. The Cancer Council South Australia, the South Australian Intellectual Disability Health Service, and other partners are committed to co-producing resources that reflect the voices of people with intellectual disability. The project has garnered significant interest and engagement, with participants expressing their eagerness to contribute to solutions that will improve healthcare for their community.

A notable outcome has been the establishment of multiple levels of engagement, including an advisory group composed of people with intellectual disability, family caregivers, service providers and health care professionals, who provide ongoing feedback and oversight. This layered structure ensures that the research remains inclusive and responsive at every stage.

Reflecting on this work, we would emphasise the importance of building strong, trusting relationships and taking the time to engage meaningfully with all partners. This work requires a strong trauma-informed approach, minimizing the risk of re-traumatisation for people with intellectual disability who may have had negative healthcare experiences in the past.

Author: Associate Professor Michelle Bellon
Acknowledgements: Dr Jennifer Baldock (Cancer Council South Australia), Tim Cahalan & Hannah Bienke (Community Researchers), Jala Burton (Flinders University), Stephanie Searle & Monica Welsh (South Australian Intellectual Disability Health Service), Professor Jullian Trollor (National Centre of Excellence in Intellectual Disability Health), Professor Catherine Patterson, Associate Professor Aileen Collier, Associate Professor Lisa Beatty (Flinders University), Emma Kemp, Drew Meehan & Bronte McQueen (Cancer Council South Australia), Felicity Crowther (South Australian Council on Intellectual Disability), Deborah Bateson (University of Sydney), Jessica Smith (Southern Adelaide Local Health Network), Karen Fullagar (Minda Inc), Alison Vivian (Our Voice South Australia), Julie Hoare (Multicultural Communities Council of South Australia)

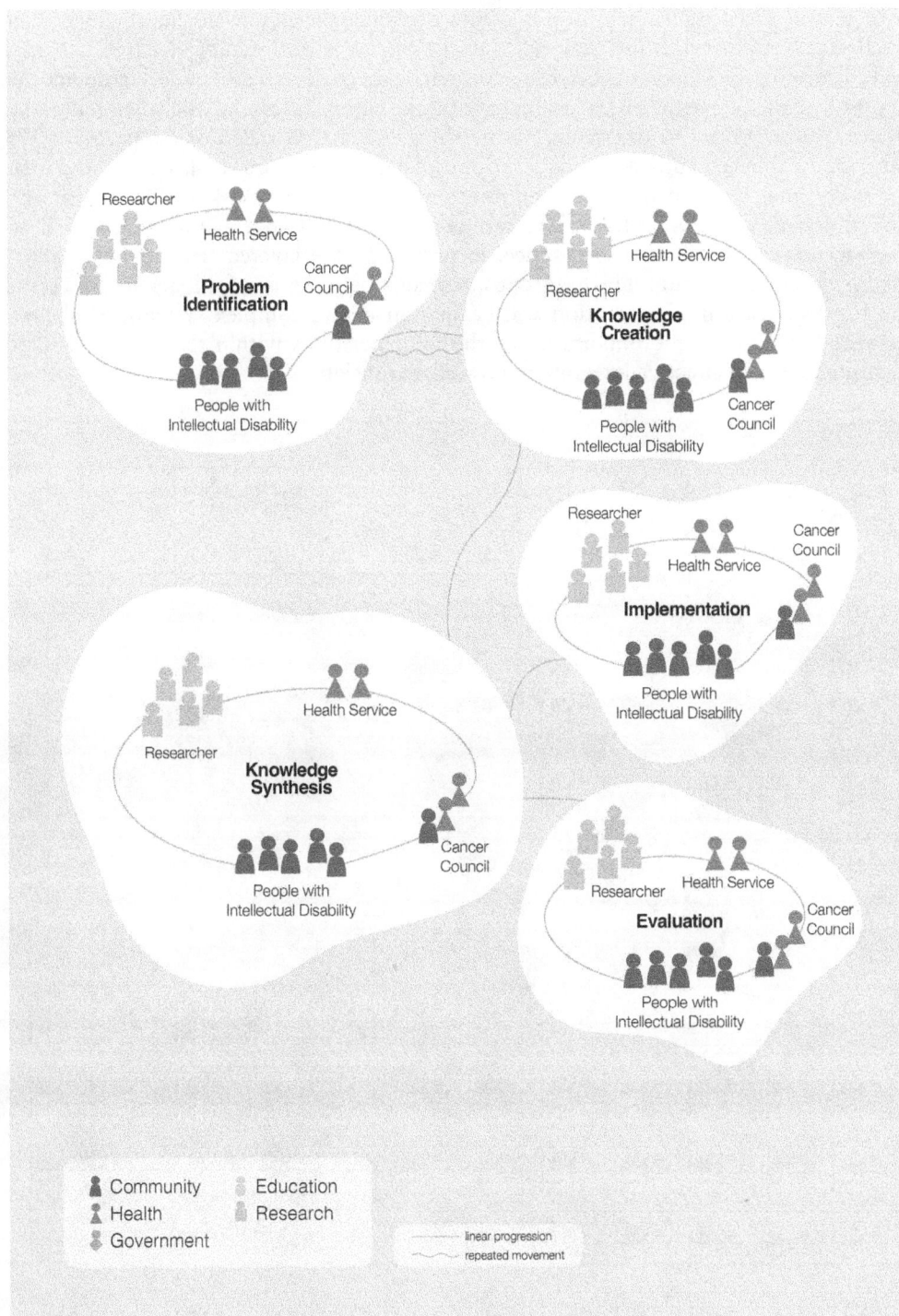

Figure 5.5 Case study 4 through the Knowledge Translation Complexity Network Model.
Source: https://doi.org/10.25451/flinders.29192750.v1

Case study 4 (Figure 5.5) demonstrates a focus on co-designing cancer care solutions with people with intellectual disabilities. As the research lead at the South Australian Intellectual Disability Health Service, Michelle's focus is on building research capacity and integrating lived experiences into research practice. This case study highlights the importance of the partnerships and collaboration within research. Michelle credits the success of the project to the strong partnerships and shared vision of the partners. We can see how through authentic collaboration and iterative exploration (as illustrated with the wavy line) between problem identification and creating new knowledge is setting this project up to generate the cancer care resources (knowledge synthesis) that will be implemented and evaluated in practice. In particular, the layered structure of engagement, with advisory and reference groups, also supports ongoing feedback loops, essential for responsive implementation and evaluation within complex systems. Michelle's case study highlights the importance of the joint positions within the Caring Futures Institute to enable effective integrated knowledge translation.

Box 5.5 *Case study 5* Developing a home care app to support end-of-life care

The ageing population in Australia has led to an increase in the number of people receiving end-of-life care at home, supported by home care workers. However, most of these workers are not qualified health professionals and may have limited training in palliative care. This means that many home care workers struggle to provide appropriate support to clients facing end-of-life issues. Our team identified a need for a solution that could provide home care workers with reliable, accessible information right at their fingertips. The goal was to create a mobile app that could help workers navigate complex care situations, offer evidence-based guidance on end-of-life issues, and improve communication between care workers and their clients. The development of this app was driven by the recognition that workers needed more support to ensure that clients could age and die with dignity at home.

To truly understand the problem, this project commenced with a comprehensive needs assessment, which included reviewing existing literature, consulting with diverse partners, and building on previous research from related initiatives like End-of-Life Directions for Aged Care. We worked closely with partners from peak bodies in aged care and palliative care. This allowed us to synthesise existing knowledge on end-of-life care and identify key gaps that the app could address.

We used a co-design approach to ensure the app would be practical and relevant for end-users. We engaged home care workers, managers, and other partners who contributed to the design and content of the app. We used various methods, including interviews, focus groups, and methods like 'closed card sorts', which helped understand how users would navigate the app logically. A key aspect of the app's development was ensuring it would be accessible to a broad range of users. This meant considering digital health literacy, visual literacy, and digital accessibility throughout the whole design process.

Since its development, the app has seen engagement from home care workers, with positive feedback validating our development approach. Several organisations have expressed interest in deploying the app across their workforce, demonstrating the demand for such a resource. While the app is currently designed for individual downloads, we are exploring ways to allow organisations to install it more broadly across their teams. International interest in the app has further highlighted its potential. We explored the app's usage patterns, which showed how users were engaging with different features and which resources were most popular. This feedback has been important for refining the app and ensuring it meets the needs of home care workers.

One of the key successes from our perspective was developing and launching the app despite the difficult circumstances of the COVID-19 pandemic, which significantly strained the aged care sector.

Overall, the project's success highlights the value of interdisciplinary collaboration. We worked collaboratively with expertise from digital design, healthcare, and user experience to create a tool that could address real-world needs in a very practical way. For us, this project demonstrates the importance of embedding knowledge translation processes into technology development. We view knowledge translation as not just about translating evidence into practice; it involves a dynamic and iterative process from identifying needs to developing solutions, testing, and evaluating outcomes. By viewing knowledge translation as a complex system, we have been able to create a more cohesive and integrated approach to our work.

Author: Professor Jennifer Tieman
Acknowledgements: Dr Amanda Adams, Dr Priyanka Vandersman

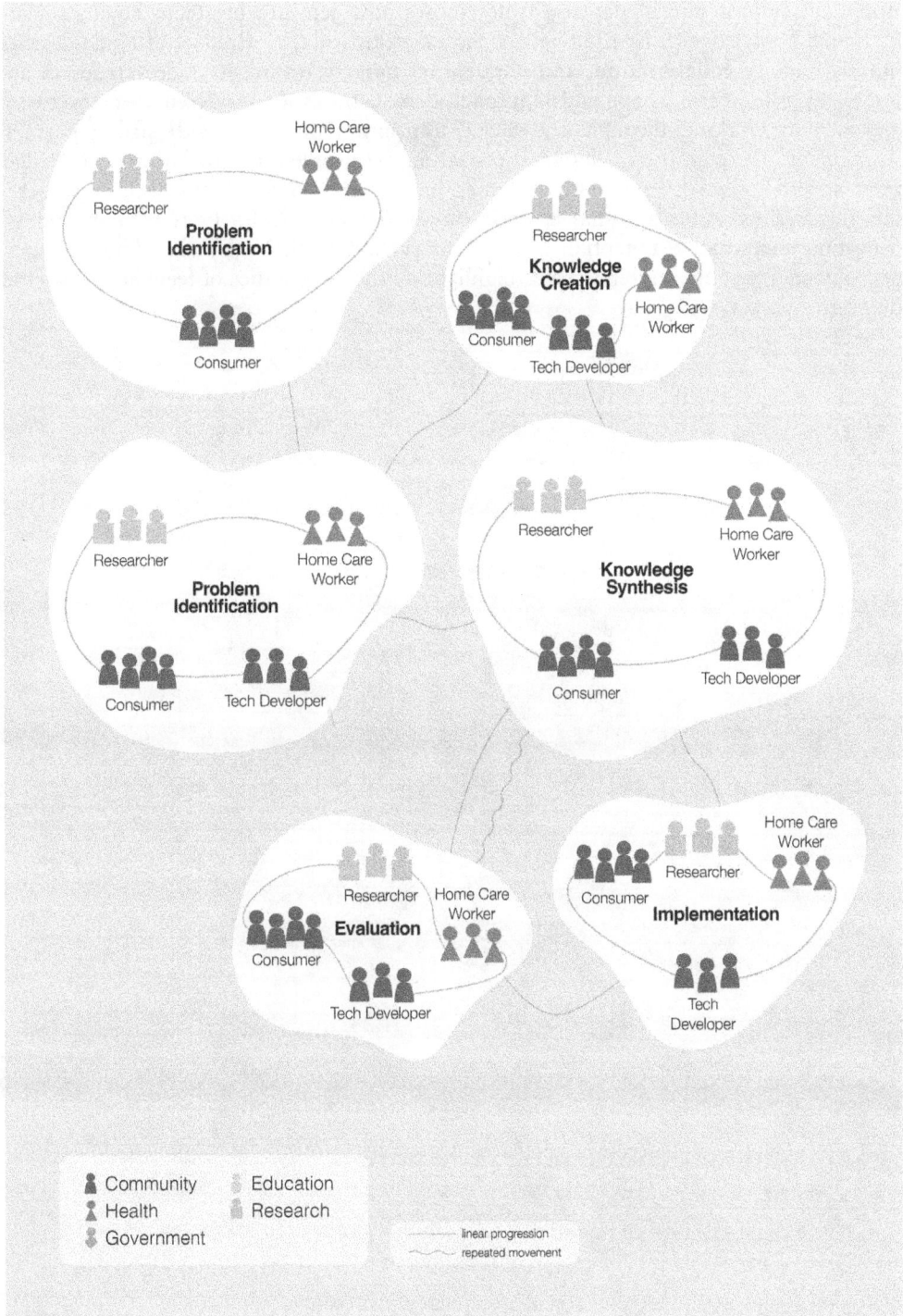

Figure 5.6 Case study 5 through the Knowledge Translation Complexity Network Model.
Source: https://doi.org/10.25451/flinders.29192753.v1

Case study 5 (Figure 5.6) demonstrates a focus on developing a home care app to support end-of-life care. This case study shows how Jen and her team have used an integrated knowledge translation approach to develop an app, demonstrating co-design, interdisciplinary collaboration, and iterative technology testing to address gaps in at-home end-of-life care. This team's approach demonstrates a considered and structured approach to working through knowledge translation processes with strong partner engagement. Through the co-design approach in the problem identification, knowledge creation, and knowledge syntheses processes, has ensured the development of a practical, relevant, and accessible app that has user buy-in. This allows for more effective implementation and scalable potential. Continuous evaluation through usage data and user feedback enables ongoing refinement, highlighting the importance of feedback loops for long-term success.

Box 5.6 *Case study 6* Developing shared care models in cancer survivorship care

People living with and beyond cancer need comprehensive, ongoing care that addresses not only their clinical needs but also their psychosocial, emotional, and practical concerns. While large tertiary care centres are traditionally responsible for on-going treatment and management of these individuals, clinicians at these centres are often time-poor with overflowing clinics and may have limited capacity to adequately provide support. Many of the symptoms and side effects experienced can be managed effectively in primary care, rather than relying on resource-limited tertiary care facilities.

Overall, our aims are to develop and implement shared-care models that can leverage the collective expertise of cancer specialists (medical and nursing), active engagement of general practitioners, and enhanced allied health offerings that are tailored to the address the care needs of people living with and beyond cancer. For example, in the current AUS-NET Survivorship trial (www.flinders.edu.au/caring-futures-institute/our-research/research-projects/aus-net) which is investigating the effectiveness and implementation of a nurse-led, shared, follow-up partnership between the acute cancer centres and general practices for people with neuroendocrine neoplasms, specialist neuroendocrine nurses develop individualised and structured survivorship care plans for each patient, considering their diagnosis, treatment history, and personal goals. The plan forms the basis for subsequent discussion with the patients' general practitioner in terms of their responsibilities of on-going care including surveillance and self-management support.

A key aspect of the design and implementation of these shared care models is the active involvement of partners, including individuals with a lived experience of cancer. Our team works closely with consumer advisory committees and not-for-profit organisations such as the McGrath Foundation (breast cancer), the Prostate Cancer Foundation of Australia (prostate cancer), and Neuroendocrine Cancer Australia (neuroendocrine tumours). These partners provide critical feedback on the model's design and help ensure that the interventions are both patient-centred and feasible within the healthcare system.

Although the models are still being evaluated, early indications are promising. The ultimate goal of these models is to demonstrate their effectiveness and cost-effectiveness through randomised controlled trials and then embed them into routine practice. A key measure of success will be whether these models are adopted beyond the trial settings and continue to be used as standard practice, providing sustainable improvements in care for people living with and beyond cancer.

Reflecting on the challenges and successes of the program of work, one of the most important factors in successful knowledge translation is meaningful partner engagement. Early and ongoing involvement of consumers, clinicians, and advocacy groups has been critical in shaping the models and ensuring that they are aligned with the real-world needs of patients and healthcare providers. For those starting out in similar projects, building strong relationships with partners and maintaining open lines of communication throughout the process are critical factors. By involving partners at every stage and focusing on practical, scalable solutions, our team are laying the groundwork for more patient-centred, efficient models of care.

Author: Dr Matthew Wallen (Co-deputy lead, on behalf of the Flinders University Cancer Survivorship Program)
Acknowledgements: Professor Raymond Chan (Co-lead), Professor Catherine Paterson (Co-lead), Dr Fiona Crawford-Williams (Co-deputy lead), Dr Carla Thamm (Clinical lead). A full list of research collaborators and project partners can be found here: www.flinders.edu.au/caring-futures-institute/cancer-care.

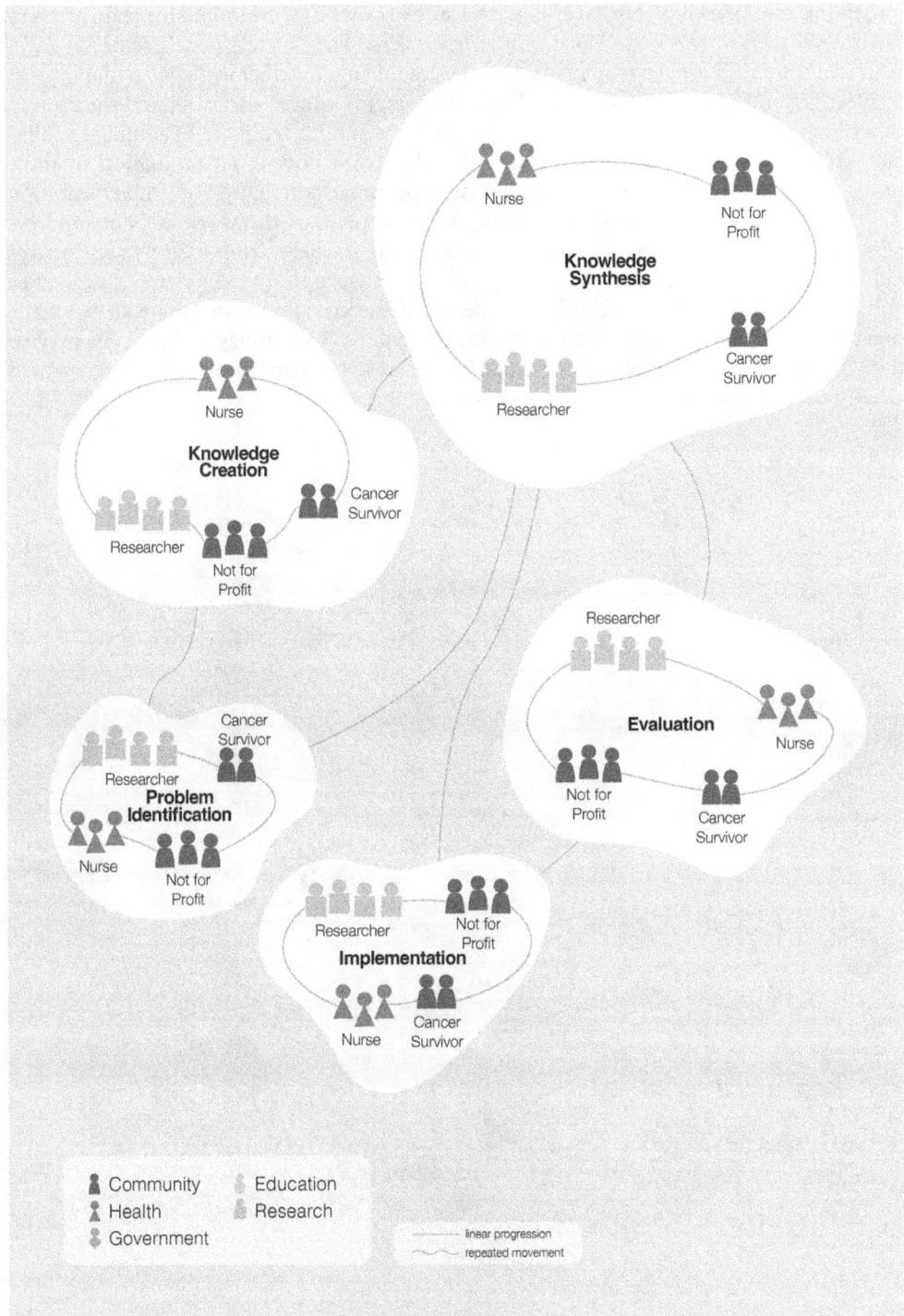

Figure 5.7 Case study 6 through the Knowledge Translation Complexity Network Model.
Source: https://doi.org/10.25451/flinders.29192759.v1

Case study 6 (Figure 5.7) demonstrates a focus on developing nurse-led shared care models in cancer survivorship care. This case study shows how Matt and his team are very much embedded in the knowledge synthesis process. They have strong partner engagement to ensure they are developing new models that bring together evidence with different perspectives and knowledge systems. Through engaging cancer survivors and their advocacy groups as well as key professional groups Matt and his team are beginning to influence broader policy processes. The focus for this team now is on evaluation of these models to generate evidence of effectiveness to aid in sustainability and implementation at scale. What will be importance for the future success of the work of Matt and his team, will be to ensure a strong understanding of the problem from various perspectives and continue the strong engagement of partners to ensure the system changes needed to embed these models of care. Until we understand the complex systems we all navigate, then the impact such evidence-based innovations will have on policy and practice may be quite limited, not because of their efficacy, but because of their failure to be implemented successfully.

Box 5.7 *Case study 7* Tackling the problem of repeated hospital presentations for older people

Frail older people are frequent presenters to hospital, both in the Emergency Department or as a patient in the hospital. About one in five older people who have had a first-time aged care eligibility assessment have an unplanned hospital presentation within the next three months. This is not ideal as hospital admission is known to expose older people to unwanted risks and can lead to a decline in their condition. It also places a lot of pressure on hospital services. So, where to begin in tackling this problem?

Understanding the problem

In a project undertaken in metropolitan South Australia, we identified older people living at home who presented at one of the major acute hospitals four or more times in one year and invited them to take part in focus group meetings to understand the problem from their perspective. We also invited staff from the hospital, from primary care and aged care to take part in similar focus group discussions. We then held a meeting with older people and service providers together so that they could hear each other's point of view. From the older person's perspective, an important point they raised was that when they went home from hospital, their social and care needs were a priority, not just their clinical care. For both older people and service providers, gaps in communication and information provision between the older person and their family, the hospital, general practitioners, aged care providers were identified. This led to the idea for a project titled 'Something Missing in the Middle' to develop and test a solution to reduce unnecessary hospital presentations for older people.

Identifying an evidence-informed solution

Creating a solution to a problem involves working together to explore approaches that could work in the local setting. In 'Something Missing in the Middle', this involved co-design workshops with older people and service providers to build on the issues identified from the initial focus group meetings. These meetings helped to really clarify what the problems were. The next step was to identify possible solutions to the problems. At this point, we reviewed the evidence to see what approaches had already been tried and tested. This did not provide us with a ready-made solution, but it did highlight the importance of developing a person-centred, locally relevant solution. Existing evidence also identified key principles that were important to consider, for example, targeting individuals most at risk, coordinating care and communication between different services, helping to navigate transitions in care and actively involving older people and their carers. This evidence was discussed in the co-design workshops, and the decision was made to focus on a care transition service supporting older people being discharged from hospital to home.

From the earlier exploration of the problem, we knew that to improve the older person's experience of leaving hospital to return home, a care transition service would need to support both their clinical and social and care needs. For example, older people had shared their experiences of returning home to an empty house and not having any food in the fridge or not being able to get to the pharmacy to collect their medicine or to a follow-up appointment with their General Practitioner. Taking these issues into consideration, older people and service providers co-designed a Care Transition Service that would be provided by a clinical nurse and an allied health assistant. These two roles would work together to support older people identified at high risk of hospital re-presentation for 6 weeks following hospital discharge.

Implementation to evaluation

The co-designed solution of a Care Transition Coordination Service was pilot tested for 6 months in one hospital. Given the small-scale nature of the project, the evaluation focused on assessing the acceptability and feasibility of the service. This involved re-visiting our key stakeholder groups: those people receiving the service (older people and their family members), staff delivering the service (the nurse and allied health assistant), and staff referring into the service (for example, other hospital clinicians). The findings highlighted that the Care Transition Coordination Service was well received by older people, their families/carers, and referrers, indicating a high level of acceptability. The service was seen to play an important role in bridging the transition from hospital to home, helping older people and their family navigate the complex aged care system, providing practical support, building confidence, and creating a set of 'eyes in the home' once the older person was discharged. Some issues with feasibility were identified from a service provider perspective, resulting in the recommendation to embed the care coordination roles within an existing community geriatric service.

Before subsequent scale-up of the Care Transition Coordination service, further research is needed to establish whether the service is effective in terms of reducing hospital re-admissions, highlighting the ongoing and iterative nature of knowledge translation.

Author: Professor Gill Harvey
Acknowledgements: Ella Bracci, Sarah Collyer

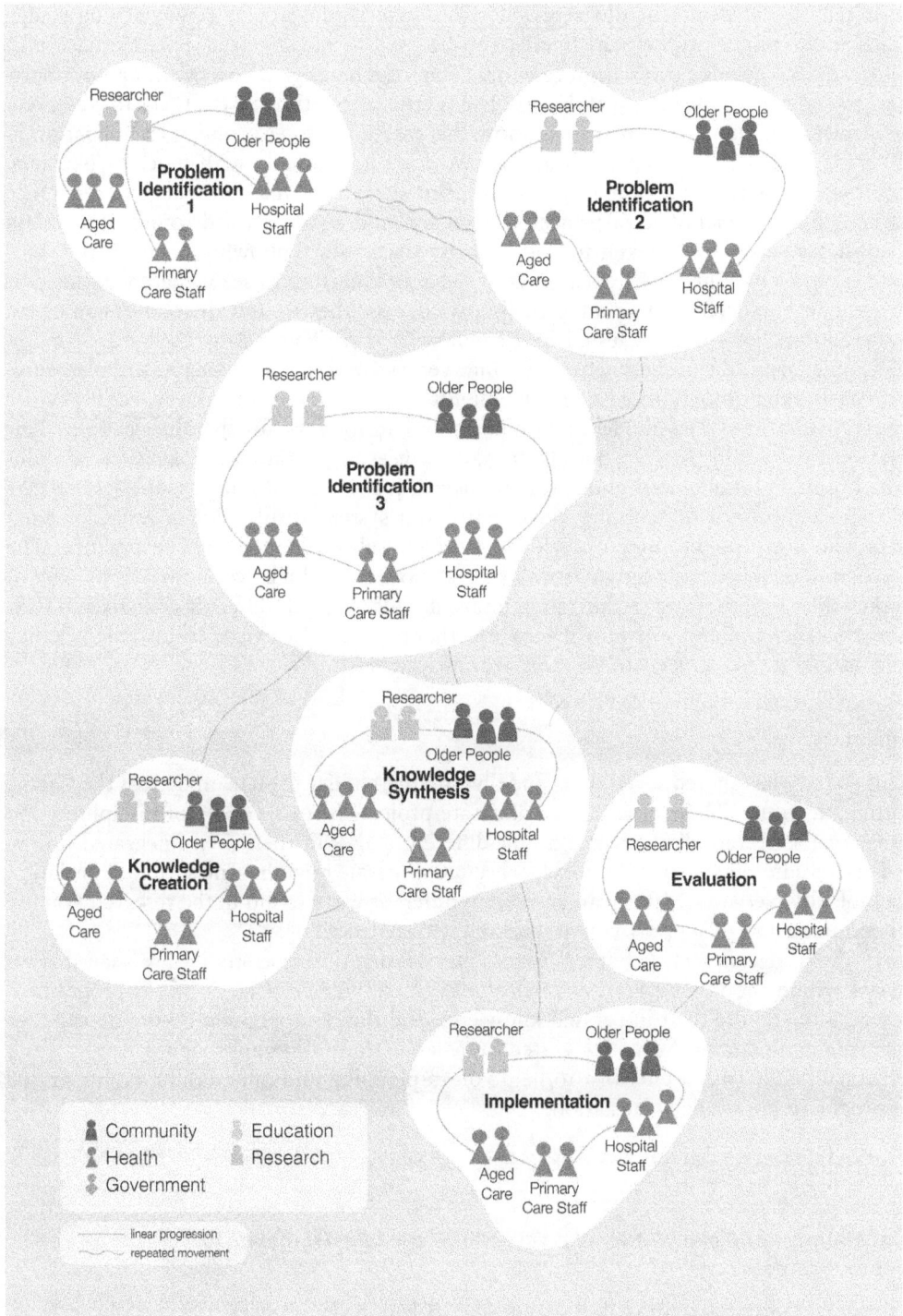

Figure 5.8 Case study 7 through the Knowledge Translation Complexity Network Model.
Source: https://doi.org/10.25451/flinders.29192765.v1

Case Study 7 (Figure 5.8) demonstrates a focus on tackling the problem of repeated hospital presentations for older people. This case study reflects how the knowledge translation complexity network model can be used to navigate the dynamic nature of integrated knowledge translation research. This case highlights how working with partners to understand the nature of the problem is critical to setting up the focus for research. As depicted in Figure 5.8, we can see how this case undertook problem identification in different ways. Firstly, by the researchers working individually with different partners, and then by bringing these partners together to share their different perspectives. Once some gaps were identified, a project was set up, and again, a third round of problem identification was undertaken to really clarify the issues. Following on from this, this case explores looking at the existing knowledge in literature to see if there was any evidence that could be used or adapted (knowledge synthesis), and then co-designing an intervention that could be tested in a small-scale way. This meant engaging teams in the implementation process where the intervention was being evaluated (implementation and evaluation). This case also highlights the importance of acknowledging wider system issues – the new model of care not only had to work for the older people, their care networks, and the staff but also it had to meet organisational goals such as reducing hospital re-admissions and saving money. Gill's work in leading this project reflects a mature approach to working consistently and systematically with a range of partners who are brought along on a journey which will lead to changes in practice. The respectful, deliberate, staged approach reflects how individuals 'volunteer' to be part of stakeholder groups, how certain 'champions' are identified in different systems and then how they build alliances that form networks that potentially can lead to sustained change and adoption of new ways of working within systems.

Summary

This chapter has shared seven short and diverse case studies from teams across the Caring Futures Institute. These case studies illustrate projects from a variety of disciplines and areas of focus, and all the teams are at different stages in their own integrated knowledge translation journey. Our goal has been to illustrate how the Knowledge Translation Complexity Network Model can be used in different ways to aid in the research you are undertaking and to support you in working with partners.

In the next chapters, (Chapters 6 and 7), two detailed case studies are shared from teams within the Caring Futures Institute. Each chapter deep dives into a program of research to explore their integrated knowledge translation approach. If you are eager to start planning out your own integrated knowledge translation approach, Chapter 8 is a practical guide, with a checklist to help you in planning and undertaking an integrated approach to knowledge translation.

Key case study references

Case Study 1 Implementation of an evidence-based model of care to improve cardiac care

Brieger, D., Amerena, J., Attia, J. R., Bajorek, B., Chan, K. H., Connell, C., ... & Zwar, N. A. (2018). National Heart Foundation of Australia and Cardiac Society of Australia and New

Zealand: Australian clinical guidelines for the diagnosis and management of atrial fibrillation 2018. *Medical Journal of Australia, 209*(8), 356–362.

Gallagher, C., Elliott, A. D., Wong, C. X., Rangnekar, G., Middeldorp, M. E., Mahajan, R., ... & Hendriks, J. M. (2017). Integrated care in atrial fibrillation: A systematic review and meta-analysis. *Heart, 103*(24), 1947–1953.

Gallagher, C., Hendriks, J. M., Nyfort-Hansen, K., Sanders, P., & Lau, D. H. (2022). Integrated care for atrial fibrillation: The heart of the matter. *European Journal of Preventive Cardiology, 29*(15), 2058–2063.

Hendriks, J. M., De Wit, R., Crijns, H. J., Vrijhoef, H. J., Prins, M. H., Pisters, R., ... & Tieleman, R. G. (2012). Nurse-led care vs. usual care for patients with atrial fibrillation: Results of a randomized trial of integrated chronic care vs. routine clinical care in ambulatory patients with atrial fibrillation. *European Heart Journal, 33*(21), 2692–2699.

Hendriks, J. M., Gallagher, C., Middeldorp, M. E., Lau, D. H., & Sanders, P. (2021). Risk factor management and atrial fibrillation. *EP Europace, 23*(Supplement_2), ii52–ii60.

Hendriks, J. M., Tieleman, R. G., Vrijhoef, H. J., Wijtvliet, P., Gallagher, C., Prins, M. H., ... & Crijns, H. J. (2019). Integrated specialized atrial fibrillation clinics reduce all-cause mortality: Post hoc analysis of a randomized clinical trial. *EP Europace, 21*(12), 1785–1792.

Kirchhof, P., Benussi, S., Kotecha, D., Ahlsson, A., Atar, D., Casadei, B., ... & Vardas, P. (2016). 2016 ESC Guidelines for the management of atrial fibrillation developed in collaboration with EACTS. *Polish Heart Journal (Kardiologia Polska), 74*(12), 1359–1469.

Linz, D., Pluymaekers, N. A., & Hendriks, J. M. (2020). TeleCheck-AF for COVID-19: A European mHealth project to facilitate atrial fibrillation management through teleconsultation during COVID19.

Case study 2 knowledge synthesis to generate a living database for the prevention of early childhood obesity

Hunter, K. E., Johnson, B. J., Askie, L., Golley, R. K., Baur, L. A., Marschner, I. C., ... & Seidler, A. L. (2022). Transforming Obesity Prevention for CHILDren (TOPCHILD) Collaboration: Protocol for a systematic review with individual participant data meta-analysis of behavioural interventions for the prevention of early childhood obesity. *BMJ Open, 12*(1), e048166.

Johnson, B. J., Chadwick, P. M., Pryde, S., Seidler, A. L., Hunter, K. E., Aberoumand, M., ... & Golley, R. K. (2025). Behavioural components and delivery features of early childhood obesity prevention interventions: Intervention coding of studies in the TOPCHILD Collaboration systematic review. *International Journal of Behavioral Nutrition and Physical Activity, 22*(1), 14.

Johnson, B. J., Hunter, K. E., Golley, R. K., Chadwick, P., Barba, A., Aberoumand, M., ... & Seidler, A. L. (2022). Unpacking the behavioural components and delivery features of early childhood obesity prevention interventions in the TOPCHILD Collaboration: A systematic review and intervention coding protocol. *BMJ Open, 12*(1), e048165.

Case study 3 co-designing implementation of clinical guideline recommendations to improve stroke rehabilitation in inpatient settings

Luker, J., Lynch, E., Bernhardsson, S., Bennett, L., & Bernhardt, J. (2015). Stroke survivors' experiences of physical rehabilitation: A systematic review of qualitative studies. *Archives of Physical Medicine and Rehabilitation, 96*(9), 1698–1708.

Luker, J., Murray, C., Lynch, E., Bernhardsson, S., Shannon, M., & Bernhardt, J. (2017). Carers' experiences, needs, and preferences during inpatient stroke rehabilitation: A systematic review of qualitative studies. *Archives of Physical Medicine and Rehabilitation, 98*(9), 1852–1862.

Lynch, E. A., Bulto, L. N., West, M., Cadilhac, D. A., Cooper, F., & Harvey, G. (2024). Codesigning implementation strategies to improve evidence-based stroke rehabilitation: A feasibility study. *Health Expectations, 27*(1), e13904.

Case study 5 developing a home care app to support end-of-life care

Adams, A., Miller-Lewis, L., & Tieman, J. (2024). Usability testing of a palliative care information resource-outcomes from the formative evaluation of the CarerHelp Toolkit prototype. *Informatics for Health and Social Care,* 1–17.

Lane, A. P., & Tieman, J. (2025). "We work in an industry where We're here to care for others, and often forget to take care of ourselves": Aged-care staff views on self-care. *Geriatrics, 10*(1), 3.

Tieman, J., & Nicholls, S. (2024). Enhancing the efficacy of healthcare information websites: A case for the development of a best practice framework. *BMJ Open, 14*(9), e088789.

Case study 6 developing shared care models in cancer survivorship care

Chan, R. J., Crawford-Williams, F., Crichton, M., Joseph, R., Hart, N. H., Milley, K., ... & Nekhlyudov, L. (2021). Effectiveness and implementation of models of cancer survivorship care: An overview of systematic reviews. *Journal of Cancer Survivorship,* 1–25.

Chan, R. J., Crawford-Williams, F., Han, C. Y., Jones, L., Chan, A., McKavanagh, D., ... & Emery, J. (2025). Implementing a nurse-enabled, integrated, shared-care model involving specialists and general practitioners in early breast cancer post-treatment follow-up (EMINENT): A single-centre, open-label, phase 2, parallel-group, pilot, randomised, controlled trial. *eClinicalMedicine,* 81.

Jefford, M., Chan, R. J., & Emery, J. D. (2024). Shared care is an appropriate model for many cancer survivors. *Journal of Clinical Oncology, 42*(17), 2105–2106.

Case study 7 tackling the problem of repeated hospital presentations for older people

Marshall, A., Rawlings, K., Zaluski, S., Gonzalez, P., & Harvey, G. (2021). What do older people want from integrated care? Experiences from a South Australian co-design case study. *Australasian Journal on Ageing, 40*(4), 406–412.

References

Graham, I. D., Logan, J., Harrison, M. B., Straus, S. E., Tetroe, J., Caswell, W., & Robinson, N. (2006). Lost in knowledge translation: Time for a map? *The Journal of Continuing Education in the Health Professions, 26*(1), 13–24. https://doi.org/10.1002/chp.47

Hendriks, J. M. L., De Wit, R., Crijns, H. J. G. M., Vrijhoef, H. J. M., Prins, M. H., Pisters, R., Pison, L. A. F. G., Blaauw, Y., & Tieleman, R. G. (2012). Nurse-led care vs. usual care for patients with atrial fibrillation: Results of a randomized trial of integrated chronic care vs. routine clinical care in ambulatory patients with atrial fibrillation. *European Heart Journal, 33*(21), 2692–2699. https://doi.org/10.1093/eurheartj/ehs071

Hendriks, J. M. L., De Wit, R., Vrijhoef, H. J. M., Tieleman, R. G., & Crijns, H. J. G. M. (2010). An integrated chronic care program for patients with atrial fibrillation. Study protocol and methodology for an ongoing prospective randomised controlled trial. *International Journal of Nursing Studies, 47*(10), 1310–1316. https://doi.org/10.1016/j.ijnurstu.2009.12.017

Hendriks, J. M. L., Tieleman, R. G., Vrijhoef, H. J. M., Wijtvliet, P., Gallagher, C., Prins, M. H., Sanders, P., & Crijns, H. J. G. M. (2019). Integrated specialized atrial fibrillation clinics reduce all-cause mortality: Post hoc analysis of a randomized clinical trial. *Europace (London, England), 21*(12), 1785–1792. https://doi.org/10.1093/europace/euz209

6 Case study

The Quality of Life – Aged Care Consumers Tool

Rachel Milte and Claire Hutchinson

Editorial introduction

In this chapter, a team from the Caring Futures Institute provide a detailed case study of how they have undertaken integrated knowledge translation. Chapters 1 and 4 provided detailed descriptions of integrated knowledge translation from a theoretical perspective and now we are illustrating how this can look in the real world. We hope this chapter illustrates that there is no 'one size fits all' approach to doing integrated knowledge translation and all projects look different. We will use the Knowledge Translation Complexity Network Model (Kitson et al., 2018) at the end of this chapter to share our reflections on how this case study has undertaken integrated knowledge translation. But first, we will recap the Knowledge Translation Complexity Network Model, as introduced in prior chapters. The model integrates five key knowledge translation processes. These five processes are: Problem Identification, Knowledge Creation, Knowledge Synthesis, Implementation, and Evaluation. Figure 6.1 provides a visual representation of the model.

Introduction

In this chapter, we share our experience of undertaking a large program of research which was funded by the Australian Research Council Linkage Project Scheme. The research was conducted between 2017 and 2022 and focused upon the development and validation of a new quality of life instrument with older people for economic evaluation and quality assessment in aged care (Project ID: LP170100664). The Australian Research Council Linkage Project Grant Scheme aims to promote 'national and international research partnerships between researchers and business, industry, community organisations and other publicly funded research agencies' to 'apply advanced knowledge to problems, acquire new knowledge and as a basis for securing commercial and other benefits of research'. The journey to translate this project into practice began not only within the period of the grant, nor while writing and submitting the grant application, but many years before. While to the naked eye successful translation of the outcomes of this project may appear to have occurred quickly (within five years of the initial awarding of the grant), this was built upon successful existing collaborations and partnerships.

Sarah Hunter, Michael Lawless, and Alison Kitson

DOI: 10.4324/9781003245995-8

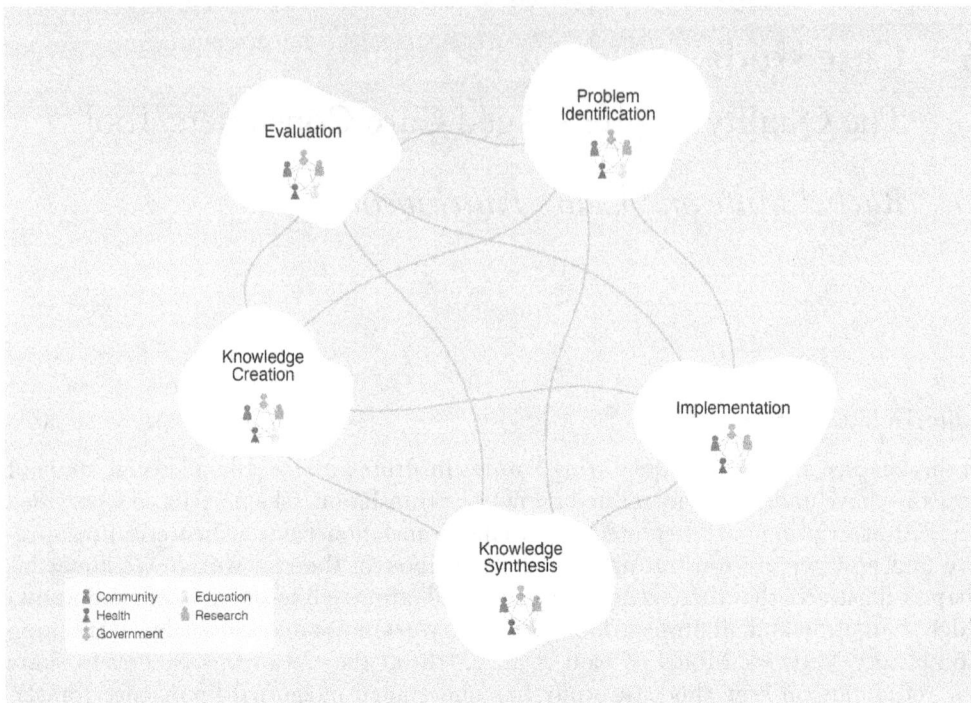

Figure 6.1 Knowledge Translation Complexity Network Model.
Source: https://doi.org/10.25451/flinders.29192585.v1

Introduction to health and social care economics

Before we begin, we want to provide some context and a brief introduction to health and social care economics. Health economics focuses on the application of economic principles to questions about the health and wellbeing of the population and the functioning of the health system which supports this. Typically, a large proportion of the work of health economists focuses on issues such as the supply of and demand for health services, the most efficient way of funding the health system, and evaluation of 'value for money' of health services. For decades, a formal structured economic evaluation has been the preferred method of assessing the value for money of a new pharmaceutical, health intervention or service. Economic evaluation is an umbrella term used to describe a range of evaluations, some of which will likely be familiar to readers even if they have not studied economics. For example, cost-minimisation analysis, cost-benefit analysis, and cost-effectiveness analysis. Excellent summaries of the different types of economic evaluation, their characteristics and examples of their application in health system setting are available for the interested reader (Brazier et al., 2016; Drummond, 2015).

Whilst an extensive knowledge of the methods of economic evaluation is not necessary to appreciate the content of this chapter, we will provide a brief summary as useful background for the project to be discussed.

All economic evaluations aim to compare two or more health or social care interventions or services in terms of their associated costs and benefits. Different methods of economic evaluation compare the costs with different ways of representing the benefits of an intervention. For example, a cost-benefit analysis presents the benefits of an intervention purely in monetary terms (for example dollars saved through reduced hospital admissions, etc). A cost-effectiveness analysis, by comparison, presents the benefits in terms of natural units most applicable to the intervention under evaluation. This often includes outcomes most familiar to and relevant for clinicians and health practitioners, such as a reduction in blood pressure for a new medication, or improvement in physical strength among patients participating in a home-rehabilitation program after discharge from hospital. Readers may be less familiar with a cost-utility analysis, which is a special type of cost-effectiveness analysis. In a cost-utility analysis, the costs associated with a new intervention are compared to a standardised unit of benefit, namely quality-adjusted life years. The consistency in measure of benefit in cost-utility analysis provides an advantage, allowing the comparison of costs and benefits of different types of interventions across different populations (at least in theory). To put it simply, a cost-utility analysis allows policy makers to compare oranges and oranges, as compared to a cost-effectiveness analysis, where policy makers comparing the findings across different interventions are asked to compare apples and oranges. In cost-utility analysis, the application of the quality-adjusted life year as a generic measure of outcome facilitates comparisons across alternative interventions, different populations, and different healthcare settings, making it easier to compare when a decision-maker is trying to decide which new health intervention they should fund. The quality-adjusted life year sounds very opaque upon first meeting, but in practice it is made of three component parts. One part is the health-related quality of life of a person at various time points, the second is how that health-related quality of life would be ranked on what is known as the 'quality-adjusted life year scale', which is a value between 0 and 1, where 1 represents full or best possible health, and 0 represents a state equivalent to death. Negative values (considered worse than death) are also possible on this scale. The final component is the length of time a person spends with health-related quality of life as described. Combining these three components will give the quality-adjusted life year over the follow up period for an individual. It is via the quality-adjusted life year and its use in cost-utility analysis that the concept of health-related quality of life becomes important in health economics.

Typically to measure health-related quality of life for use in cost-utility analysis standardised questionnaires are used, namely Generic-Preference Based Measures. Generic-preference based measures are made of two component parts: the first is a descriptive system, which is typically a multiple choice questionnaire which patients use to describe their health status across specified domains (for example mobility, level of pain experienced, mental health, level of sensory impairments), and secondly an 'off the shelf' scoring algorithm which is developed which can convert the health state to a utility value on the 'quality-adjusted life year scale', usually based on the opinions of members of the general population. There are many different generic-preference based measures which are available which can be used to generate utility values. Investigation of the validity and reliability of the measures, and which are the best measures to use for cost-utility analysis is an area of much debate and investigation among health economists.

The problem

Most of the development in the methodology and application of economic evaluation has typically been undertaken in the tertiary healthcare sector. Less common has been the application of health economics to broader social and supportive care systems, such as care in the community for people with a disability, or for older people via the aged care system. In fact, most health economists have tended to ignore the aged care system, despite the fact it forms a major component of government spending in many high-income countries across the world and is increasingly forming part of the care systems in low- and middle-income countries. Government spending on aged care for 2022–23 reached over $27 billion in Australia. With this increase in spending, there have been increasing calls for greater monitoring of the quality-of-care participants receive, and consideration of the value for money of the services provided by the health and social care sectors. This has seen a slow but steady increase in evaluation and research within the sector.

The remainder of this chapter goes on to describe a case study of one research project undertaken in the aged care setting during a period of unprecedented change, and the factors which led to successful implementation into practice. We will look at the project chronologically, and describe the key practical considerations, challenges, learnings, and factors which we believe contributed to the project's success.

Preparation and pre-grant phase

As we described in the introduction to this chapter, the journey to translate this project into practice began many years before receiving grant funding. For us, this time before funding was spent building partnerships and building credibility.

Building partnerships takes time

Building authentic, collaborative, and respectful partnerships will form an ongoing theme throughout the discussion of this project. They are the strong foundation which can make your path to translation so much easier. Crucially this takes time, energy, and investment, with no guarantee of tangible success. Developing these partnerships over time is key, as it allows you to then have working partnerships ready to start for unexpected opportunities that come up. From our own experience, our team members drew on partnerships with Aged Care Providers which had been developed several years prior to the development and submission of this ARC linkage grant. Part of our approach to developing these partnerships has been authentic engagement – which we conceptualise as a genuine 'two-way street'. Too often researchers wish to engage with industry in a transactional way – where the researcher prioritises their needs over and above the needs and priorities of the partner and views the partner as a source of resources (e.g. money, staff, participants, ideas) which can be gouged to achieve their aims. This may be deliberate on the part of the researcher (i.e. they may believe that their needs are more important) but we also believe that this can be implicit (i.e. where the researcher is so focused on the importance of the research, they are undertaking that they behave as if their needs are more important). For success, it is important that relationships are built on a foundation of mutual respect. Clear and frequent communication is important, so that all parties can clearly understand each other's perspectives, what each other's priorities are and why. This process takes time, and while it is so important, not all researchers invest in this stage. It will involve asking your partners about their priorities in their organisation and listening to their responses. An ideal scenario would be where your research is able to address one or more of these priorities, directly or indirectly. We were able to do this with the current project.

The relationships for this project began many years before, during the development process for a previous Australian Research Council funded linkage project led by

Professor Julie Ratcliffe and conducted between 2012 and 2016. The project (*A health economic model for the development and evaluation of innovations in aged care: an application to Consumer Directed Care*, Project ID LP110200079) was focused on a major policy reform challenge that aged care providers were experiencing at the time – namely the implementation of consumer directed care into the aged care sector. As part of that project, aged care industry partnerships were formed with several Australian provider organisations including the ACH Group, Helping Hand, Resthaven, Hamondcare, and Catholic Community Services. This project was a success, completed within 5 years and met all the proposed aims. The relationships built during this project formed the foundations for the partnerships for the subsequent 'Quality of Life – Aged Care Consumers Tool' project.

Building evidence that you are leaders in the field takes time

Once the relationships with industry were formed, it also took time to build the recognition that we were the leaders in the field to undertake the work and to find funding for the proposed work. While this project was successful in its first submission under the Australian Research Council Linkage scheme, it was previously submitted on two separate occasions to the National Health and Medical Research Council but was unsuccessful. It was through this process that Professor Ratcliffe realised that the idea and the partnerships were strong, but that aged care was not a priority for the National Health and Medical Research Council at that time, due to its strong focus on healthcare. By comparison, the Australian Research Council focuses on a broader range of research and aged care (whilst somewhat under-researched at the time) did fall under their remit.

Professor Ratcliffe also used this time between successive grant application submissions to undertake more pilot work to provide better evidence of the need for a new quality of life instrument for older people. This work was published in two manuscripts (Milte et al., 2014; Ratcliffe et al., 2017). A study by Milte et al. (2014) identified through a mixed methods approach that older people highly valued broad components of quality of life such as independence and control, safety and dignity, as contributing to their quality of life. This was further supported by the findings of Ratcliffe et al. (2017). This was the first study to directly compare the relative importance of the components of quality of life among older and younger people. The study evaluated a wide-range of components of quality of life, including aspects of physical and mental health, mobility, absence of pain, quality of sleep, any vision or hearing loss, as well as broader aspects of quality of life which have not been included in traditional generic-preference based measures, such as control over your own life, quality of social relationships, and independence. This study found that older people and younger people did value these components of quality of life differently. For example, older people highly valued the ability to be independent, manage their self-care, and have control over their lives. For younger people, feeling safe, having good social relationships, and mental health were the most important components of a good quality of life. Crucially, the vast majority of generic-preference based measures used in practice to evaluate the impact of health interventions on quality of life for use in cost-utility analysis did not include all these broader components of quality of life that were important to older people. This fact is unsurprising, given that older people themselves were typically excluded from the development and validation of these existing Generic-preference based measures. The combined findings of these two pilot studies indicated a need for a quality-of-life instrument developed from its inception with older people who were using aged care services.

Early stages of Australian Research Council Linkage

In 2018, we were very excited to discover that the Australian Research Council Linkage application had been successful and was funded. However, were also aware that the hard work was just beginning. From the beginning of the project, partially due to the links with the partners, we focused on the implementation into practice for the Quality of Life-Aged Care Consumers instrument, however we understood that this would not be easy to achieve. We focused our efforts for implementation on two goals. One goal, was that the Quality of Life-Aged Care Consumers instrument could be used to as a measure of quality of care in the aged care sector more broadly, however given the challenges we believed this would entail we did not believe the chances of this were likely. Secondly, we aimed for the Quality of Life-Aged Care Consumers instrument to be able to generate quality-adjusted life years for economic evaluation of new models of care and interventions with older people. To give ourselves the best chance of achieving these aims, we made implementation a focus from the start of the project.

Engage early and often with partners

From our previous experience in working with partners, we decided the best approach was to engage early and often. One of our first activities was to set up a website, which we specifically targeted at industry and policy makers to help them stay abreast of new developments and informed about our project. Our website was external to any of our organisations or universities, and therefore, we had more control over the look and layout of the website, and it also gave the appearance that the website 'belonged' to the project, rather than any one partner or institution. We also committed to keep the website updated along the way, including publications and updates on progress. While updating the website took some time and money, as compared to a 'set and forget approach' we considered it essential to ensure the project looked 'alive' online. The website became a vehicle for interested parties to contact the research team about the project and for forming new collaborations including three aged care organisations who eventually joined the team as associated partners to assist with recruitment for the Quality of Life-Aged Care Consumers evaluation study.

We found regular meetings with our partners through our Steering Group essential. We initially aimed to meet every 3 months with our Steering Group, but this was changed to every 2 months during the mid-stages of the grant at their request. Our Steering Group performed two main functions. One was to allow all members of the research team across Australia and our formal partners on the project (who were named on the research grant and/or contributed funding to the research) to meet regularly and keep up to date on the progress of the project and to help with making governance decisions for the grant as needed. We also used our Steering Group to give advice on practical decisions on the day-to-day running of the project, for example commenting on proposed methodology, methods for recruitment and data collection. A second function was to contribute to higher level planning – for example maintaining the relevance of the project to industry, informing the research team about relevant changes within the industry, and keeping the project focused on the implementation into practice. Our Steering Group was formed with this in mind.

We included, as Steering Group members, the researchers working on the project, including all the named Chief Investigators (including Rachel), the Project Manager (Claire), and a representative from all the Aged Care Industry partners and Consumer Representative group named as formal partners for the project. These members had primary responsibility for the first function of the Steering Group. To meet the secondary function of the Steering Group (higher level planning and maintaining the relevance of the project to a rapidly changing industry), we invited others onto the Steering Group, including representatives from the State and the Commonwealth government health and aging policy portfolios. While these people are extremely busy, and may not attend all the meetings, having their participation can keep them informed about the project, which can make sharing your research findings later easier given they have a basic knowledge of your project.

Mid stages of the Australian Research Council Linkage

Be open to sharing the research

As we moved into the mid-point of our project, we continued to share our research findings with our Steering Group to keep them informed and engaged in the project. As the project progressed, we found our Aged Care partners maintained their engagement and that their feedback was invaluable to the success of the project. Sharing the research journey with them, asking for their input, and considering and respecting their point of view positively benefited the project. They were able to highlight elements for the project as important that we didn't initially consider, but which have been essential for implementation. For example, we initially focused on self-completion for the Quality of Life-Aged Care Consumers instrument as part of our project. Our industry partners asked for a version of the tool suitable to be completed by proxies (for example a close family member) or an interviewer-facilitated version for cases where the person themselves was unable to complete. This has been essential for the widespread roll-out of the Quality of Life-Aged Care Consumers instrument as a quality-of-care instrument in residential aged care, where large numbers of older people have significant cognitive impairment or dementia and need someone to complete on their behalf. Having a proxy version available ensures that the wording used is consistent among proxies and makes it easier for providers to get a perspective regarding people with cognitive impairment. We were also asked about our plans for how data would be collected in practice, for example about the resources which would be available to help organisations collect the Quality of Life-Aged Care Consumers instrument data. Whilst the research team at that time were deeply embedded in the data collection process, we took the comments of our Steering Group on board and began to consult with them more broadly about what would be needed for implementation into practice. Our partners were useful in drawing the research team out of the daily business of research, and focusing on the bigger picture, namely where we wanted to be when we had completed our project and the real purpose of our research – to solve a significant real-world problem and implement it successfully into practice.

This is an ongoing process, as our original budget for the project was limited and did not include large scale resources for developing digital versions, guides, videos, or translations of our new instrument. Our relationships with our partners also pushed us outside of our comfort zones as researchers. At their request, we began piloting the draft instrument with our industry partners internally 12 months prior to the project end. This process was very useful, by allowing us to trial the instrument in practice, and begin testing administration methods. In the fast-paced environment of aged care at the time, where much change was occurring, this pushed us to keep focus on implementation, despite our desires to sometimes just focus on the research agenda, and in the end, this was critical to our success.

Demystifying research to support authentic involvement

To ensure that partners can give valuable input, it is important to 'de-academic' the research process wherever possible. One example from our own study is as follows. We knew that we wanted to make sure that our partners could be involved in selecting the final items for inclusion as the questions of the Quality of Life-Aged Care Consumers instrument. However, for scientific rigour, it was important that the selection of items was based upon a combination of complex psychometric and validity statistics and as well as detailed data on the feasibility and acceptability of the items for older people themselves. Following on from work by Keetharuth et al. (2018), we used a 'traffic-light system' to summarise the data visually to allow partners without detailed understanding or experience of psychometrics (as well as researchers without this experience for that matter!) to usefully interpret the data and contribute to the item selection. Further details on this approach can be found in Hutchinson et al. (2021). Importantly, this allowed our partners to contribute to selecting the final items to be used in the Quality of Life-Aged Care Consumers instrument, increasing their investment in the instrument.

We were also open to sharing our research with our partners and the industry more broadly in real-time. In traditional research paradigms, it is more usual for researchers to keep the research close to their chests until it is published in an academic publication – which may not be until years down the track. However, this also slows the implementation of the research into practice, as industry or policy makers are likely not aware of the research and its findings. In the current research, we shared our research findings with our partners throughout our research process, which increased their engagement with the research, as they could see its progress in real-time. This involved sharing findings before they were finalised but allowed us to receive feedback. We used confidentiality agreements where needed to protect the unique research findings. This then resulted in our industry partners being ready to implement even before the research project had finished.

Royal Commission into Aged Care

Successful translation of research into practice also has an 'unknown' factor. This is a factor that cannot be predicted but assists in pushing the translation of the research to another level. While you cannot predict when or how this will occur, it is important to be ready to launch into action when opportunity arises. For our project, one of these factors was the Royal Commission into Aged Care Quality and Safety (Australian Government, 2021). The Royal Commission was launched by the Australian Government in 2018 in response to intense media scrutiny on the aged care sector in Australia, and after a crescendo of damming media reports of serious neglect and poor-quality care. A Royal Commission is a form of public enquiry in Australia, focusing on answering questions of key public importance. To do this it has broad and far-reaching powers to gather information, including the ability to compel witnesses to appear before it, and to request organisations to produce documents as evidence. They are relatively rare, being called when a serious matter of public interest is at stake.

Practically, a Royal Commission concentrates public and professional interest on a matter, focusing public and media attention on a subject, and are usually associated with increased transparency and reporting of information on a topic. A Royal Commission is governed by terms of reference which must be completed within a particular timeline, after which a report and series of recommendations are prepared and released to the government. This may include recommendations of changes to policy or practice within government, or suggestions for new or amended legislation. There is usually public expectation for the government to act upon recommendations from a Royal Commission. In fact, often a government will begin to act before a Royal Commission releases their recommendations, to try and limit any fall out from criticism of government programs that make occur. They therefore are a unique and rare opportunity to make large scale change to government policy and practice during a Royal Commission.

The Royal Commission into Aged Care Quality and Safety (hereafter referred to as 'the Royal Commission') terms of reference included a remit to advise on the quality of aged care services provided to all Australians, including 'what the Australian Government, aged care industry, Australian families and the wider community can do to strengthen the system of aged care services to ensure that the services provided are of high quality and safe'. Our research project was just getting started at this time, but we recognised that the Royal Commission would likely provide a once in a lifetime opportunity for our research to contribute to largescale reform in the aged care sector. This led to several implications: we needed to keep in touch with the Royal Commission in case any alignment between our research and their aims became evident, and we needed to act quickly to ensure that if our research could be useful to them, it would be available at the right time. Because of their strict timelines, they would need to report by a pre-determined date, whether our research was ready or not, we wanted to ensure our research could be included. And finally, the government would likely be looking for solutions to problems in the aged care sector throughout the inquiry period and beyond. If we could anticipate what their needs might be after the Royal Commission, we could have available research which could help them.

There were several potential ways we could contribute to the Royal Commission. As part of the process there are calls for submissions (usually written). Researchers were able to lead a submission or contribute to submissions written by others. Additionally, they called upon a range of 'witnesses' to give evidence in public hearings. Witnesses could include people with lived experience, industry or sector employees, representatives from peak bodies, as well as researchers. As part of the Royal Commission, Professor Ratcliffe was part of a written submission from the Caring Futures Institute, as well as being called upon subsequently as an expert witness in public hearings.

Another option was for researchers to contribute to the Royal Commission via undertaking targeted research requested by the Commission. A Royal Commission will typically have a program of research alongside it as part of the information gathering to allow the Commissioners to make informed recommendations to government in their final report. This can include literature reviews consolidating current available evidence, reviews of policy and practice in Australia and internationally, as well as primary data collection and surveys to answer key questions to inform policy. This research can be performed by the Royal Commission staff, government agencies, or external researchers commissioned by the Royal Commission. Professor Ratcliffe was commissioned by the Royal Commission to undertake specific projects relating to investigating preferences of the general population for quality of aged care as well as their opinions regarding future funding mechanisms and willingness to pay for improvements to the sector. Professor Ratcliffe was approached by the Royal Commission because of our engagement with the broader aged care sector about the Quality of Life-Aged Care Consumers project. While we were not expecting this, she jumped at the chance to connect with the Royal Commission and to contribute to their research program.

The research period was intense, as it needed to be undertaken within a specific time frame, to be provided to the Commissioners to inform their processes and decisions. We managed this by drawing on all the resources available to us at the time to get this research done. However, there was an opportunity cost, in that it meant that Professor Ratcliffe had to focus a significant amount of time on Royal Commission projects, while also trying to keep the Australian Research Council Linkage project moving, as well as her other projects. Similarly other staff had to manage multiple priorities while working on this research. However, we framed this as a unique opportunity which would not last forever, therefore, it was worth putting in a lot of hard work for the relatively short amount of time of the project. It is worth noting that there are a number of challenges which University researchers face to making the most of these opportunities. Universities are large organisations, with many layers of bureaucracy. They are not renowned for their speed or flexibility of processes. Additionally, the usual funding model for university research impacts upon their ability to respond to opportunities. University research is primarily funded through grant schemes, which have become highly competitive over the past few years. Even when grants are successful, researchers will be funded for only a few years on a grant, and to undertake a specific project. Therefore, any staff which need to work on a new research opportunity will need to be moved from another project or alternatively new staff recruited and employed by the organisation. Attracting new staff with the specific skills needed for a project may be time consuming. Additionally, there are several internal processes for employing a new staff member, and this is after you have organised a contract for undertaking the research project with an external body like the Royal Commission, which needs to occur before you can request any money to be transferred to fund these employees. While Universities are beginning to recognise the difficulties with their internal processes slowing down researchers and limiting their abilities to act flexibly and quickly to make the most of contract-style research opportunities such as those presented by the Royal Commission – however we feel there is still a long way to go! And we believe it is worth continuing to streamline processes and support researchers undertaking contract-style research, given the high potential for translation into practice when you are undertaking research which has been directly requested by the government or industry.

Despite these challenges, we experienced an enormous range of benefits from undertaking this Royal Commission research. It hugely assisted us in making connections with government policy makers. However, tit can be very difficult for people outside of government to break into their circles. It can be difficult to get in contact directly with people making decisions, and they are so busy that reaching out through generic contact points can lead to 'radio silence'. Yet, undertaking this research allowed us to make our work known to a government audience. Once we were better known to people in government, it allowed us to connect with them more easily. Additionally, undertaking this research was another opportunity to engage with the government and those advising government on what they considered the key questions and problems they were facing. This then gave us reassurance that we were on the right track with our research to provide useful solutions, or the opportunity to tweak the focus of our research to better fit their needs. For example, our engagement with the Royal Commission provided support to the message we received from our industry partners, which use as a quality indicator was a key use for the Quality of Life-Aged Care Consumers instrument. Therefore, we focused our energy on ensuring it was fit for this purpose, as well as for use in economic evaluation as a utility measure, which was our original priority coming from a health economic researcher perspective.

Finalising research project

Challenges along the way

As we progressed towards project completion, there were several challenges along the way. We wish to comment on some the challenges we faced to reassure any person moving into this space that this work can be difficult, time consuming, frustrating, and make you feel like you are going around in circles. This is how it was for us at times, and we are sure that future projects will also feel this way. This is not a sign that you are not doing things right or well. Rather, we take it as an indicator of the complexity and difficulty of the problem you are trying to solve.

One of the ongoing challenges we faced was maintaining engagement among the partners. A main feature of the Aged Care industry over the life of our project has been change. There have been changes to funding, changes to policy, organisational restructures, changes to executive leadership, and even a pandemic. As a result of these changes, we experienced a large amount of turnover of key staff within our partners organisations and partners on the project. Personnel who had been a key contact for project governance, input in the Steering Group, or to facilitate approvals for project activities within the aged care organisations would change roles or leave the organisation, leaving us to form relationships with new individuals. Overall, engagement from partners, partner organisations, and personnel within those organisations fluctuated throughout the project. Keeping in mind the amount of change we were aware was occurring within the sector, we accommodated any changes in personnel, and dedicated time to bringing new personnel up to speed on the project.

Another challenge which we experienced was burden on the aged care organisations who had signed up to the research. We had originally five partner organisations for the research who formed the core of our source of participants for the project. While we aimed to reduce burden on them where possible, as the project progressed into its quantitative phase, the sheer number of participants we needed to recruit for a strong sample made it challenging for our original partners to find all the participants we needed. So, we made the decision to expand our partners to include more organisations to share the burden of recruitment. We made a conscious decision to do this transparently, and with the agreement of our original partners. Thankfully, this strategy worked well, and we ended the project with good relationships maintained with all our partners.

Future work and sustainability

A key learning from this work was that translation and implementation are never complete, there is always more work to be done. From engaging with our partners, we have continued to find opportunities to learn more about their needs in practice and how we can better support the implementation of the Quality of Life-Aged Care Consumers instrument into practice. One aspect that was highlighted by our aged care industry partners, was the importance of digitisation of the tools. They highlighted that increasingly their records, and data collection is electronic not via paper. If we wanted our tools to be taken up widely, we would need them to be able to be integrated into electronic data collection systems. Challengingly, there is no consistent electronic system used across aged care, a number of commercial providers implement their systems into aged care. This work is still ongoing. Another key ongoing aspect of implementation is investment in research. From an implementation perspective, ongoing research into population norms (i.e. identifying 'normal' or usual scores for populations such as home care recipients and resident) is useful to provide explanation and interpretation of scores when the Quality of Life-Aged Care Consumers instrument is used as a wide-spread quality indicator. Another key factor in the successful translation of the Quality of Life-Aged Care Consumers instrument has been in linking with relevant people to understand how to properly licence and administer the tool into practice. We did not have the necessary expertise to do this. Luckily, through the University we had ability to link into expertise in these areas – through advice from specialists in contracting, and licencing.

We also feel that there is much more to do in this field to fully implement into practice. We have so far focused on developing the Quality of Life-Aged Care Consumers and Quality of Care Experience-Aged Care Consumers instruments as traditional text-based instruments. However, there are a wider range of methods to convey concepts and collect responses available. Particularly from the disability sector, researchers have investigated using alternative communication strategies, such as using pictorial representations of concepts alongside text, and easy-read language modifications. These methods could enable the collection of important self-reported quality of care data from people who traditionally have been excluded, such as people with dementia or cognitive impairment, people from a culturally and linguistically diverse backgrounds, people with communication impairments, or with low literacy. Additionally, over a quarter of the population of Australia was born overseas, with 23% reporting using a language other than English at home (Australian Bureau of Statistics, 2022). This is a significant portion of the population who may need to respond to the Quality of Life-Aged Care Consumers and Quality of Care Experience-Aged Care Consumers instruments in a language other than English. The most common languages spoken in Australia other than English are Mandarin, Arabic, Vietnamese, Cantonese, and Punjabi. Among older Australians specifically, the most commonly spoke languages other than English are Italian, Chinese (Cantonese and Mandarin), and Greek (Australian Institute of Health and Welfare, 2024). We have commenced work with colleagues at the University of Hong Kong to translate the Quality of Life-Aged Care Consumers and Quality of Care Experience-Aged Care Consumers instruments into Chinese using a robust backwards and forwards translation approach, and we hope to continue working to translate the instruments to ensure a large proportion of Australia's older people who speak a language other than English are able to self-report their quality of life in their preferred language.

Finally, in the past there has been a tendency for the health system to drive changes in research and development, with the aged care sector less known for driving innovative research. However, we plan to turn this approach around, with plans to expand the use of the Quality of Life-Aged Care Consumers and Quality of Care Experience-Aged Care Consumers instruments into areas of the health system where older people are a large proportion of users and they share similar objectives to the aged care program, for example supporting older people to maintain their independence, quality of life, and wellbeing. We have commenced work to evaluate the feasibility and validity of using the Quality of Life-Aged Care Consumers and Quality of Care Experience-Aged Care Consumers instruments as outcome measures in subacute care focused on older people, such as transition care. The use of these instruments in transition care with older people has advantages in allowing consistent measurement of outcomes across the aged care and health systems, given the interactions between these two. Over 40% of hospitalisations among older people are also associated with use of the aged care system either before and/or afterwards (Australian Institute of Health and Welfare, 2020). A large proportion of older people who are hospitalised are discharged using a higher level of aged care services than they were on admission, indicating a potential for improving the care across the two systems.

In summary, we have shared our experiences of a research program which has been successfully implemented into practice. Our experience has been a mix of deliberate and conscious choices to support implementation, in addition to a range of choices made in response to a rapidly evolving policy environment over the period of the research. Flexibility and ability to see and have respect for multiple viewpoints and come to a shared decision about the way forward has been critical for our project. We hope that by sharing our experience we have been able to express the dynamic nature of knowledge translation and although it can be challenging, how worthwhile a part of research it can be.

Editorial Reflection

In this chapter, we have seen how researchers in the Caring Futures Institute's Healthy Ageing and Aged Care Area of Focus engaged in knowledge translation to develop and validate new quality of life instruments for economic evaluation and quality assessment in aged care. This is an example of where policy reform can be utilised if you have a long-term collaborative network of researchers and industry partners who have been working together to build a foundational evidence base. In Figure 6.2 we use the Knowledge Translation Complexity Network Model to illustrate the team's journey and how they engaged with their partners to move through the key knowledge translation processes.

Sarah Hunter, Michael Lawless, and Alison Kitson

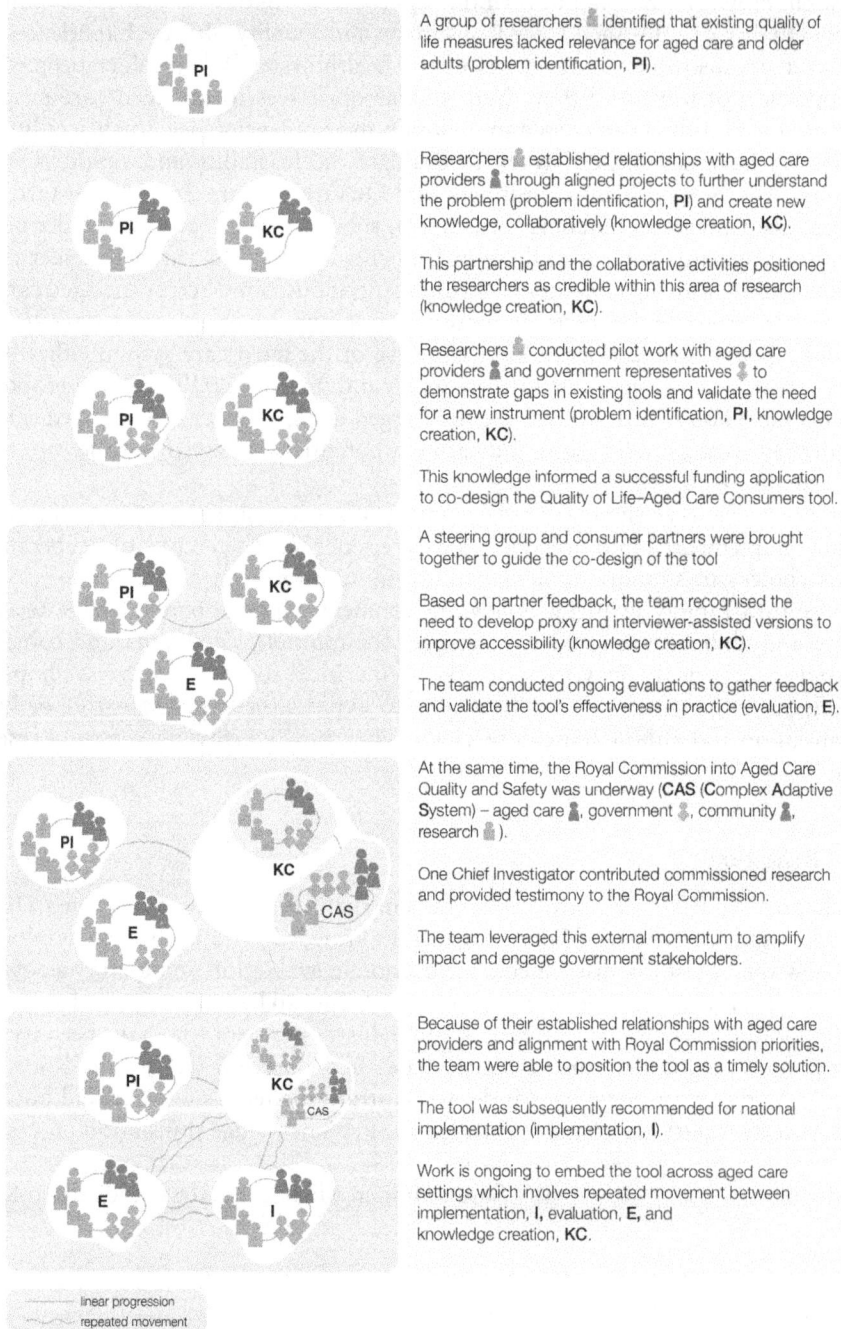

A group of researchers 👥 identified that existing quality of life measures lacked relevance for aged care and older adults (problem identification, **PI**).

Researchers 👥 established relationships with aged care providers 🧍 through aligned projects to further understand the problem (problem identification, **PI**) and create new knowledge, collaboratively (knowledge creation, **KC**).

This partnership and the collaborative activities positioned the researchers as credible within this area of research (knowledge creation, **KC**).

Researchers 👥 conducted pilot work with aged care providers 🧍 and government representatives 🧍 to demonstrate gaps in existing tools and validate the need for a new instrument (problem identification, **PI**, knowledge creation, **KC**).

This knowledge informed a successful funding application to co-design the Quality of Life–Aged Care Consumers tool.

A steering group and consumer partners were brought together to guide the co-design of the tool

Based on partner feedback, the team recognised the need to develop proxy and interviewer-assisted versions to improve accessibility (knowledge creation, **KC**).

The team conducted ongoing evaluations to gather feedback and validate the tool's effectiveness in practice (evaluation, **E**).

At the same time, the Royal Commission into Aged Care Quality and Safety was underway (**CAS** (Complex Adaptive System) – aged care 🧍, government 🧍, community 🧍, research 👥).

One Chief Investigator contributed commissioned research and provided testimony to the Royal Commission.

The team leveraged this external momentum to amplify impact and engage government stakeholders.

Because of their established relationships with aged care providers and alignment with Royal Commission priorities, the team were able to position the tool as a timely solution.

The tool was subsequently recommended for national implementation (implementation, **I**).

Work is ongoing to embed the tool across aged care settings which involves repeated movement between implementation, **I**, evaluation, **E**, and knowledge creation, **KC**.

———— linear progression
~~~~~~ repeated movement

Figure 6.2 Case study through the Knowledge Translation Complexity Network Model.
Source: https://doi.org/10.25451/flinders.29192777.v1

References

Australian Bureau of Statistics. (2022). *Cultural diversity of Australia*. Retrieved 16 August from www.abs.gov.au/articles/cultural-diversity-australia

Australian Government. (2021). *Aged care quality and safety*. Retrieved 1 April from www.roya lcommission.gov.au/aged-care

Australian Institute of Health and Welfare. (2020). *Interfaces between the aged care and health systems in Australia—movements between aged care and hospital 2016–17*. Retrieved 16 August from www.aihw.gov.au/reports/aged-care/movements-between-aged-care-and-hospital/contents/ summary

Australian Institute of Health and Welfare. (2024). *Older Australians*. Retrieved 16 August from www.aihw.gov.au/reports/older-people/older-australians/contents/population-groups-of-interest/ culturally-linguistically-diverse-people

Brazier, J., Ratcliffe, J., Saloman, J., & Tsuchiya, A. (2016). *Measuring and Valuing Health Benefits for Economic Evaluation* (2nd Edition). Oxford University Press. https://doi.org/10.1093/med/ 9780198725923.001.0001

Drummond, M. (2015). *Methods for the Economic Evaluation of Health Care Programmes* (4th Edition). Oxford University Press.

Hutchinson, C., Ratcliffe, J., Cleland, J., Walker, R., Milte, R., McBain, C., Corlis, M., Cornell, V., & Khadka, J. (2021). The integration of mixed methods data to develop the quality of life – aged care consumers (QOL-ACC) instrument. *BMC Geriatrics*, *21*(1), 702. https://doi.org/10.1186/ s12877-021-02614-y

Keetharuth, A. D., Taylor Buck, E., Acquadro, C., Conway, K., Connell, J., Barkham, M., Carlton, J., Ricketts, T., Barber, R., & Brazier, J. (2018). Integrating qualitative and quantitative data in the development of outcome measures: The case of the Recovering Quality of Life (ReQoL) Measures in mental health populations. *International Journal of Environmental Research Public Health*, *15*(7). https://doi.org/10.3390/ijerph15071342

Kitson, A., Brook, A., Harvey, G., Jordan, Z., Marshall, R., O'Shea, R., & Wilson, D. (2018). Using complexity and network concepts to inform healthcare knowledge translation. *International Journal of Health Policy and Management*, *7*(3), 231–243. https://doi.org/ 10.15171/ijhpm.2017.79

Milte, R., Ratcliffe, J., Chen, G., Lancsar, E., Miller, M., & Crotty, M. (2014). Cognitive overload? An exploration of the potential impact of cognitive functioning in discrete choice experiments with older people in health care. *Value in Health*, *17*(5), 655–659. https://doi.org/https://doi.org/ 10.1016/j.jval.2014.05.005

Ratcliffe, J., Lancsar, E., Flint, T., Kaambwa, B., Walker, R., Lewin, G., Luszcz, M., & Cameron, I. D. (2017). Does one size fit all? Assessing the preferences of older and younger people for attributes of quality of life. *Quality of Life Research*, *26*(2), 299–309. https://doi.org/10.1007/ s11136-016-1391-6

7 Case study

The iSupport for dementia program

Lily Xiao

Editorial introduction

Similar to Chapter 6, in this chapter, another team from the Caring Futures Institute provide a detailed case study of how they have undertaken integrated knowledge translation. Previous chapters (Chapters 1 and 4) provided detailed descriptions of integrated knowledge translation from a theoretical perspective and now we are illustrating how this can look in the real world. Along with Chapter 6, we hope this chapter illustrates that there is no "one size fits all" approach to doing integrated knowledge translation and all projects look different. We will use the Knowledge Translation Complexity Network Model (Kitson et al., 2018) at the end of this chapter to share our reflections on how this case study has undertaken integrated knowledge translation. But first, we again recap the Knowledge Translation Complexity Network Model, as introduced in prior chapters. The model integrates five key knowledge translation processes. These five processes are: Problem Identification, Knowledge Creation, Knowledge Synthesis, Implementation, and Evaluation. Figure 7.1 provides a visual representation of the model.

Sarah Hunter, Michael Lawless, and Alison Kitson

Introduction

In this chapter, I share my experience in leading two large research projects related to the iSupport for Dementia program, a skills training program for informal carers of people with dementia originally developed by the World Health Organization to support the Global Action Plan on the Public Health Response to Dementia (World Health Organization, 2021). The first project is entitled 'Creating partnership in iSupport program to optimise carers' impact on dementia care' and was funded by the 2020 Medical Research Future Fund Dementia Ageing and Aged Care Mission. This scheme was set up by the Australian Government under the auspices of the National Health and Medical Research Council to support implementation research focused on addressing gaps in access to high-quality care for older Australians from diverse and disadvantaged backgrounds. The second project is entitled 'Optimising support for Chinese carers of people with dementia by embedding iSupport in routine dementia care services in Australia and Greater China'. This project was funded by the 2020 and 2022 National Foundation for Australia-China Relations grants (two grants) and the 2022 Aged Care Research & Industry Innovation Australia grant.

Both projects began in 2020 and were ongoing at the time when this chapter was developed. Therefore, this chapter focuses on my team's understanding of knowledge

DOI: 10.4324/9781003245995-9

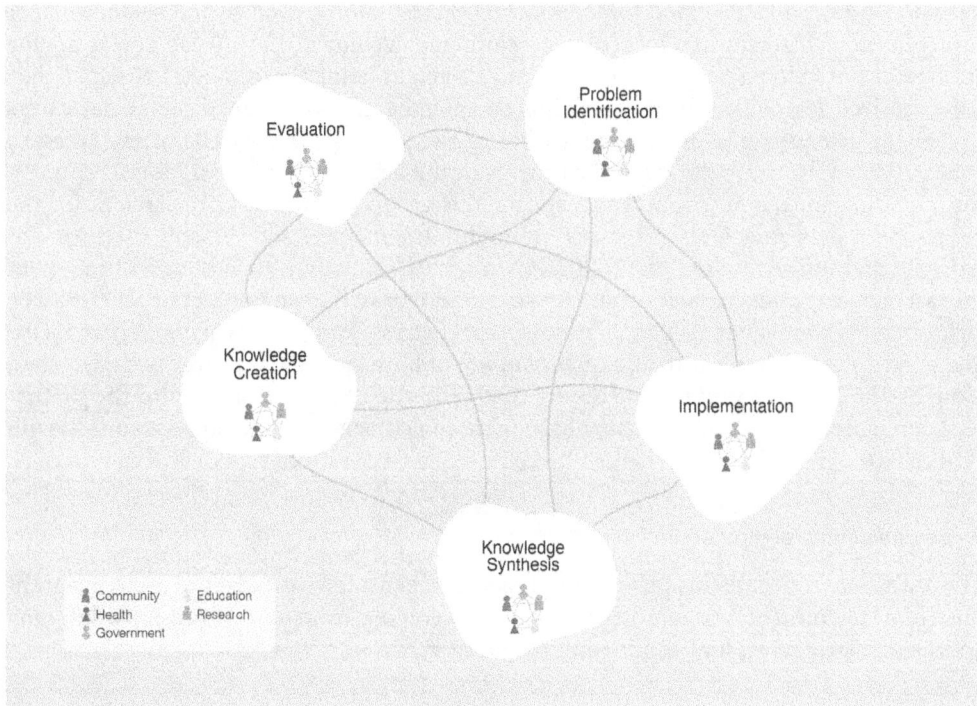

Figure 7.1 Knowledge Translation Complexity Network Model.
Source: https://doi.org/10.25451/flinders.29192585.v1

translation and shares our experiences of applying theory-informed knowledge translation and in facilitating industry-driven initiatives to embed the adapted iSupport program
into routine care services in Australia. We embrace the definition of knowledge translation
by the Canadian Institutes of Health Research described as 'Knowledge Translation is
defined as a dynamic and iterative process that includes synthesis, dissemination, exchange
and ethically-sound application of knowledge to improve the health of Canadians, provide more effective health services and products and strengthen the health care system'
(Canadian Institutes of Health Research, 2016). However, we also believe that knowledge creation through the engagement with the knowledge users across all study phases
of a project should be seen as part of knowledge translation. Therefore, we have begun
to embrace principles of integrated knowledge translation. Through this chapter, I will
unpack the non-linear, networked, and complex nature of integrated knowledge translation and how our plan ultimately changed throughout the project due to partners' engagement, the influence of contextual factors, and the unexpected challenges we encountered.

Project one: Creating partnership in iSupport program to optimise carers' impact on dementia care

The problem

In Australia, over 421,000 people live with dementia and two third of them live in the
community (Dementia Australia, 2024). The majority of people with dementia live in

their own homes and are cared for by informal carers (family, friends, and neighbours, or carers hereafter) (Australian Institute of Health and Welfare, 2024). While carers are the cornerstone of helping people with dementia remain at home for as long as possible, they have received less education preparation and limited support than professional carers to manage dementia and other complex health issues for people with dementia (Bressan et al., 2020). Carers are not viewed as clients in the health and aged care services; therefore, funding sources to support or care for this group is limited. Care services for the people with dementia after diagnosis are highly fragmented and difficult for carers to navigate and utilise (Steiner et al., 2020). Carers feel socially isolated due to time spent on care, stigma, and the lack of quality social networks (Greenwood et al., 2018). The lack of ability to manage dementia at home, carer stress, and distress are widely reported and contribute to poor health and quality of life of both carers and people with dementia (Stall et al., 2019), hospital admissions, emergency department uses and to the premature permanent admission to nursing home care of people with dementia (Cepoiu-Martin et al., 2016).

Preparation and pre-grant phase

The journey to translate this project into practice began a few years before receiving grant funding. This time before funding was spent leveraging existing relationships, building governance structures, and conducting preparatory work.

Leveraging existing relationships

The World Health Organization agreed to take action to achieve the goal stated as '75% of countries will provide support and training programmes for carers and families of people with dementia by 2025' (World Health Organization, 2021, p. 183). At the time, I served on the World Health Organization Expert Panel for development of their iSupport program (World Health Organization, 2019a). I was acutely aware of the gap in carer support services within the Australian context based on my long-term engagement with carers and care service providers in dementia research.

To maximise impact of the iSupport program within the Australian environment, I led a team to propose a 'Partnership in iSupport program' built on collaboration between dementia care service providers and informal carers of people with dementia in Australian hospital and community aged care settings.

Incorporating governance as a mechanism for engagement and impact

To build the collaboration, we followed an integrated knowledge translation approach, as described by Graham et al. (2018) which highlighted the importance of engaging knowledge users in the whole research process. Therefore, we wanted to engage knowledge users from the planning phase of grant application and in development of research questions. The ultimate knowledge users of the iSupport for Dementia program are carers of people with dementia. However, health and social care professionals who support people with dementia and their carers, are also knowledge users, as they deliver the iSupport program to carers in a complex health and aged care organisation and system.

To engage these knowledge users, we drew on co-design frameworks introduced by the World Health Organization (2019b) and Goeman et al. (2019) to develop a governance structure that engaged various knowledge users in the research. Following this approach, we developed a Steering Committee that included researchers and representatives of partner organisations. Additionally, we established a Reference Group consisting of representatives of carers, people with early stages of dementia, health and social care professionals, dementia care researchers or experts, policy makers or decision makers at an organisation level and a national level. Members in this group were selected for their knowledge and experiences to ensure they could advise on strategies to implement the iSupport program and provide feedback on core resources and guidelines for the Australian context.

Preparatory work

We engaged knowledge users in the preparation phase to discuss how to adapt and implement the iSupport program in an Australian social context before applying for the Medical Research Future Fund grants (Xiao et al., 2021). Through co-design with representatives of carers, and clinicians we identified the research questions and developed the research proposal. One of our partner sites was chosen to participate in a small-scale study focused on identifying feasibility and acceptability of implementation of the World Health Organization iSupport manual (Xiao, 2020). Insights gained from this work as well as through two systematic reviews by one of our PhD students, also contributed to the co-design of our grant applications. The systematic reviews increased our understanding of 1) the effectiveness of internet-based psychoeducation programs for carers of people with dementia (Yu, Xiao, Ullah, Meyer, Wang, Pot, & He, 2023); and 2) the experiences of carers of people with dementia in web-based psychoeducation programs (Yu, Xiao, Ullah, Meyer, Wang, Pot, & Shifaza, 2023). These systematic reviews informed the project team of the most effective way to implement the iSupport program to support carers.

Additionally, findings from this preparatory work informed refinement of our project proposal. We ended up outlining three interrelated phases of work to implement the iSupport program into routine care services. **Phase 1** focuses on co-designing with stakeholders to identify new services to be delivered by an iSupport program facilitator to enhance support for carers of people with dementia in the program. **Phase 2** comprises a randomised controlled trial to determine the intervention effectiveness, establish the intervention cost-effectiveness; and understand carers' experiences in the program. **Phase 3** aims to embed the 'Partnership in iSupport program' to routine services in the four participating organisations.

Based on our experiences in the project, we suggest that engagement with the knowledge users should be considered as a crucial element of integrated knowledge translation. Doing so, allows you to be aware of and address the influence of contextual factors in embedding and sustaining interventions in care services (Damschroder et al., 2022; Kitson et al., 2017). Below we explore the phases we have completed so far.

Phase 1

Knowledge creation and synthesis through the engagement with partners

Having employed some elements of the iSupport program in a small-scale study during the preparation phase, in phase 1 we progressed investigation of an implementation strategy for the iSupport program using a multi-method study design.

This design included a pre-workshop survey, workshops (or interviews) and post-workshop survey with stakeholders to identify and reach a consensus on activities to be delivered and strategies to be applied by the iSupport facilitators to achieve the expected innovation outcomes (Yu, Hunter, et al., 2023; Yu, Hunter, et al., 2024). Findings from this study generated new knowledge to better understand the role of an iSupport facilitator and enabled the project team to detail the pathway to achieve intervention outcomes in phase 2 and to develop a project implementation manual which included the iSupport facilitator's roles and responsibilities, a training program for the facilitators, and other aspects relating to project implementation in the real world. The project implementation manual to be tested in phase 2 will then be adapted in phase 3 to facilitate the knowledge translation process. From this work, we published a study protocol to guide the planned trial in phase 2 (Xiao, Yu, et al., 2022).

Phase 2

Understand your stakeholders and their needs

In phase 2, we invited two tertiary hospitals and two aged care organisations to participate in a randomised controlled trial to take part in the iSupport program (Xiao, Wang, et al., 2022). We also added a qualitative evaluation alongside the trial to understand partner perspectives of the enablers and barriers of implementing the iSupport program. The qualitative evaluation encompasses interviews with site leaders, facilitators, and carers. Findings from this part of study will also inform the project team of an iSupport implementation plan to enable scale-up of the iSupport program into other organisations.

To unpack the contextual factors that may impact implementation of the iSupport program, we used the Consolidated Framework for Implementation Research framework (Damschroder et al., 2022). This framework enabled us to structure the qualitative interview questions to determine:

- **Outer Setting factors**: the health and aged care policies, standards, and financing
- **Inner Setting factors**: the health and aged care organisation factors such as the governance structure, leadership, resources, staffing, culture
- **Individual**: the individual factors such as the characteristics of carers of people with dementia, carers' willingness and capability and capacity to support their peers, the characteristics of staff who work with carers of people with dementia, teamwork, networks, and relationships with their peers and with carers, and
- **Implementation Process**: the project factors comprising the study on the gap in supporting carers of people with dementia, the design of the iSupport program to address the gap, the co-design with stakeholders to implement the iSupport program, monitoring the contextual factors affecting the implementation and evaluating the effectiveness of the iSupport innovation and knowledge translation.

Knowledge created from phase 2, and the use of the Consolidated Framework for Implementation Research will inform phase 3 focused on scaling up implementation. We have commenced the planning for phase 3 which was involved comprehensive consultations with key partners.

Future work and sustainability

Enabler partners to take the lead

Throughout the project, what we have learned most is the importance of enabling industry partners to lead their initiatives in tailoring the iSupport program to suit their needs and fit it to their workflow. In other words, industry-driven initiatives will largely decide the adaptation and sustainability of the iSupport program. However, researchers in the project still need to work alongside industry partners by providing evidence of successful implementation in similar projects, training facilitators and staff to deliver the program, observing, and evaluating the process and outcomes.

In our original plan for phase 3 of the project, we demonstrated a straightforward approach to embed all intervention components according to a protocol in the iSupport program including:

1) Managing transitions for people with dementia
2) Managing dementia progression
3) Psychoeducation using the iSupport program
4) Care support group led by the iSupport facilitator
5) Feedback on services to improve dementia care services (Xiao, Yu, et al., 2022).

In the consultations we undertook to prepare for phase 3, our industry partners questioned the adaptability of the iSupport program into their routine services. They were not sure if the whole program would fit within their existing workflow, staffing level and resources. In addition, industry partners also questioned the feasibility of the research design that required the recruitment of a large sample size of carers of people with dementia in a relatively short period.

Our approach to resolving these unexpected challenges included a focused literature review to identify strategies used in other successful knowledge translation projects in the dementia caregiver research field such as the Resources for Enhancing Alzheimer's Caregiver Health II project (Berwig et al., 2017; Cho et al., 2019a, 2019b; Nichols et al., 2016). The Resources for Enhancing Alzheimer's Caregiver Health II program is an evidence-based carer support program originally developed in the long-term care environment in the United States of America, and has been successfully scaled up and sustained in routine care services in various care settings including community aged care (Cho et al., 2019b; Nichols et al., 2016), and hospital settings (Stevens et al., 2012). The adaptation involved co-design and consultations with knowledge translation experts and other stakeholders, the assessment of the contextual factors in the care settings and the rationale for tailoring the program for the care settings. The tailored program included, but was not limited to, changes to the intervention elements and the length of the intervention based on the carers' needs assessment and the organisation's capacity and capability to deliver the innovation. Through conducting this literature review, this enabled discussions with our industry partners about how to make the iSupport innovation adaptable and implementable.

We supplied the evidence-based strategies reported in the literature to the site leaders of our industry partners; this supported them in discussions with their staff to identify site-specific strategies to fit the iSupport program within their organisation's environment. We also reassured the industry partners of the flexibility for each organisation to undertake the program in their own way and that we would not impose a unified implementation protocol for the four organisations.

During this planning period for phase 3, the project team also approached knowledge translation experts to gain their advice on industry partner-led integrated knowledge translation, the research design to monitor and evaluate the processes and outcomes, education and training for staff involved in the knowledge translation, as well as adaptation and implementation strategies based on other successful projects within the Caring Futures Institute, Flinders University.

Although we are still working through the plan for the translation phase, our preliminary experience in this project's planning activities underscores the need for co-design, and engagement of all levels of staff in that co-design, due to the complexity, relationships, and networks existing in the whole process of knowledge translation. Our experiences in this project also support the need to facilitate an industry partner-driven integrated knowledge translation approach to tailor, adapt, scale up and sustain implementation in the real world.

Project two: Optimising support for Chinese carers of people with dementia by embedding iSupport in routine dementia care services in Australia and Greater China

The problem

It is estimated that over 11 million people live with dementia in greater China including Mainland China, Taiwan, Hong Kong and Macau, making up to 25% of the total population with dementia globally (Jia et al., 2020). This number is expected to triple by 2050, predicting increased demand for dementia care services and support for family carers (Alzheimer's Disease International, 2018). Furthermore, over 40 million family carers are involved in dementia care in these regions (Alzheimer's Disease Chinese, 2020; Taiwan Association of Family Caregivers, 2020). As caring for older people is viewed as the family's responsibility in Chinese filial piety culture, carers in these regions may be less likely to seek help outside their family. Therefore, they may experience more adverse impacts of caregiving on their health and wellbeing compared with those from Western cultures (World Health Organization, 2015). Dementia care services are also shaped by social and economic factors. The development of dementia care policies, guidelines, standards, and services in these regions varies (Wang et al., 2019; Xiao et al., 2014). Therefore, facilitating knowledge translation of the World Health Organization iSupport program in Greater China may be a strategy to address the disparities in supporting carers in Greater China.

Additionally, Australia is recognised for its pursuit of excellence in dementia care policies, resources, and care services. However, disparities in dementia care exist between the mainstream cultural group and those from culturally and linguistically diverse communities (Xiao et al., 2013; Xiao et al., 2016). Addressing these disparities is a priority in Australian Government dementia care policies (National Ageing Research Institute & National Health and Medical Research Council National Institute for Dementia Research, 2020). Chinese-Australians are one of the largest culturally and linguistically diverse groups and Chinese is the second most common language spoken at home in Australia (Australian Bureau of Statistics, 2021). The tailoring of the iSupport program is an opportunity to engage other culturally and linguistically diverse communities in Australia through the development of a "Culturally tailored iSupport model" of care (National Institute for Dementia Research, 2023).

Preparation phase

To address the lack of support for carers of people with dementia in greater China and the Chinese-Australian community, I am leading a large team across Australia and China in a four-phase project.

- **Phase 1** focuses on culturally adapting the iSupport program using a qualitative approach and partner consultations
- **Phase 2** determines the effectiveness and cost-effectiveness of a 'Tailored Chinese iSupport program' via a randomised controlled trial
- **Phase 3** embeds the iSupport program in routine care services of aged care and hospital care settings using a type 2 hybrid effectiveness-implementation randomised controlled trial (Curran et al., 2012)
- **Phase 4** aims to disseminate the evidence-based Chinese iSupport resources to carers of people with dementia using a mixed methods study.

Our industry partners in the project include Chinese-ethno-specific aged care organisations in Australia, primary care organisations, hospital memory clinics, and dementia and aged care organisations in Greater China. Researchers in the project team are from three universities and a research institute in Australia and nine universities in Great China.

Use of theoretical frameworks to inform study design and partner engagement

We have established a governance structure described by Goeman et al. (2019) to ensure partners' engagement in the project and we have applied the 'Ecological Validity Framework' described by Bernal and Domenech Rodríguez to ensure the culturally tailored iSupport program for Chinese carers (Bernal & Domenech Rodríguez, 2012). We have also applied the integrated knowledge translation framework described by Graham et al. (2018) to ensure that the experiences and experts of carers for people with dementia and frontline staff who care for them have been integrated into the research questions, study designs, findings, and recommendations. Furthermore, we have employed the Consolidated Framework for Implementation Research framework (Damschroder et al., 2022) to analyse qualitative data we previously collected via co-design workshops and interviews with key partners to identify enablers and barriers and possible solutions when embedding a Chines iSupport program into routine care services.

We have embraced integrated knowledge translation throughout the project by hosting regular webinars with partners and by establishing an iSupport community of practice. Already, we have hosted nine webinars, with project team members providing an interactive presentation on a relevant topic to the project. The webinars are provided in both English and Mandarin, and have attracted over 600 audience members who were health professionals, aged care workers, health professional students, researchers, and academics. We recorded the webinars and disseminated those recordings via Flinders University Caring Futures Institute website, our iSupport program website, and YouTube. The number of people who visited the Chinese iSupport website across the study site has reached 8,396 by 2024.

Phase 1

Knowledge creation through the engagement with partners

In this phase, we engaged representatives of Chinese-ethno-specific aged care organisations, Chinese-Australian carers of people with dementia and care workers who provide direct care for Chinese-Australians living with dementia to understand their perspectives on the cultural and linguistic appropriateness of a Chinese iSupport program. We also explored factors affecting the implementation of the Chinese iSupport program in Australia with these partners. In total, 18 Chinese-Australian carers and 17 care workers reviewed a translated Chinese iSupport manual, documented their comments and, through focus groups, elaborated on their comments relating to the manual. Findings informed our team of further revisions needed for the translated Chinese iSupport contents, the online Chinese iSupport program design and layout, the strategies to motivate and engage carers, care workers and Chinese-ethno-specific aged care organisations in the iSupport program. The findings also enabled the team to design a bilingual and bicultural iSupport facilitator-enabled peer support for carers. In addition, findings helped the research team to identify facilitator-enabled access to needs-based care services in the intervention.

The elements included in the 'Tailored Chinese iSupport program' comprise: 1) carers' self-directed learning using the Chinese iSupport manual online, e-book or hardcopy; 2) participation in a peer support group to overcome social isolation and exchange experiences in dementia care and 3) tailored assistance provided by the iSupport facilitator in accessing and utilising resources and services. More detailed findings from this study phase are available from our publication on this study phase (Che et al., 2024; Xiao et al., 2022).

Phase 2

Establishing effectiveness

We published a trial protocol (Xiao, Wang, et al., 2022) and a manuscript to report the effectiveness of the iSupport program (Xiao et al., 2024). In summary, we recruited 266 caregivers of people with dementia in the trial and 212 of them completed the 6-month intervention including 104 in the intervention group and 108 in the usual care group. Results indicated that the intervention group showed statistically improved 1) mental-health related quality of life, 2) Self-Efficacy for Controlling Upsetting Thoughts, and 3) carers' reactions to changed behaviours of people with dementia, compared to the usual care group. However, there were no statistically significant differences between the intervention group and the usual care group in: 1) physical-health related quality of life, 2) quality of life of people with dementia, 3) quality of social support, 4) self-efficacy for obtaining respite, 5) Self-Efficacy for Responding to Disruptive Patient Behaviours, and 6) the changed behaviours of people with dementia. Carers in the intervention group had positive experiences in sharing dementia care and supporting peers. The economic analysis to determine whether the intervention is cost-effective is in progress at the time of writing.

Phase 3

Implementation through knowledge creation, synthesis, and partner engagement

Following cultural adaptation of the iSupport program in phase 1, we undertook a systematic review to synthesise research evidence on Chinese caregivers' experiences in dementia care (Zhang et al., 2023). This review investigated system factors, organisation factors and individual factors, and the findings informed planning for the phase 3 trial.

In addition, we undertook a qualitative study to co-design implementation strategies with partners, using the RE-AIM framework (Glasgow et al., 2019). The RE-AIM framework includes five dimensions described as Reach, Effectiveness, Adoption, Implementation, and Maintenance and have been widely recognised as five indicators of a successful implementation project (Glasgow et al., 2019). We interpret each dimension as follows:

1) **Reach** means the representativeness of carers in the Chinese iSupport program
2) **Effectiveness** indicates the impact of iSupport on carers, people with dementia and frontline staff
3) **Adoption** refers to the number of sites that initiate the Chinese iSupport program after the trial within or outside the participating organisations
4) **Implementation** emphasizes the adherence to the study protocol by carers, frontline staff and facilitators
5) **Maintenance** underscores the sustainability of the Chinese iSupport program after the project.

The RE-AIM framework informed the semi-structured questions to better understand partners' thoughts and ideas about 1) factors affecting implementation and 2) to identify possible solutions. We also applied the RE-AIM framework to identify qualitative and quantitative data to collect to analyse the effectiveness of the Chinese iSupport program and the effectiveness of the implementation strategies we used. For example, for the 'Reach' indicator we would collect social-cultural demographic data of carers and their care recipients to assess whether the Chinese iSupport program was reaching those with various literacy level and digital literacy levels. Moreover, for the 'Effectiveness' indicator we would collect quantitative data to measure quality of life of carers and their care recipients, and qualitative data via interviews to understand the perceptions of carers, frontline staff, and facilitators on the effectiveness of implementation strategies.

Having been informed by the systematic review and the qualitative study, we proceeded to plan the type 2 hybrid effectiveness-implementation randomised controlled trial (Curran et al., 2012) to evaluate implementation and effectiveness of the Chinese iSupport program in routine care services. For this trial, participating organisations will include three ethno-specific aged care organisations in Australia, and hospital memory clinics and primary care organisations in mainland China. The trial will last 6 months with 158 carers of people with dementia who are clients of the participating organisations. Carers have been randomly assigned to either the 'Usual iSupport' group or 'Tailored iSupport' group with the ratio of 1:1. Carers in the 'Usual iSupport' group are guided by frontline staff in accessing the resources to perform self-directed learning. Carers in the 'Tailored iSupport' group are assigned to a trained iSupport facilitator and engage in the following activities: 1) individualised learning using iSupport, 2) peer support to overcome social isolation and 3) assistance to access and utilise resource and care services tailored to the needs of people with dementia and carers. Further details of the planned trial are in our published trial protocol (Xiao et al., 2025).

In this phase, we will support the leadership/management and iSupport facilitators to lead the implementation in their organisation to sustain the iSupport program beyond the life of the project. We will provide a train-the-trainer program for iSupport facilitators appointed by the industry partners. We also provide consultations for them during the implementation. We have developed the 'iSupport Facilitator Implementation Manual' (or a playbook) that includes principles, guidelines, case scenarios and resources for them to implement the iSupport innovation in their organisations' context. The project will enable the facilitators to develop leadership, knowledge, and skills to work with carers of people with dementia and staff in their organisation to implement the two intervention strategies and to train new facilitators to adopt the iSupport services in new sites. Our role as researchers in this phase is to observe the processes and outcomes of the knowledge translation.

Future work and sustainability

Have a clear plan

The Dissemination and Implementation framework clearly explains seven key action steps for successful knowledge dissemination (Patient-centered Outcomes Research Institute, 2015). Therefore, we consider this framework suitable for our planned phase 4 of the project which will be focused on dissemination of the Chinese iSupport.

Train the workforce, so that they can train others

Additionally, we have designed phase 4 of the project to publish and disseminate iSupport multimedia resources to partners. This is informed by our stakeholder consultations on the implementation of the Chinese iSupport program in phase 1 (Xiao et al., 2022) and a study we undertook to assess carers' needs when scaling up the iSupport program in Australia and China (Yu, Xiao, et al., 2024). We have already published a web-based iSupport program, iSupport e-book, iSupport audiobooks, iSupport lite posters and iSupport lite videos. These resources consider the various literacy and digital literacy levels and other circumstances that prevent carers from using a single format of the iSupport manual. For example, the 'lite' versions are simplified and shorter versions of the resources. We have also designed a four-session train-the-trainer program to train 20 expert trainers across 10 study sites and ongoing support to enable them to co-design dissemination plans with identified health and aged care organisations and stakeholders via their networks. Moreover, these expert trainers will train more iSupport trainers nominated by dementia and aged care organisations, hospital memory clinics, geriatric wards and primary care organisations and support them to develop their action plan to disseminate the iSupport multimedia resources to carers of people with dementia and staff involved in dementia care.

We have also established a Chinese iSupport community of practice which includes iSupport facilitators, iSupport project team members, researchers, and partners who are interested in the project. For example, health professional students, health and social care professionals, informal carers of people with dementia. We have organised monthly community of practice webinars over the four-month implementation period during phase 3 to enable people involved in the Chinese iSupport multimedia resources dissemination to share their experiences and support each other. So far, our community of practice webinars have attracted over 200 participants. We will publish the recorded webinars on our websites across all study sites to further disseminate the evidence-based Chinese iSupport resources.

Partnering to sustain the Chinese iSupport program in the aged care system

We recognise that the most challenging aspect in this project is to identify funding sources to sustain the Chinese iSupport program in the aged care and health care systems. Currently, there is no funding source to support aged care organisations in Australia and health care organisations in China to deliver the Chinese iSupport program to carers of people with dementia.

In Australia, our partnership with the three Chinese ethno-specific aged care organisations enables the identification of the "Carer Gateway" as a platform to integrate the Chinese iSupport program into the aged care system. The Carer Gateway is funded by the Department of Health and Ageing, Australian Government and provide free services and support for carers from all groups and all care areas (Department of Health and Ageing & Australian Government, 2023). Services and support include: 1) peer support groups; 2) tailored support for carers to access and utilise care services; 3) counselling services; 4) coaching for carers to improve their capability in their carer's role; 5) skills courses for carers to undertake their carer's role; and 6) access to emergency respite.

We have been supporting our industry partners to contact and negotiate with key informants at the Carer Gateway who are knowledgeable about policies and procedures to apply for contracts with the Carer Gateway. Our role in this crucial part of knowledge translation includes the provision of written report on the evidence-based Chinese iSupport program with recommendations on how to fit the program within the Carer Gateway environment. In addition, we also have a responsibility to work with industry partners to estimate the cost on the services and the ongoing education and consultation support for the Chinese iSupport facilitators to deliver high-quality services to carers.

Conclusion

Based on our experiences in undertaking the two projects presented in this case study chapter, we suggest that every researcher needs to develop a knowledge translation plan within their projects to optimise the positive research impact on the population we care for, the health and aged care workforce and the health and social care systems. Our experiences support that knowledge translation needs to be built on a co-design approach to enable authentic partnership and engagement with partners throughout the project. Researchers will need to build adequate budget to support partner engagement in their projects. Moreover, knowledge translation is theory informed and evidence-based practice. Therefore, researchers will need to learn and interact with knowledge translation experts and demonstrate capability to critique and select relevant theories to inform their knowledge translation practice. They also have an obligation to contribute to the knowledge creation or theory development in the knowledge translation research field.

Editorial Reflection

In this chapter, we have seen how researchers in the Caring Futures Institute's Healthy Ageing and Aged Care Area of Focus engaged in knowledge translation processes to implement a program to support informal carers of people with dementia (iSupport) into routine care services in Australia. This is an example of how utilising international evidence-based programs developed by peak and credible bodies such as the World Health Organization can be effective to focus efforts on understanding the problem at a local level and influencing interest at a local level to optimise implementation efforts. In Figure 7.2 we use the Knowledge Translation Complexity Network Model to illustrate the team's journey and how they engaged with their partners to move through the key knowledge translation processes.

Sarah Hunter, Michael Lawless, and Alison Kitson

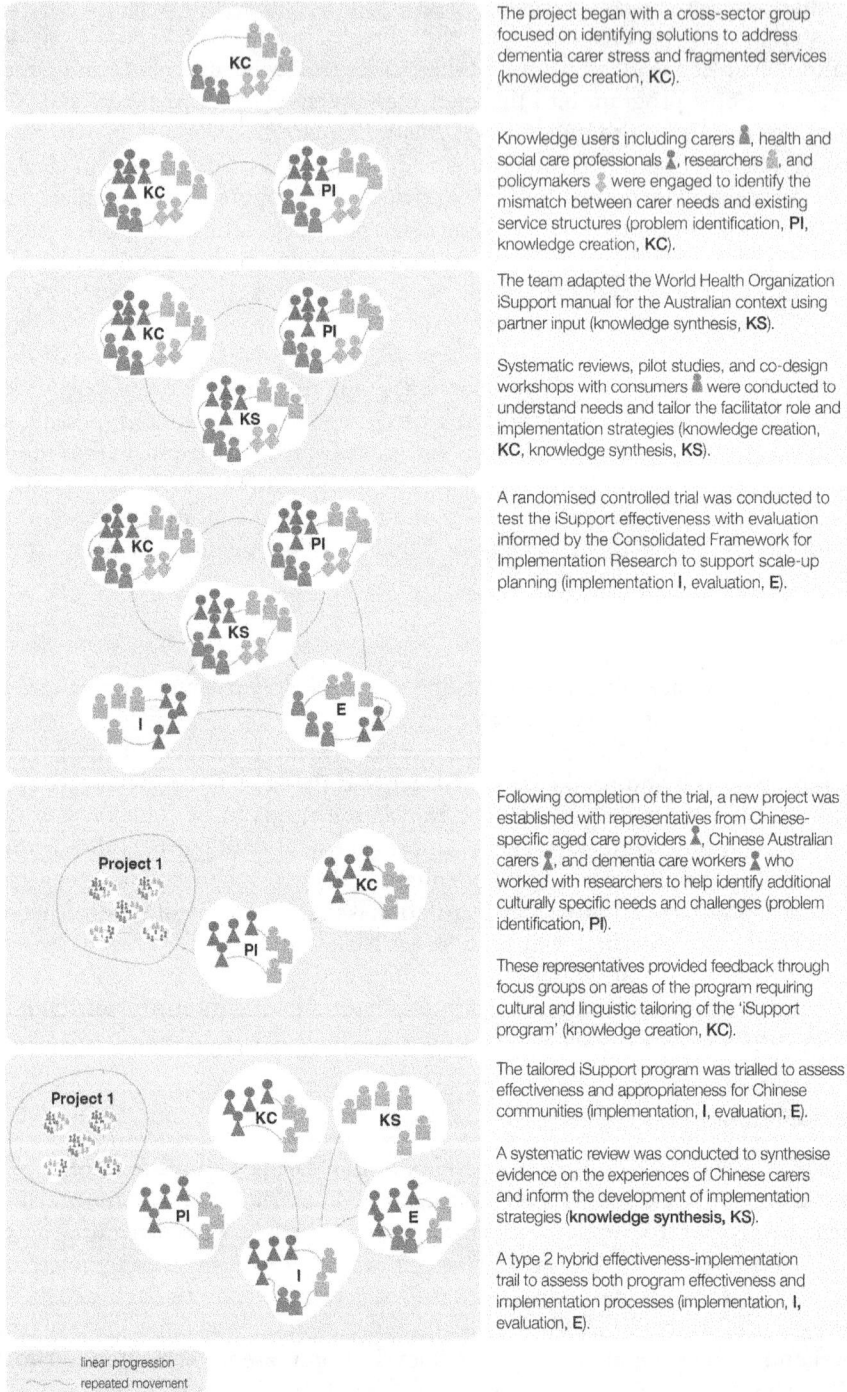

The project began with a cross-sector group focused on identifying solutions to address dementia carer stress and fragmented services (knowledge creation, **KC**).

Knowledge users including carers, health and social care professionals, researchers, and policymakers were engaged to identify the mismatch between carer needs and existing service structures (problem identification, **PI**, knowledge creation, **KC**).

The team adapted the World Health Organization iSupport manual for the Australian context using partner input (knowledge synthesis, **KS**).

Systematic reviews, pilot studies, and co-design workshops with consumers were conducted to understand needs and tailor the facilitator role and implementation strategies (knowledge creation, **KC**, knowledge synthesis, **KS**).

A randomised controlled trial was conducted to test the iSupport effectiveness with evaluation informed by the Consolidated Framework for Implementation Research to support scale-up planning (implementation **I**, evaluation, **E**).

Following completion of the trial, a new project was established with representatives from Chinese-specific aged care providers, Chinese Australian carers, and dementia care workers who worked with researchers to help identify additional culturally specific needs and challenges (problem identification, **PI**).

These representatives provided feedback through focus groups on areas of the program requiring cultural and linguistic tailoring of the 'iSupport program' (knowledge creation, **KC**).

The tailored iSupport program was trialled to assess effectiveness and appropriateness for Chinese communities (implementation, **I**, evaluation, **E**).

A systematic review was conducted to synthesise evidence on the experiences of Chinese carers and inform the development of implementation strategies (**knowledge synthesis, KS**).

A type 2 hybrid effectiveness-implementation trail to assess both program effectiveness and implementation processes (implementation, **I**, evaluation, **E**).

Figure 7.2 Case study through the Knowledge Translation Complexity Network Model.
Source: https://doi.org/10.25451/flinders.29192786.v1

References

Alzheimer's Disease Chinese. (2020). *Chinese Family Caregiver*. Retrieved 12 July 2024, from www.adc.org.cn/

Alzheimer's Disease International. (2018). *World Alzheimer Report 2018. The state of the art of dementia research: New frontiers*. www.alzint.org/resource/world-alzheimer-report-2018/

Australian Bureau of Statistics. (2021). *Cultural diversity: Census*. www.abs.gov.au/statistics/peo ple/people-and-communities/cultural-diversity-census/latest-release

Australian Institute of Health and Welfare. (2024). *Dementia in Australia*. AIHW. www.aihw.gov. au/reports/dementia/dementia-in-aus/contents/summary

Bernal, G., & Domenech Rodríguez, M. M. (2012). *Cultural adaptations: Tools for evidence-based practice with diverse populations*. American Psychological Association. https://doi.org/10.1037/ 13752-000

Berwig, M., Heinrich, S., Spahlholz, J., Hallensleben, N., Brahler, E., & Gertz, H. J. (2017). Individualized support for informal caregivers of people with dementia-effectiveness of the German adaptation of REACH II. *BMC Geriatrics, 17*(286) https://doi.org/10.1186/s12 877-017-0678-y

Bressan, V., Visintini, C., & Palese, A. (2020). What do family caregivers of people with dementia need? *Health & Social Care in the Community, 28*(6), 1942–1960. https://doi.org/10.1111/ hsc.13048

Canadian Institutes of Health Research. (2016). *Knowledge translation: Definition*. Canadian Institutes of Health Research. Retrieved 22 August 2022 from https://cihr-irsc.gc.ca/e/29418. html#1

Cepoiu-Martin, M., Tam-Tham, H., Patten, S., Maxwell, C. J., & Hogan, D. B. (2016). Predictors of long-term care placement in persons with dementia. *International Journal of Geriatric Psychiatry, 31*(11), 1151–1171. https://doi.org/doi:10.1002/gps.4449

Che, S. L., Wu, J., Lei, W. I., Xiao, L. D., & Zhu, M. (2024). Perspectives on dementia care self-learning platform: A focus group study of family and professional caregivers. *Geriatric Nursing, 58*, 282–289. https://doi.org/https://doi.org/10.1016/j.gerinurse.2024.05.027

Cho, J., Luk-Jones, S., Smith, D. R., & Stevens, A. B. (2019a). Erratum to: Evaluation of REACH-TX: A community-based approach to the REACH II intervention. *Innovation in aging, 3*(3), igz041. https://doi.org/10.1093/geroni/igz041

Cho, J., Luk-Jones, S., Smith, D. R., & Stevens, A. B. (2019b). Evaluation of REACH-TX: A community-based approach to the REACH II Intervention. *Innovation in Aging, 3*(3), igz022. https://doi.org/10.1093/geroni/igz022

Curran, G. M., Bauer, M., Mittman, B., Pyne, J. M., & Stetler, C. (2012). Effectiveness-implementation hybrid designs: Combining elements of clinical effectiveness and implementation research to enhance public health impact. *Medical Care, 50*(3), 217–226. https://doi.org/ 10.1097/MLR.0b013e3182408812

Damschroder, L. J., Reardon, C. M., Widerquist, M. A. O., & Lowery, J. (2022). The updated consolidated framework for implementation research based on user feedback. *Implementation Science: IS, 17*(1), 1–75. https://doi.org/10.1186/s13012-022-01245-0

Dementia Australia. (2024). *Dementia facts and figures*. Dementia Australia. www.dementia.org. au/about-dementia/dementia-facts-and-figures?utm_campaign=&utm_source=google&utm_ medium=search&gad_source=1&gclid=Cj0KCQjw2uiwBhCXARIsACMvIU2A6zJg0YVBoG Aku-4uF123n1T7Ltm8p0eVDlaT27EumvwZ6E2v2xoaAjoyEALw_wcB

Department of Health and Ageing, & Australian Government. (2023). *Carer Gateway*. Department of Health and Ageing. Retrieved 28 August 2023 from www.carergateway.gov.au/

Glasgow, R. E., Harden, S. M., Gaglio, B., Rabin, B., Smith, M. L., Porter, G. C., Ory, M. G., & Estabrooks, P. A. (2019). RE-AIM planning and evaluation framework: Adapting to new science and practice with a 20-Year review. *Frontiers in Public Health, 7*, 64–64. https://doi.org/ 10.3389/fpubh.2019.00064

Goeman, D. P., Corlis, M., Swaffer, K., Jenner, V., Thompson, J. F., Renehan, E., & Koch, S. (2019). Partnering with people with dementia and their care partners, aged care service experts, policymakers and academics: A co-design process. *Australasian Journal on Ageing, 38*(2), 53–58. https://doi.org/10.1111/ajag.12635

Graham, I. D., Kothari, A., McCutcheon, C., & Integrated Knowledge, T. (2018). Moving knowledge into action for more effective practice, programmes and policy: Protocol for a research programme on integrated knowledge translation. *Implementation Science, 13.* https://doi.org/10.1186/s13012-017-0700-y

Greenwood, N., Mezey, G., & Smith, R. (2018). Social exclusion in adult informal carers. *Maturitas, 112,* 39–45. https://doi.org/10.1016/j.maturitas.2018.03.011

Jia, L., Quan, M., Fu, Y., Zhao, T., Li, Y., Wei, C., Tang, Y., Qin, Q., Wang, F., Qiao, Y., Shi, S., Wang, Y.-J., Du, Y., Zhang, J., Zhang, J., Luo, B., Qu, Q., Zhou, C., Gauthier, S., & Jia, J. (2020). Dementia in China: Epidemiology, clinical management, and research advances. *The Lancet Neurology, 19*(1), 81–92. https://doi.org/10.1016/S1474-4422(19)30290-X

Kitson, A., Brook, A., Harvey, G., Jordan, Z., Marshall, R., O'Shea, R., & Wilson, D. (2017). Using complexity and network concepts to inform healthcare knowledge translation. *International Journal of Health Policy and Management, 7*(3), 231–243. https://doi.org/10.15171/ijhpm.2017.79

Kitson, A., Brook, A., Harvey, G., Jordan, Z., Marshall, R., O'Shea, R., & Wilson, D. (2018). Using complexity and network concepts to inform healthcare knowledge translation. *International Journal of Health Policy and Management, 7*(3), 231–243. https://doi.org/10.15171/ijhpm.2017.79

National Ageing Research Institute, & National Health and Medical Research Council National Institute for Dementia Research. (2020). *Culturally and Linguistically Diverse (CALD) Dementia Research Action Plan.* National Ageing Research Institute.

National Institute for Dementia Research. (2023, 10th July 2023). *$3.5 million in targeted research funding to improve dementia care in culturally diverse communities.* National Institute for Dementia Research.

Nichols, L. O., Martindale-Adams, J., Burns, R., Zuber, J., & Graney, M. J. (2016). REACH VA: Moving from translation to system implementation. *The Gerontologist, 56*(1), 135–144. https://doi.org/10.1093/geront/gnu112

Patient-centered Outcomes Research Institute. (2015). *Implementation and Dissemination Toolkit.* Retrieved 10 July 2023 from www.pcori.org/sites/default/files/PCORI-DI-Toolkit-February-2015.pdf

Stall, N. M., Kim, S. J., Hardacre, K. A., Shah, P. S., Straus, S. E., Bronskill, S. E., Lix, L. M., Bell, C. M., & Rochon, P. A. (2019). Association of informal caregiver distress with health outcomes of community-dwelling dementia care recipients. *Journal of the American Geriatrics Society, 67*(3), 609–617. https://doi.org/10.1111/jgs.15690

Steiner, G. Z., Ee, C., Dubois, S., MacMillan, F., George, E. S., McBride, K. A., Karamacoska, D., McDonald, K., Harley, A., Abramov, G., Andrews-Marney, E. R., Cave, A. E., & Hohenberg, M. I. (2020). We need a one-stop-shop. *BMC Geriatrics, 20*(1), 49. https://doi.org/10.1186/s12877-019-1410-x

Stevens, A. B., Smith, E. R., Trickett, L. R. A., & McGhee, R. (2012). Implementing an evidence-based caregiver intervention within an integrated healthcare system. *Translational Behavioral Medicine, 2*(2), 218–227. https://doi.org/10.1007/s13142-012-0132-9

Taiwan Association of Family Caregivers. (2020). *Caregivers in Taiwan.* Taiwan Association of Family Caregivers. Retrieved 1 August 2020 from www.familycare.org.tw

Wang, J., Xiao, L. D., & Li, X. (2019). Health professionals' perceptions of developing dementia services in primary care settings in China: A qualitative study. *Aging & Mental Health, 23*(4), 447–454. https://doi.org/10.1080/13607863.2018.1426717

World Health Organization. (2015). *China country assessment report on ageing and health.* World Health Organization.

World Health Organization. (2019a). *iSupport for Dementia*. World Health Organization. Retrieved 21 March 2025 from www.who.int/publications/i/item/9789241515863

World Health Organization. (2019b). *iSupport for Dementia: Training and support manual for carers of people with dementia*. World Health Organization. www.who.int/publications/i/item/9789241515863

World Health Organization. (2021). *Global status report on the public health response to dementia*. World Health Organization. Retrieved 27 October from www.who.int/publications/i/item/9789240033245

Xiao, L. (2020). Adapting iSupport for Australian carers. *Australian Journal of Dementia Care, 8*(6), 12–13.

Xiao, L., Cheng, A., Xie, C., Chiu, K., Yu, Y., Ullah, S., Wang, J., Hu, R., Xu, D., Pan, X., & Zhang, A. R. Y. (2025). Evaluating an evidence-based iSupport for Dementia programme in routine care services: Study protocol for a hybrid type II trial. *BMJ Open, 15*(2), e086667. https://doi.org/10.1136/bmjopen-2024-086667

Xiao, L., De Bellis, A., Habel, L., & Kyriazopoulos, H. (2013). The experiences of culturally and linguistically diverse family caregivers in utilising dementia services in Australia. *BMC Health Services Research, 13*(427) https://doi.org/10.1186/1472-6963-13-427

Xiao, L., De Bellis, A., Kyriazopoulos, H., Draper, B., & Ullah, S. (2016). The effect of a personalized dementia care intervention for caregivers from Australian minority groups. *American Journal of Alzheimer's Disease and other Dementias, 31*(1), 57–67. https://doi.org/10.1177/1533317515578256

Xiao, L., McKechnie, S., Jeffers, L., De Bellis, A., Beattie, E., Low, L.-F., Draper, B., Messent, P., & Pot, A. M. (2021). Stakeholders' perspectives on adapting the World Health Organization iSupport for Dementia in Australia. *Dementia, 20*(5), 1536–1552. https://doi.org/10.1177/1471301220954675

Xiao, L., Ullah, S., Rujun, H. U., Wang, J., Wang, H., Chang, C.-C., Kwok, T., Zhu, M., Ratcliffe, J., Brodaty, H., Brijnath, B., Chang, H.-C., Wong, B., Zhou, Y., Jinjie, H. E., Xia, M., Hong, J.-Y., Che, S., & Milte, R. (2024). The effects of a facilitator-enabled online multicomponent iSupport for dementia program: A multicentre randomised controlled trial. *International Journal of Nursing Studies*, 104868. https://doi.org/https://doi.org/10.1016/j.ijnurstu.2024.104868

Xiao, L., Wang, J., He, G.-P., DeBellis, A., Verbeeck, J., & Kyriazopoulos, H. (2014). Family caregiver challenges in dementia care in Australia and China: A critical perspective. *BMC Geriatrics, 14*(6) https://doi.org/doi: 10.1186/1471-2318-14-6

Xiao, L., Wang, J., Ratcliffe, J., Ullah, S., Brodaty, H., Brijnath, B., Chang, H. C., Wang, H., Chang, C. C., Kwok, T., & Zhu, M. (2022). A nurse-led multicentre randomized controlled trial on effectiveness and cost-effectiveness of Chinese iSupport for dementia program: A study protocol. *Journal of Advanced Nursing, 78*(5), 1524–1533. https://doi.org/10.1111/jan.15216

Xiao, L., Ye, M., Zhou, Y., Chang, H.-C., Brodaty, H., Ratcliffe, J., Brijnath, B., & Ullah, S. (2022). Cultural adaptation of World Health Organization iSupport for Dementia program for Chinese-Australian caregivers. *Dementia (London, England), 21*(6), 2035–2052. https://doi.org/10.1177/14713012221110003

Xiao, L., Yu, Y., Ratcliffe, J., Milte, R., Meyer, C., Chapman, M., Chen, L., Ullah, S., Kitson, A., De Andrade, A. Q., Beattie, E., Brodaty, H., McKechnie, S., Low, L.-F., Nguyen, T. A., Whitehead, C., Brijnath, B., Sinclair, R., & Voss, D. (2022). Creating 'Partnership in iSupport program' to optimise family carers' impact on dementia care: A randomised controlled trial protocol. *BMC Health Services Research, 22*(1), 762. https://doi.org/10.1186/s12913-022-08148-2

Yu, Y., Hunter, S. C., Xiao, L., Meyer, C., Chapman, M., Tan, K. P., Chen, L., McKechnie, S., Ratcliffe, J., Ullah, S., Kitson, A., Andrade, A. Q., & Whitehead, C. (2023). Exploring the role of a facilitator in supporting family carers when embedding the iSupport for Dementia programme in care services: A qualitative study. *Journal of Clinical Nursing, 32*, 7358–7371. https://doi.org/10.1111/jocn.16836

Yu, Y., Hunter, S. C., Xiao, L., Meyer, C., Chapman, M., Tan, K. P., Chen, L., McKechnie, S., Ratcliffe, J., Ullah, S., Kitson, A., Andrade, A. Q., Whitehead, C., & Bierer, P. (2025). Stakeholder's consensus on activities to be delivered by the facilitators in a planned iSupport program in Australia: A mixed-methods study. *Geriatric Nursing, 64,* 103412. https://doi.org/10.1016/j.gerinurse.2025.103412

Yu, Y., Xiao, L., Cheng, A., Wang, I., Chiu, K., Chan, E., Xie, C., Zhou, Y., Zhuang, Z., & Wang, J. (2024). Chinese-Australian carers' perceived needs and preferences in planning to embed an iSupport for Dementia program in aged care services. *Australasian Journal on Ageing, 43*(3), 512-22. https://doi.org/10.1111/ajag.13287

Yu, Y., Xiao, L., Ullah, S., Meyer, C., Wang, J., Pot, A. M., & He, J. J. (2023). The effectiveness of internet-based psychoeducation programs for caregivers of people living with dementia: A systematic review and meta-analysis. *Aging Ment Health, 27*(10), 1895–1911. https://doi.org/10.1080/13607863.2023.2190082

Yu, Y., Xiao, L., Ullah, S., Meyer, C., Wang, J., Pot, A. M., & Shifaza, F. (2023). The experiences of informal caregivers of people with Dementia in Web-Based Psychoeducation Programs: Systematic review and metasynthesis. *JMIR Aging, 6.* https://doi.org/10.2196/47152

Zhang, Y., Xiao, L., & Wang, J. (2023). Chinese diaspora caregivers' experiences in dementia care in high-income countries: A systematic review. *Dementia (London, England), 22*(5), 1115–1137. https://doi.org/10.1177/14713012231169830

8   Getting started with integrated knowledge translation

Michael Lawless, Alison Kitson, Sarah Hunter and Tiffany Conroy

Introduction

This chapter offers a practical guide to getting started with integrated knowledge translation, drawing on the Knowledge Translation Complexity Network Model (Kitson et al., 2018). We have talked about this model in detail in Chapter 4.

The ideas shared in this chapter came from our own experiences of doing integrated knowledge translation. These projects had us working across different disciplines and partnering with people and teams within various organisations, states, and countries, all the while managing multiple knowledge translation processes at once. We had to bring together knowledge from systematic reviews, lived experience, professional practice, and various academic disciplines. Most of us were launched rather unexpectedly into the world of knowledge translation. We had to figure it out as we went along, learning on the job with guidance and support from those who have gone before us. Along the way, our mentors and colleagues helped us reflect on what we were doing and learning. It was through thinking about our experiences and plans through the lens of different theories, models, and frameworks that our thinking about knowledge translation really began to take shape.

Many of us were first introduced to knowledge translation through our involvement in implementation projects or by working in partnership with practitioners, community members, and policymakers to co-design solutions. Along the way, we came across challenges related to managing different expectations, priorities, and contextual factors. Over time, and through discussions with colleagues from different disciplines navigating similar challenges, we realised that concepts from complexity and network science, encapsulated in the Knowledge Translation Complexity Network Model, might help us make better sense of these processes and relationships. They offered a new lens to structure our work – not just for planning forward, but also for looking back to reflect on what worked, what didn't, and what we could do differently next time. At the same time, we came to see that the Knowledge Translation Complexity Network Model can be challenging to understand and apply in practice, even for those already familiar with knowledge translation.

Integrated knowledge translation core elements

To make things simpler, we carried out our own knowledge synthesis. Our goal in doing this was to distil the basic ideas or **Core Elements** of knowledge translation. These are the elements that researchers and their teams can use as a sense-check to make sure the

DOI: 10.4324/9781003245995-10

Table 8.1 Core elements, their definitions, and alignment with knowledge translation concepts

Core element	Definition	How it aligns with knowledge translation concepts
Connect	'Connect' in knowledge translation is about navigating and facilitating relationships across different people, groups, organisations, and disciplines. It involves engaging people early and throughout different knowledge translation processes, facilitating ongoing dialogue, and bringing together diverse perspectives. Integrating these varied perspectives helps create strong networks and deepens our understanding of contextual factors, so that knowledge can move more effectively through systems to make a timely impact.	Recipients, Facilitation, Leadership (i-PARIHS), Opinion leaders/change agents, champions, implementation leads, Leadership engagement, commitment, involvement, accountability (CFIR), Collective action, reflexive monitoring (NPT), Build trust and shared vision (SAR)
Clarify	'Clarify' means ensuring that focus, goals, key messages, and rationale of a knowledge translation project are clear and understood by everyone involved, according to their role and context. It involves bringing together different types of knowledge, such as research evidence, lived experience, and practice-based viewpoints, to build a shared understanding that continually guides the direction of the work. By making sure everyone is on the same page, clarifying activities help frame shared goals and collaborative processes in a way that is understood and relevant to all involved.	Innovation (i-PARIHS), Intervention characteristics (CFIR), Implementation object, Evidence (CICI), Coherence, Cognitive Participation (NPT)
Customise	'Customise' means adapting knowledge translation approaches to fit the specific needs, contextual barriers and enablers, and priorities of the different parties involved. This could involve adapting intervention components or implementation strategies to fit with the constraints of a particular practice setting. It could also involve using plain language, visual aids, or digital tools, and tailoring strategies to suit local conditions, cultural norms, organisational culture, and available resources. Customising helps ensure that the knowledge being shared, created, or implemented is feasible, relevant, accessible, and equitable, with ongoing feedback loops allowing for adjustments as needed.	Context (i-PARIHS, CICI), Compatibility (CFIR), Inner and outer context/setting (CICI, NASSS, CFIR), Wider system (political, policy, regulatory, professional, socio-cultural), Organisational capacity/readiness (NASSS), Organisational commitment (CFIR), Culture (i-PARIHS), Policy (BCW)

Core element	Definition	How it algins with knowledge translation concepts
Co-create	'Co-create' involves working closely with people, teams, and organisations to share knowledge and and develop solutions together. It focuses on ensuring partnership and developing capacity for integrating contributions from diverse partners at every step, from creating tools and interventions to co-designing implementation and evaluation strategies. It encourages continuous learning and adaptation, with participants' feedback helping to shape and refine outcomes. 'Co-create' fosters shared ownership, leading to solutions that are more effective and sustainable because they are developed with input and commitment from all involved.	Implementation drivers/strategies [i-PARIHS, CFIR, NIRN], Establish imperative [SAR], Tension for Change [CICI], Incentives and rewards [CFIR], Competency drivers, Leadership drivers, Organisation drivers [NIRN], Sustainability, embedding, and adaptation over time [MRE, NASSS, MAY, CICI]
Confirm	'Confirm' is about using systematic methods to make sure that knowledge translation efforts lead to meaningful and measurable change. It involves embedding evaluation throughout different knowledge translation processes to see how well things worked and where things could be improved in the future. This includes assessing aspects like clinical outcomes, feasibility, acceptability, implementation processes, scalability, and cost-effectiveness, as well as considerations like equity and sustainability. Teams can use this information to make more informed decisions about how best to move forward. 'Confirm' supports accountability, guides evidence-informed decision-making, and helps foster continuous learning.	Intervention characteristics (e.g., innovation, stakeholder perceptions, strength and quality of evidence, relative advantage, trialability, adaptability, compatibility, complexity, cost) [i-PARIHS, CFIR], Context [i-PARIHS, CICI], Implementation outcomes (e.g., fidelity, uptake, acceptability, penetration, cost) [CICI], Spread, scale up [NASSS]

Note. BCW: Behaviour Change Wheel (Michie, van Stralen et al. 2011); CICI: Context and Implementation of Complex Interventions framework (Pfadenhauer, Gerhardus et al. 2017); CFIR: Consolidated Framework for Implementation Research (Damschroder, Reardon et al. 2022); i-PARIHS: integrated-Promoting Action on Research in Health Services (Harvey and Kitson 2016); MAY: Implementation, Context and Complexity framework (May, Johnson et al. 2016); MRE: Definition of Sustainability (Moore, Mascarenhas et al. 2017); NASSS: Non-adoption, Abandonment, Scale-up, Spread and Sustainability of Health and Care Technologies (Greenhalgh, Wherton et al. 2018); NIRN: National Implementation Research Network (Bertram, Blase et al. 2015); NPT: Normalisation Process Theory (May, Mair et al. 2009); SAR: Model of Implementation Strategy design (Sarkies, Bowles et al. 2017).

key ingredients of an integrated knowledge translation approach are being considered. We came up with these elements by identifying and extracting common constructs from widely used knowledge translation theories, models, and frameworks (Chapter 4), comparing these constructs, and then synthesising them to form higher-order categories. From there, we grouped and refined these constructs into five core elements: **Connect, Clarify, Customise, Co-create,** and **Confirm.**

To validate these elements, we applied them retrospectively to the case studies featured in this book, asking ourselves what kinds of questions research teams might use to guide their decision-making. Table 8.1 introduces the core elements, along with a short definition and how they align with concepts from some widely used knowledge translation theories, models, and frameworks.

The five core elements can be used as simple rules of thumb to help guide individuals and teams to do knowledge translation in a more purposeful and integrated way. They are not meant to replace established theories, models, and frameworks, but to sit alongside them as a practical starting point. In a field with a lot of terms, tools, and theoretical approaches, it is easy to feel overwhelmed. The core elements are intended to help cut through the noise and support anyone, from beginners to experts, to focus on what matters when getting started with knowledge translation.

It is also important to remember that these elements are **interconnected**. They are not linear steps to work through in order, and they don't map neatly on to the specific processes of the Knowledge Translation Complexity Network Model: Problem Identification, Knowledge Creation, Knowledge Synthesis, Implementation, and Evaluation. In fact, each element shows up across multiple processes. You can think of them as familiar ingredients or flavour combinations that can be combined in different ways to create an entirely new recipe (Figure 8.1). While they provide a basic reference point, as we've discussed in previous chapters, knowledge translation always happens within complex social systems. You will need to remain flexible, and keep in mind both the local and broader system context to put these ideas into practice effectively. There's

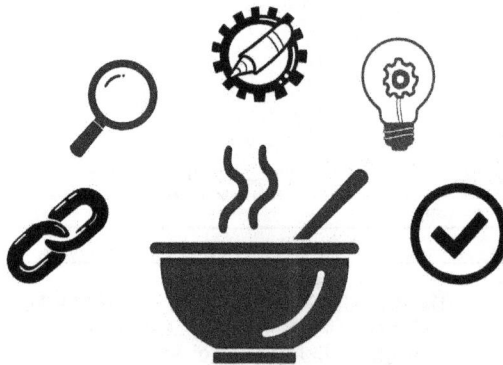

Figure 8.1 The five core elements are like familiar ingredients that can be combined to create a new recipe.
Source: https://doi.org/10.25451/flinders.29192825.v1

no one-size-fits-all recipe. Your methods should be shaped by your setting, your team, and your shared goals.

How to use this chapter

We hope this chapter will help you get your head around doing knowledge translation in an integrated way with clarity and confidence.

The chapter follows the five core elements of **Connect, Clarify, Customise, Co-create,** and **Confirm.** It explores how each can help keep the basic ingredients of knowledge translation in mind while working through with dynamic knowledge translation processes and systems. The core elements can help by:

- Supporting teams to plan and stay on track by consistently thinking about the five core elements throughout their work
- Guiding effective collaboration with partners and bringing together diverse perspectives
- Providing flexibility so that strategies can adapt to new information, shifting contexts, and evolving needs
- Offering a simple tool for checking progress, identifying gaps, and refining goals over time
- Acting as guideposts to help prioritise next steps and navigate challenges as they come up.

For each of the core elements, we have included a checklist to help guide individuals and teams in planning and undertaking an integrated approach to knowledge translation. These questions are not meant to be rigid or prescriptive. You don't need to answer them all to get started. Instead, think of them as prompts to spark reflection, facilitate discussions, and support decision-making. These checklists serve a few purposes, they:

- Help teams identify the people, organisations, and systems that might be involved in or affected by different knowledge translation processes at various timepoints in their work.
- Can be used as conversation starters to encourage teams to explore integrated knowledge translation from new angles, shifting discussions from abstract concepts to practical actions.
- Provide an informal evaluative framework, supporting teams in planning actions, tracking progress, and assessing impacts over time.

First, let's take another look at the Knowledge Translation Complexity Network Model (Figure 8.2):

We encourage you to start by thinking about the Knowledge Translation Complexity Network Model (for more information about this model, see Chapter 4) as a roadmap, and work out which research process(es) – Problem Identification, Knowledge Creation, Knowledge Synthesis, Implementation, Evaluation – map on to your project. Next, think about the different people and groups you need to engage across the various systems you might be working with. From there, think about the ways you can **Connect** the different people operating within these systems, work together to **Clarify** the problem and what

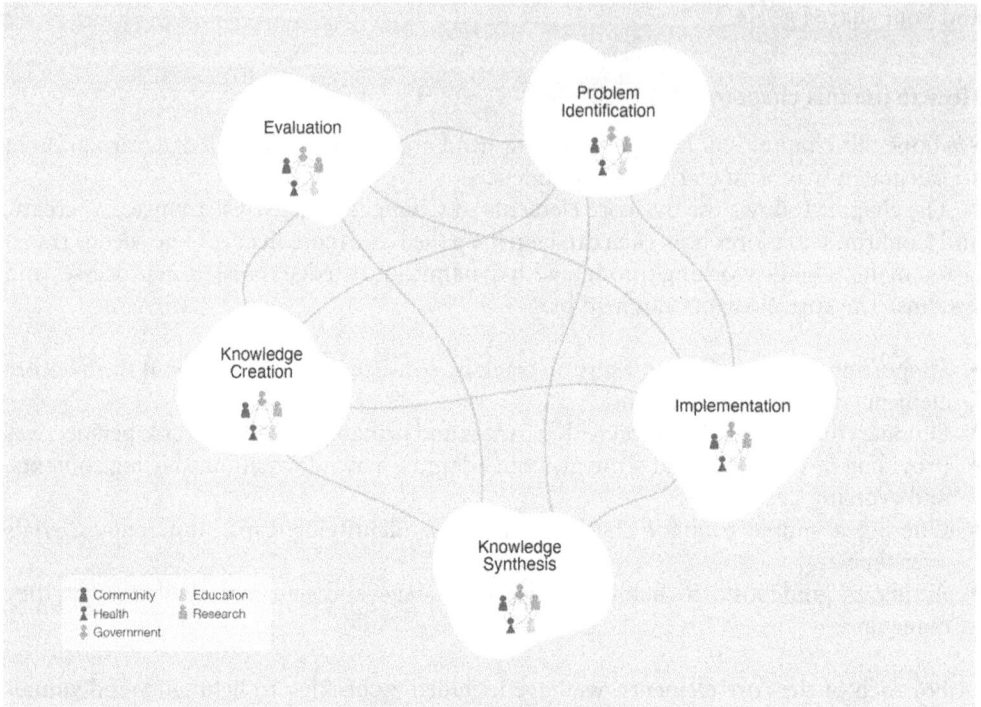

Figure 8.2 Knowledge Translation Complexity Network Model.
Source: https://doi.org/10.25451/flinders.29192585.v1

needs to be done, and **Customise** testable solutions that account for the variability in local contexts and cultures. You can then **Co-create** solutions while systematically keeping track of the processes of developing, testing, and refining those solutions. Finally, you can **Confirm** whether these solutions are achieving the desired impact, ensuring they are relevant to those using them, feasible to implement, cost-effective, scalable, and sustainable.

Core element 1: connect

Taking an integrated approach to knowledge translation means connecting with partners early and check in with them regularly. Establishing shared understandings from the outset helps to build trust, align expectations, and create a strong foundation for collaborative knowledge translation approach.

1 Identifying and engaging partners:

Effective knowledge translation begins with identifying and engaging with partners who have a stake or interest in the problem, recognising that their specific concerns might vary. Identifying the right combination of partners helps make sure that the research problem is relevant and grounded in real-world experiences and priorities.

Practical steps:

- Use a range of **Problem Identification** methods (e.g., audits, document reviews, focus groups, interviews, system mapping, root cause analysis, Delphi panels, journey mapping, and ethnographic observation) to define the shared problem(s). Work collaboratively to explore different perspectives and describe the problem(s) in terms and frameworks that resonate with various partners. Using forums, communities of practice, or knowledge brokers can facilitate exchange and discussion between disciplines or sectors to define and frame the problem.
- Reflect on the priorities and lived realities of each group. Are they aligned in how they see the problem and pathways to generate and embed potential solutions? How much do they vary in their interests and concerns, skills, resources, preferred strategies, and definitions of success? Co-design processes, along with other knowledge exchange and networking approaches, offer a valuable way to bring diverse groups together to make sense of the issue collectively and support shared decision-making.

2 *Establishing a network:*

Building a strong collaborative network early is essential for sharing knowledge and building trust. Networks function dynamically, with **nodes** (single agents that interact with other agents, e.g., an individual clinician or researcher), **hubs** (single agents that interact more extensively with other single agents and become the champion within and between groups, e.g., a knowledge broker or boundary spanner), and **clusters** (sub-networks made up of single agents and the wider group of single agents being led by single agents who have taken on the role as leaders and boundary spanners all pursuing the same goals, e.g., an implementation team) facilitating the movement of knowledge in the system.

Practical steps:

- Map your stakeholders to identify **nodes** (i.e., individuals), **hubs** (e.g., key players who influence many individuals) and **clusters** (e.g., teams focused on specific knowledge translation processes like knowledge creation or knowledge synthesis). You can use simple network mapping approaches such as Mendelow's Matrix, or more sophisticated and interactive approaches, including network visualisations (see Chapter 3).
- Next, consider how you will support the team to understand and **navigate** their networks to spot opportunities and barriers; **negotiate** roles, expectations, and resources; and **mobilise** people and teams together to act collectively and work towards shared goals
- Finally, think about how you will check that there is trust and shared understanding, and facilitate connections between people and groups. This could involve informal conversations and team-building activities or more structured approaches like facilitated workshops. These conversations need to be revisited regularly as the team matures and the project progresses.

BOX 8.1 Connect – Checklist Items

Are there any individuals or groups who may not have been obvious at first but could bring valuable perspectives or resources to the project? Consider reaching out to less visible or non-traditional partners who might offer perspectives that are not immediately apparent but could enrich the project.

How will you ensure ongoing engagement with partners, rather than just at the beginning of the project? Building and maintaining connections requires consistent communication. Plan regular check-ins or updates to keep everyone informed and involved throughout the process.

How will feedback from partners will be gathered, processed, and acted upon? Effective collaboration involves listening respectfully to partners' input and showing how their contributions influence decisions. Make sure there is a mechanism in place for this.

How are different partners' interests, values, and concerns being balanced? Identify any potential conflicts early and think about how to negotiate compromises that respect diverse viewpoints while still moving towards project goals.

Do partners feel they have a meaningful role and influence in the project? It's important that partners see themselves as active contributors, not just as passive participants. Assess whether they feel empowered to voice their opinions and ideas.

Are there existing networks or partnerships that can be leveraged to strengthen knowledge translation processes? Look for opportunities to tap into established communities of practice, professional networks, or collaborations to broaden the project's reach and impact.

How will you ensure that knowledge exchange is two-way and inclusive of all partners? Consider creating opportunities for all partners to share their expertise and learn from each other, such as through co-design processes and collaborative brainstorming sessions.

Have you considered the role of knowledge brokers or other intermediaries to facilitate connections across different teams, sectors, or disciplines? Knowledge brokers and similar boundary spanning roles can help bridge gaps between groups that may not usually interact, making it easier to integrate diverse perspectives into the project.

What strategies are in place to build trust within the network, especially among groups that may not have worked together before? Trust is essential for effective collaboration. Think about how you can establish trust-building activities, such as informal meet-and-greets, team-building exercises, or transparent communication practices.

Are there cultural or contextual factors that might affect how partners interact and communicate? Be mindful of differences in communication styles, organisational culture, or professional norms that could influence how partners engage. Adapt your strategies to accommodate these factors.

Core element 2: clarify

Successful knowledge translation relies on working collaboratively to clarify project goals and processes by integrating diverse sources of knowledge. Establishing a shared understanding early on helps ensure that research is relevant, lining up with partner priorities and grounded in the best available evidence.

1 Clarifying the problem and goals:

Once the initial problem(s) are identified, it's important to clarify what the team will focus on and how the research questions or interventions will be framed. Clarifying goals ensures that the research reflects both the needs expressed by partner and matching it up with relevant research-based knowledge.

Practical steps:

- Use knowledge translation theories, models, and frameworks to structure early conversations. These can help ensure that everyone understands the scope of the problem and agrees on the key questions and approaches moving forward. Bear in mind, you might need to use a combination of different theories, models, and frameworks to guide specific processes like co-design, implementation, or evaluation for large-scale projects.
- Bring together different sources of knowledge – research evidence, professional judgment, lived experience, and local information (e.g., documents, databases). With your team, discuss how much importance or 'weight' should be given to each source.
- Ask: Is the available evidence from all sources adequate? How do partners receive and value this evidence? What other sources of knowledge will you need to gather or create?
- Work out a strategy or way of reaching agreement from the different partners. Ideally, you should have these principles agreed from the beginning of your engagement process.

2 Knowledge synthesis for shared understanding:

Synthesis is about integrating evidence from multiple sources (research, experience, local context) into a coherent, shared understanding that guides decision-making, including the development of evidence-informed interventions, strategies, and products (e.g., guidelines, decision aids, or creative resources like videos or infographics).

Practical steps:

- Facilitate discussions on how best to synthesise available knowledge, considering the nature of the evidence and partners involved. For example, you might run a workshop where partners review research evidence alongside their professional and lived experiences, identifying where they align or diverge.
- Ensure that all partners contribute to shaping the intervention or knowledge translation strategy. Use reflective tools to evaluate the collective understanding and identify gaps in knowledge or areas for further inquiry.

BOX 8.2 Clarify – Checklist Items

Have the research goals been clearly communicated to all partners, and do they understand how their input will shape the project? It's important to ensure that everyone knows the intended outcomes and how their contributions will help achieve them. Clear communication can prevent misunderstandings and sets a common direction.

Are there any gaps or inconsistencies in the information gathered from different knowledge sources? Identifying and addressing gaps early can help refine the research focus and ensure a more comprehensive approach. Consider if further information needs to be gathered to bridge these gaps.

Have the key questions and goals been framed in a way that resonate with all partners, including those with lived experience? Make sure the language and approach used to frame the research questions are inclusive and understandable for everyone involved, not just those with technical expertise.

How will you prioritise different sources of knowledge when they offer conflicting information or perspectives? Developing a clear strategy for handling conflicts between sources (e.g., lived experience vs. research evidence) will help maintain focus and balance in decision-making.

Do partners agree on the importance given to different types of evidence? Clarify how different sources of knowledge will be valued in the decision-making process, ensuring transparency and mutual understanding.

Has the project's scope been clearly defined and communicated? Ensuring that everyone understands what the project will and will not address helps set realistic expectations and keeps the team focused.

Are there mechanisms in place for ongoing clarification and adjustments as new information emerges? The need to clarify does not end once the project starts. Make sure there is flexibility to revisit and refine goals, questions, and strategies as new insights come up.

How will you ensure that complex concepts are broken down into simpler, more accessible ideas for all partners Use analogies, visual aids, or straightforward language to make sure that everyone, regardless of their background, can engage with the key concepts.

Is there a shared understanding of how success will be measured, and do all partners agree on the criteria? Clarifying how success is defined and assessed ensures that everyone is working toward the same targets and knows how progress will be tracked.

Have you considered how the context (e.g., cultural, organisational, geographical) might affect the interpretation of different knowledge sources? Being mindful of contextual factors can help prevent misinterpretations and ensure that knowledge is applied appropriately within different settings.

Core element 3: customise

Effective knowledge translation requires tailoring the approach to the specific context, partners, and local conditions to ensure knowledge is communicated effectively and applied in practice. Adapting knowledge translation strategies to fit real-world opportunities and constraints, such as organisational culture, available resources, and partners priorities, can improve relevance, feasibility, and impact.

1 Adapting the knowledge translation approach to the context:

The success of knowledge translation efforts often depends on how well they are tailored to the context, including both the organisational culture and the needs of partners. Customising your approach is about ensuring that the intervention, communication, and methods resonate with the people involved and the setting.

Practical steps:

- Customise the language, format, and medium of communication for each group. Consider whether partners need visual aids, plain language summaries, or digital tools to grasp the concepts effectively.
- Tailor knowledge translation strategies to local factors such as resources, time constraints, and regulations. For example, if resources are limited, focus on incremental, achievable changes first rather than going straight for large-scale interventions.
- Use ongoing feedback loops during implementation and evaluation to continuously refine and adapt the strategy based on what is working and what is not.

2 Understanding the study context:

Customisation also involves understanding the different knowledge systems, assumptions, and values that partners bring to the table. Think about their standard routines and existing organisational processes and how the knowledge translation strategy fits.

Practical steps:

- Regularly engage partners in reflective discussions about how the intervention fits their professional and personal realities. Encourage them to voice their challenges and suggest adjustments.
- Use and revisit **network maps** (these can be simple illustrations/grids like Mendelow's Matrix) to visualise how different actors in the network are interacting, and whether there are gaps or misunderstandings that need to be addressed.

BOX 8.3 Customise – Checklist Items

Have you identified and considered cultural, linguistic, or regional factors that might affect how knowledge is shared and received? Customising the knowledge translation approach means being sensitive to cultural norms, language preferences, and regional contexts that could impact how effectively information is communicated.

Are there specific communication preferences or tools that would help engage partners more effectively? Different groups may respond better to certain formats (e.g., workshops, webinars, infographics). Identifying these preferences can improve engagement and understanding.

Have you ensured that the knowledge translation strategy aligns with partners' existing workflows and routines? Introducing new practices or information should ideally complement, not disrupt, partners' regular activities. Consider how best to integrate new ideas into their existing processes.

How will you handle feedback to refine the knowledge translation approach and is there a system for acting on that feedback in a timely way? Effective customisation relies on being adaptable. Regularly gathering and acting on feedback can help you make timely adjustments to improve the relevance and impact of the knowledge translation strategy.

Are there external factors (e.g., policy changes, funding limitations, technological access) that might require adapting your knowledge translation strategy? Being aware of broader external influences ensures that your approach remains realistic and adaptable to changing conditions.

How are you addressing potential barriers to understanding, such as technical jargon or complex concepts? Simplify language where possible, use analogies or metaphors, and offer visual aids or hands-on examples to make complex information more accessible. Make sure you have lots of stories to share.

Have you established a clear plan for scaling the knowledge translation approach if successful, or is it designed to remain local and specific? Customising also involves deciding whether an approach is scalable or if it should be tailored to a specific context. Consider how the strategy might be adapted for wider use or scaled up or back as needed.

Are you considering the different ways partners process information (e.g., visual learners, hands-on practitioners)? Adapting to different learning styles can make knowledge translation more effective. Ensure that materials and presentations cater to various ways of understanding and engaging with content.

Have you checked whether your knowledge translation strategy is aligned with the broader goals of the organisation or community? Customisation includes making sure that your approach supports the long-term goals and values of the community or institution you are working with.

Are you prepared to revise the knowledge translation strategy if unexpected challenges or opportunities arise during implementation? Building in flexibility allows you to pivot and adjust when things don't go as planned or when new opportunities present themselves.

Core element 4: co-create

Knowledge translation is inherently a collaborative process that involves co-creating knowledge, interventions, and evaluation processes with partners. Engaging partners throughout these processes fosters shared ownership, enhances relevance, and increases the likelihood of relevant and sustained impact.

1 Collaborative knowledge creation and action:

Co-design processes can help ensure that knowledge is developed *with* knowledge users, rather than *for* them. This collaborative approach strengthens ownership of the intervention, tool, or knowledge translation strategy, increasing the chance that it will be introduced and sustained in practice.

Practical Steps:

- Engage partners in the **Knowledge Creation** process by using participatory approaches such as co-design processes to capture diverse perspectives
- Use adaptive methods for **Implementation** (Chapter 2) – adapt and co-create new routines or processes that align with the partners' workflows and values. Build in flexibility to adapt these routines as the project evolves.

2 Co-creating the evaluation process:

Evaluation approaches should be co-created, giving partners a say in how success is defined and measured. This helps ensure that the metrics used are meaningful, relevant, and match up with what matters most to those involved.

Practical steps:

- Use both formative and summative evaluation methods to ensure partners have an ongoing role in shaping the evaluation process. For example, you might develop evaluation criteria through consensus-building exercises or partner-led scoring activities.
- Reflect on outcomes together with partners to surface key lessons, identify challenges, and explore opportunities for improvement.

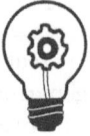

BOX 8.4 Co-Create – Checklist Items

Are partners involved from the earliest stages and do they have a meaningful role in decision-making throughout the co-creation process? Co-creation starts with early engagement. Ensure partners are not just consulted but actively participate in defining the goals, strategies, and processes from the beginning.

Have you set up mechanisms to facilitate ongoing communication between all partners during the co-creation process? Co-creation relies on ongoing dialogue, not just occasional check-ins. Make sure there are regular opportunities for partners to share their insights and feedback and for you to respond to them.

How are you ensuring that all voices, including less dominant or less vocal individuals, are heard and valued? Co-creation should be inclusive. Consider using facilitation techniques to draw out perspectives from those who might otherwise be overlooked, ensuring a diverse range of inputs.

Is there clear agreement on how decisions will be made, especially when there are differing opinions? Establishing transparent decision-making processes, such as consensus-building or voting, can help manage conflicts and ensure that the co-creation process moves forward smoothly.

Have you considered how partners' diverse skills, experiences, and knowledge systems can be integrated into the co-creation process? Each participant brings unique strengths. Think about how to leverage these differences to enrich the knowledge creation, implementation, and evaluation efforts.

Are there shared goals and mutual benefits for all participants in the co-creation process? Co-creation is more successful when everyone sees clear benefits from the collaboration. Make sure there is alignment on what success looks like and that all partners feel they will gain value from their involvement.

Do you have a plan for managing changes and adapting strategies as new insights emerge from partners? Co-creation should be flexible and adaptive. Be prepared to revisit and adjust plans based on feedback and new information that arises during the project.

How will you handle conflicts or disagreements that may arise during co-creation? Address potential conflicts by setting up clear communication channels and conflict resolution strategies that allow for respectful and constructive dialogue.

Are you providing partners with the tools, resources, and training they need to contribute effectively? Ensure that everyone has the necessary skills and knowledge to engage fully in the co-creation process. This might involve training sessions, preparatory materials, or orientation workshops.

Is there a plan to celebrate and share successes with all partners as the project progresses? Acknowledging and celebrating progress, even small wins, can build momentum and strengthen the sense of ownership and commitment among partners.

Core element 5: confirm

Successful knowledge translation requires systematically evaluating the impact of the strategies used, including interventions, tools, and products, to check that they achieve their intended outcomes and making evidence-based adjustments along the way. Evaluation isn't just something that happens at the end. It's an ongoing process that helps teams measure success, refine strategies, and sustain impact over time. This section focuses on Confirm as the process of checking out what's been done, learning from it, staying accountable, and improving things as you go.

1 Embedding evaluation throughout the process:

Evaluation should be integrated into all stages of knowledge translation, not just as a final step. A well-designed evaluation process helps teams assess whether the intervention is relevant, feasible, cost-effective, scalable, and sustainable.

Practical steps:

- Define clear evaluation criteria that reflect partner priorities, organisational goals, and policy considerations. These criteria should go beyond research outcomes to include practical measures of success, such as engagement levels, usability, implementation fidelity, and long-term sustainability.
- Use mixed evaluation methods, including formative (ongoing feedback loops) and summative (final impact assessment) approaches, to capture both process and outcome data in the short- and long-term.
- Engage partners in defining success by incorporating their perspectives on what matters most, ensuring that evaluation methods align with their experiences and priorities.

2 Measuring and adapting for impact:

Knowledge translation is an iterative process, meaning that evaluation findings should inform ongoing refinements and adaptations to maximise effectiveness.

Practical steps:

- Collect and analyse data regularly to assess progress and identify areas needing adjustment. Consider using both qualitative (e.g., interviews, focus groups) and quantitative (e.g., surveys) data to capture a full picture of impact.
- Track implementation fidelity – how closely the intervention follows the intended design – while allowing for necessary adaptations based on local needs.
- Establish structured feedback loops where partners are given the opportunity to review findings and contribute to decisions on refining or scaling the intervention.
- Ensure transparency in how evaluation findings are used, avoiding 'tick-box' assessments by embedding a culture of reflective practice and learning.

> ✓   BOX 8.5 Confirm – Checklist Items
>
> **Have you identified key evaluation criteria that align with research, partner priorities, and system-level considerations?**
>
> Evaluation should reflect what success looks like in both academic and non-academic contexts, ensuring findings are actionable.
>
> **Are you using a combination of formative and summative evaluation methods to support ongoing learning and adaptation?**
>
> An iterative approach allows for timely improvements rather than waiting for end-of-project reviews.
>
> **Have you planned for how evaluation findings will be used to refine, adapt, and sustain the intervention?**
>
> Evaluation should be a mechanism for continuous improvement, not just a reporting requirement.
>
> **Are there mechanisms for partners to contribute to defining success and interpreting evaluation data?** Co-designed evaluation criteria ensure that what is measured aligns with partners priorities.
>
> **Is there a strategy for sharing evaluation results in accessible, actionable ways?** Different audiences (e.g., policymakers, practitioners, funders) require different formats, such as infographics, executive summaries, or interactive dashboards.
>
> **Have you considered potential unintended consequences, or equity impacts in your evaluation?** Understanding who benefits, who is excluded, and why can help refine implementation and ensure greater equity and accessibility.
>
> **Are there systems in place to track long-term sustainability beyond the initial implementation phase?** Ensuring continued leadership, funding pathways, and integration into routine practice will increase the likelihood of lasting impact.
>
> **How are findings being translated into practice, policy, or ongoing research initiatives?** Evaluation should serve as a decision-making tool that informs scaling, policy recommendations, and resource allocation.

Chapter summary

This chapter provides readers with a set of practical reflective questions that can help with navigating new ways of thinking about integrated knowledge translation. They are not meant to be prescriptive or rigidly followed but they will help to guide conversations with other research team members, key partners and other people who need to know about the work. Whether your project is about implementing existing evidence into a practice context, or working with partners to refine ways to improve access to new evidence or knowledge (knowledge synthesis) you will find yourself reflecting on who you need to **Connect** with, what you need to make sure you all have a shared understanding about (**Clarify**), how you modify and shape the task (whether it's implementing new evidence, refining existing evidence or generating new understanding) to make sure it fits with existing norms and practices (**Customise**). Once you have checked out these areas you will feel more confident that you are enroute to work with your partners to do the job (**Co-create** – whether it's implementing evidence, refining evidence, generating new evidence, or understanding the problem) following rigorous and transparent research methods. All that work will help you ensure that your choices around how you are going to evaluate what you have done will be appropriate (**Confirm**). So, in terms of acquiring new skills to help you navigate your knowledge translation journey, your 'compass' will help you check out whether, when and how you need to focus on **Connecting, Clarifying, Customising, Co-creating,** and **Confirming** the work you are doing.

References

Bertram, R. M., Blase, K. A., & Fixsen, D. L. (2015). Improving programs and outcomes: Implementation frameworks and organization change. *Research on Social Work Practice, 25*(4), 477–487.

Damschroder, L. J., Reardon, C. M., Widerquist, M. A. O., & Lowery, J. (2022). The updated Consolidated Framework for Implementation Research based on user feedback. *Implementation science, 17*(1), 75.

Harvey, G., & Kitson, A. (2016). PARIHS revisited: from heuristic to integrated framework for the successful implementation of knowledge into practice. *Implementation science, 11*(1), 33.

Greenhalgh, T., Wherton, J., Papoutsi, C., Lynch, J., Hughes, G., A'Court, C., ... & Shaw, S. (2018). Analysing the role of complexity in explaining the fortunes of technology programmes: empirical application of the NASSS framework. *BMC medicine, 16*(1), 66.

Kitson, A., Brook, A., Harvey, G., Jordan, Z., Marshall, R., O'Shea, R., & Wilson, D. (2018). Using complexity and network concepts to inform healthcare knowledge translation. *International Journal of Health Policy and Management, 7*(3), 231–243. https://doi.org/10.15171/ijhpm.2017.79

May, C. R., Johnson, M., & Finch, T. (2016). Implementation, context and complexity. *Implementation science, 11*(1), 141.

May, C. R., Mair, F., Finch, T., MacFarlane, A., Dowrick, C., Treweek, S., ... & Montori, V. M. (2009). Development of a theory of implementation and integration: Normalization Process Theory. *Implementation science, 4*(1), 29.

Michie, S., Van Stralen, M. M., & West, R. (2011). The behaviour change wheel: a new method for characterising and designing behaviour change interventions. *Implementation science, 6*(1), 42.

Moore, J. E., Mascarenhas, A., Bain, J., & Straus, S. E. (2017). Developing a comprehensive definition of sustainability. *Implementation Science, 12*(1), 110.

Pfadenhauer, L. M., Gerhardus, A., Mozygemba, K., Lysdahl, K. B., Booth, A., Hofmann, B., ... & Rehfuess, E. (2017). Making sense of complexity in context and implementation: the Context and Implementation of Complex Interventions (CICI) framework. *Implementation science, 12*(1), 21.

Sarkies, M. N., Bowles, K. A., Skinner, E. H., Haas, R., Lane, H., & Haines, T. P. (2017). The effectiveness of research implementation strategies for promoting evidence-informed policy and management decisions in healthcare: a systematic review. *Implementation Science, 12*(1), 132.

Section III

Facilitating the journey

9 Leadership reflections for integrated knowledge translation

Alison Kitson

Introduction

The purpose of this chapter is to provide some personal reflections on how we can facilitate the alignment of research leadership with leadership for integrated knowledge translation. It's a reflective journey for several reasons. First, it draws on my own experiential journey as a researcher and leader who stumbled into the world of evidence-based practice and (integrated) knowledge translation. My journey has shaped my theoretical and practical understanding of the mechanisms that optimise knowledge translation success. Next, I will provide some reflections on what knowledge translation success looks like at individual, team, and organisational levels, again drawing on both experiential knowledge as well as empirical research. The chapter finishes with thoughts about leadership and capacity development for integrated knowledge translation from the lens of the research leader who is also facilitating integrated knowledge translation.

Research leaders play a key role in knowledge translation by enabling a culture that embraces working with partners, emphasising the values of evidence-based practice, and that supports implementation and evaluation strategies. They set the strategic direction for knowledge translation and ensure that research efforts reflect the needs of healthcare users and other partners. Their role extends to capacity building across traditional research and practice areas and engaging with partners. They can function as champions of the creation and use of new knowledge, and they can support novel ways to implement new knowledge into policy and practice and evaluate its success. Effective research leaders act as role models to junior researchers and promote an inquiry-driven culture (Chan et al., 2023).

Despite these acknowledgements of the importance of the research leader's role, there has been little focused attention paid to understanding how they learn how to do this. Spyridonidis et al. (2015) examined the sort of leadership qualities that were required when researchers and service leaders worked together to promote better integrated knowledge translation activity. Their findings indicated that both research and service leaders had to shift from a 'top-down', hierarchical approach and move towards more collaborative leadership approaches, where influence is shared, and leadership is distributed across different levels.

Generic leadership capability is acknowledged as an important enabler for integrated knowledge translation (Gagliardi & Dobrow, 2016) at individual, team and organisational levels. While team science (Begerowski et al., 2021) approaches have helped clarify the need for research leaders to move beyond single discipline thinking and embrace transdisciplinary collaboration (Aarons et al., 2020; Lawless et al., 2024) there is still

DOI: 10.4324/9781003245995-12

limited understanding of how leaders actually make this shift. Specifically, we know little about how they move from disciple-specific mindsets to embracing integrated ways of thinking that actively includes a wider range of partner groups.

Leadership capacity and capability at what is often termed the 'research-user' level have been given more attention in the implementation science literature. Aarons and colleagues' work on developing the Implementation Leadership Scale (Aarons, Ehrhart, & Farahnak, 2014) has shaped the way teams can prepare for implementing new evidence-based practice processes. In addition, Birkin et al. (2016) have looked at leadership attributes in the context of organisational readiness, while Kitson et al. (2021) and Harvey et al. (2019) have explored leadership as a key enabler for effective implementation at unit level.

However, less is known about how research leaders lead integrated knowledge translation approaches across research teams and research institutes, how they establish the right culture and how they evaluate the success of integrated knowledge translation. Additionally, the integrated knowledge translation literature tends to distinguish between knowledge producers and knowledge users. Most of the focus has been on how knowledge producers can engage knowledge users in collaborative activities focusing on concepts such as research partnerships (Bowen et al., 2019; Hoekstra et al., 2020) and how such partnerships are initiated (Zych et al., 2020).

But how does a researcher from a traditional clinical or biomedical background begin to engage more broadly beyond the boundaries of their specific discipline? As Greenhalgh and Wieringa (2011) articulate, there is a need to embrace a broader conceptualisation of 'knowledge', recognising the contributions of disciplines such as philosophy, sociology, and organisational science. They argue for a shift from a narrow focus of the 'know-do' gap to a deeper exploration of the context-specific practical wisdom that underpins clinical judgement and actions. This includes understanding how tacit knowledge (knowledge gained through experience and practice) is generated and shared amongst practitioners, how complex links between power and knowledge are negotiated, and how these dynamics inform approaches to facilitating partnerships between researchers, practitioners, policy makers and other partners.

Such advice has been around in the literature for nearly two decades. Yet, we still don't have a clear roadmap to help research leaders know how to work more effectively with their teams and other partners to apply integrated knowledge translation principles. Spyridonidis et al. (2015) and Kislov et al. (2018) identified the lack of empirical understanding of the link between leadership *and* knowledge translation and leadership *for* knowledge translation from their work on Collaboration for Leadership in Applied Health Research and Care programs. This distinction is important for how we can better understand what needs to happen to equip research leaders to become more effective champions for and facilitators of integrated knowledge translation. So, how do researchers become leaders for knowledge translation?

Where my integrated knowledge translation journey began

Becoming a researcher and leader

My initiation to research happened early, when I was awarded a PhD scholarship to study the therapeutic role of the nurse in caring for older hospitalised people across

---

Box 9.1 Proposition of the PARIHS framework (adapted from Harvey & Kitson, 2015)

SI = f (E, C, F)

SI = Successful implementation
f = function (of)
E= Evidence
C = Context
F = Facilitation

Northern Ireland (Kitson, 1991). I found that the role of the ward or unit leader was key to determining the quality of the care patients received (Kitson, 1986, 1987). That work led to setting up and running a national program on improving standards of nursing care for the Royal College of Nursing in the United Kingdom (Kitson, Harvey, Hyndman, Sindhu, et al., 1994; Kitson, Harvey, Hyndman, & Yerrell, 1994).

In the 1990s, efforts to improve nursing care standards were largely based on clinical experience (or tacit knowledge), patient feedback, and relatively small amounts of research evidence (Kitson et al., 1996). At the time, the evidence base informing clinical nursing interventions was still emerging, which prompted a broader movement within the profession. There was growing interest in making tacit knowledge more explicit, setting up clinical research units, and developing roles that facilitated the adoption of new standards of care into clinical practice (Ward et al., 1998).

It was from this context that we developed the Promoting Action into Research Implementation in Health Services (PARIHS) Framework (Kitson et al., 1998). This co-designed approach to understanding successful implementation of evidence into practice was developed to help applied researchers work with clinicians to get evidence into practice. The PARIHS Framework argued that a conscious and deliberate intervention shaped by active facilitation was required at local level to work out what mechanisms were needed to enhance the potential for successful implementation. The proposition of the PARIHS framework can be seen in Box 9.1

Uptake use and refinement of PARIHS

The PARIHS Framework was one of the first frameworks to explicitly identify context as an influencing factor on implementation success (Kitson et al., 1998). The framework was used and tested by international research teams and across a decade we received feedback on the framework's ability to achieve implementation success.

This led to the refinement of the framework and the integrated PARIHS or i-PARIHS framework was published (Harvey & Kitson, 2015; Harvey & Kitson, 2016). The proposition of the i-PARIHS framework can be seen in Box 9.2

Work has continued developing support tools for using i-PARIHS (Hunter, Kim, & Kitson, 2020; Hunter et al., 2023; Hunter, Kim, Mudge, et al., 2020) as well as ongoing evaluation of the way facilitation and facilitators can influence successful implementation (Baloh et al., 2018; Bidassie et al., 2015; Dogherty et al., 2010; Harvey et al., 2023; Kitson & Harvey, 2016; Ritchie et al., 2021; Stetler et al., 2006).

Box 9.2 Proposition of the i-PARIHS framework (adapted from Harvey & Kitson, 2015)

$SI = Fac^n (I + R + C)$

SI = Successful implementation
Fac^n = Facilitation
I = Innovation
R = Recipients (individual and collective)
C = Context (inner and outer)

How the i-PARIHS approach connects to integrated knowledge translation

PARIHS and i-PARIHS have had strong support from knowledge or research-users, including managers and clinicians, as they could understand it and use it in practice (Hunter, Kim, & Kitson, 2020; Hunter, Kim, Mudge, et al., 2020). From the research-producer community there are still questions about how effective facilitation is as an intervention and how big a 'dose' is needed for the implementation to be successful (Bucknall et al., 2022; Fasugba et al., 2025). Additionally, we worked on deepening our understanding of how PARIHS and i-PARIHS were used for different stages of the implementation research process (Bergström et al., 2020; Hunter et al., 2025) to create more consistent guidance on how to use the framework. We explored how different implementation research teams made decisions about which implementation theory, model or framework to use (Lynch et al., 2018)) as well as how to combine them across studies (Hunter et al., 2025).

Less has been written about the respective roles of the research producers, the research users and the 'facilitators' or linkage roles. These are three separate but interrelated roles in the implementation phase of the research process, but they have key roles to play in the other stages of the research process, namely problem identification, knowledge creation, knowledge synthesis, and evaluation. It was in having the opportunity to systematically explore how each of the research steps or processes could be enriched by using the principles of integrated knowledge translation that the next phase of my learning journey began.

From i-PARIHS to co-creating knowledge translation

The opportunity to further test the link between research processes and knowledge translation came when I became the knowledge translation lead in a National Health and Medical Research Council-funded population health study (Hoon-Leahy et al., 2012). My task was to work with the rest of the interdisciplinary team to construct a systematic approach to working with a local community to identify the most pressing health needs of the community and to co-design ways to provide better health services that would meet their needs (Kitson et al., 2013).

This project was one of the first integrated knowledge translation projects undertaken by this interdisciplinary team. It comprised health service researchers, epidemiologists, general practitioners, allied health professionals, economists, nurses, and knowledge translation experts as well as key community partners. The Co-creating Knowledge

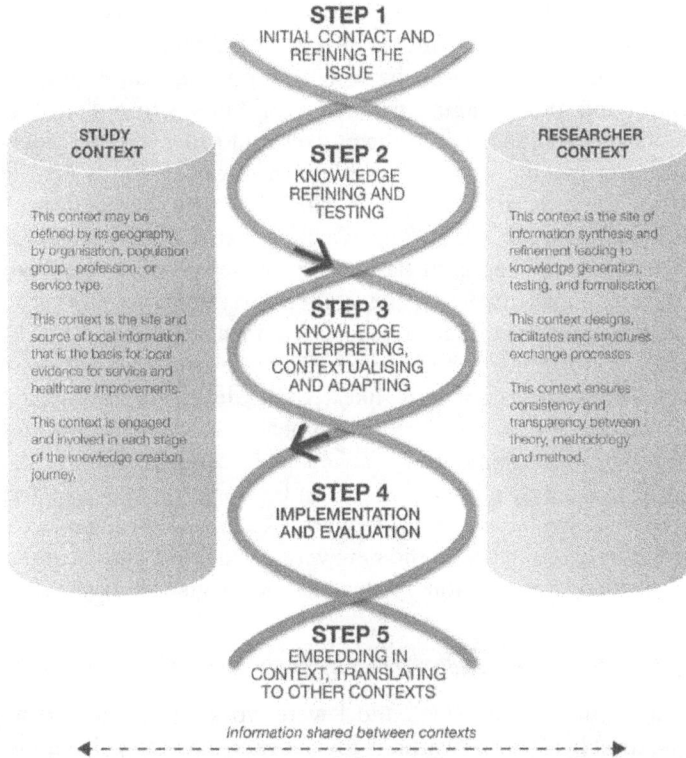

STEP 1
INITIAL CONTACT AND
REFINING THE
ISSUE

STUDY CONTEXT

This context may be defined by its geography, by organisation, population group, profession, or service type.

This context is the site and source of local information that is the basis for local evidence for service and healthcare improvements.

This context is engaged and involved in each stage of the knowledge creation journey.

STEP 2
KNOWLEDGE
REFINING AND
TESTING

RESEARCHER CONTEXT

This context is the site of information synthesis and refinement leading to knowledge generation, testing, and formalisation.

This context designs, facilitates and structures exchange processes.

This context ensures consistency and transparency between theory, methodology and method.

STEP 3
KNOWLEDGE
INTERPRETING,
CONTEXTUALISING
AND ADAPTING

STEP 4
IMPLEMENTATION
AND EVALUATION

STEP 5
EMBEDDING IN
CONTEXT, TRANSLATING
TO OTHER CONTEXTS

Information shared between contexts

Figure 9.1 Co-KT framework.
Source: Kitson et al. (2013).

Translation framework (Figure 9.1) was used to shape the way that a rural based population health intervention was co-designed, implemented, and evaluated.

The five steps in the process included collecting and analysing local data (initial contact and refining the issue); developing partner relationships and deepening understandings (knowledge refining and testing); co-designing the evidence-based intervention using existing best practice literature together with partner experiences (knowledge interpreting, contextualising, and adapting); an implementing and evaluation phase and taking learnings from the implementation phase into broader policy and practice changes (embedding in context, translating to other contexts).

Findings showed that the community of around 14,000 people identified the need for improved musculoskeletal healthcare, in particular access to general practice and physiotherapy services. The project was limited in its success related to finding lasting solutions to these needs because of lack of a locally accessible policy, financial and service delivery model; lack of continued engagement with local partners; access challenges and poor working relations between general practitioners and allied health professionals. Even though key outcome measures of peoples' pain relief and general functional ability improved over the course of the study this was not sustained because of the broader organisational and systems challenges encountered (Dent et al., 2016).

The Co-creating Knowledge Translation framework was then used in another National Health and Medical Research Council study as part of a Centre of Research Excellence in Frailty and Healthy Ageing (Archibald, Ambagtsheer, et al., 2017). The knowledge translation team took on the role of supporting the interdisciplinary team members in identifying and engaging partners and coming to a shared understanding on what frailty meant to older people themselves and other partners including general practitioners and orthopaedic surgeons (Ambagtsheer et al., 2019; Ambagtsheer et al., 2017; Archibald, Kitson, et al., 2017; Archibald, Lawless, Ambagtsheer, et al., 2020; Archibald, Lawless, Gill, et al., 2020). This work was particularly impactful as it ensured that the whole focus of the research had a consumer lens from the beginning. Novel approaches to partner engagement were developed and tested as well as studies exploring how members of the interdisciplinary research team learned how to work together and shift their thinking from multi- or interdisciplinary collaboration to recognising what transdisciplinary teamwork might look like (Archibald et al., 2023; Archibald et al., 2018; Lawless et al., 2024). Overall, the project generated multiple new insights into the management of frailty in the community as well as deepening our understanding of new methodologies to engage patients' views of complex constructs such as frailty (Lawless, Archibald, Pinero de Plaza, et al., 2020; Lawless, Archibald, Ambagtsheer, et al., 2020; Lawless, Drioli-Phillips, et al., 2020) and new ways to tackle transdisciplinary leadership and integrated knowledge translation approaches (Ambagtsheer et al., 2019).

From co-creating knowledge translation to complexity thinking

At around the same time as my teams and I were working on the two major research projects on population health interventions for a rural community and understanding the nature of frailty, we got involved in a university-led initiative that was trying to understand how to optimise research impact (Harvey et al., 2015). We facilitated a series of events and workshops across a large interdisciplinary health and medical sciences faculty in a research-intensive university and worked with a partner group to generate a shared understanding of what an integrated knowledge translation approach to research activity would look like in such an organisation. The first piece of work involved interviewing key leaders about their understanding of, and interest in, knowledge translation (Harvey et al., 2015), which then shaped the emerging Knowledge Translation Complexity Network Model (Brook et al., 2016; Kitson et al., 2018).

From these discussions, the Knowledge Translation Complexity Network Model (which you will hopefully now be familiar with; Figure 9.2) was co-designed by an interdisciplinary team to take account of the discourse emerging in the knowledge translation and implementation science communities around complexity thinking. As was clear from the findings of our own work using the Co-creating Knowledge Translation framework, we had to extend our thinking about the mediating effect of multiple systems and processes within complex social networks on local actions to try and solve local problems. This meant that instead of looking at systems in isolation we needed ways to show the interdependencies and impacts of multiple systems and processes operating within networks.

Reflecting on my own knowledge translation journey I could summarise it by saying that I started off in a traditional health service, mixed methods way (PhD), then I was

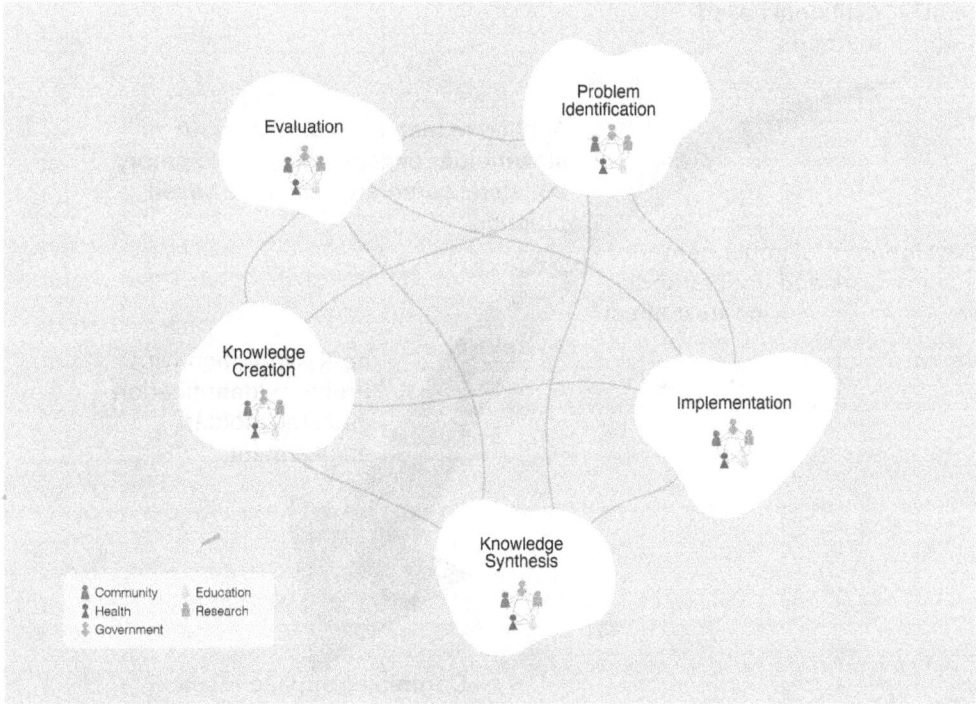

Figure 9.2 Knowledge Translation Complexity Network Model.
Source: https://doi.org/10.25451/flinders.29192585.v1

thrown into an applied research project that required me to develop partner engage-ment and implementation skills. I then connected these to the evidence-based practice movement and developed a conceptual framework to help make sense of what was happening in the real world. Then I discovered the need to focus as much on problem identification through partner engagement at every step of the knowledge translation journey and finally my journey has ended up trying to understand how applied research, integrated knowledge translation, and complexity science connect. Figure 9.3 represents what my journey looked like.

In the next section of this chapter, I will outline three key mechanisms, namely the role of the individual in the research and knowledge translation processes; how teams work together to build knowledge translation capacity; and how systems and organisations can build on and draw from the energy and self-determining activity of individuals and teams within their structures. In describing how these interrelated processes overlap, engage and react with each other I will also be making observations about the leadership requirements, from research leaders in particular who have a role to play in developing the next generation of knowledge translation scientists and practitioners.

PhD - traditional mixed
methods

Applied research - learning about
stakeholder engagement, participatory
action research and evidence based
practice

Development of implementation
framework and understanding
context effect

co-KT approach with
Problem Identification
and stakeholder
engagement

Combining applied research,
implementation research and
complexity science

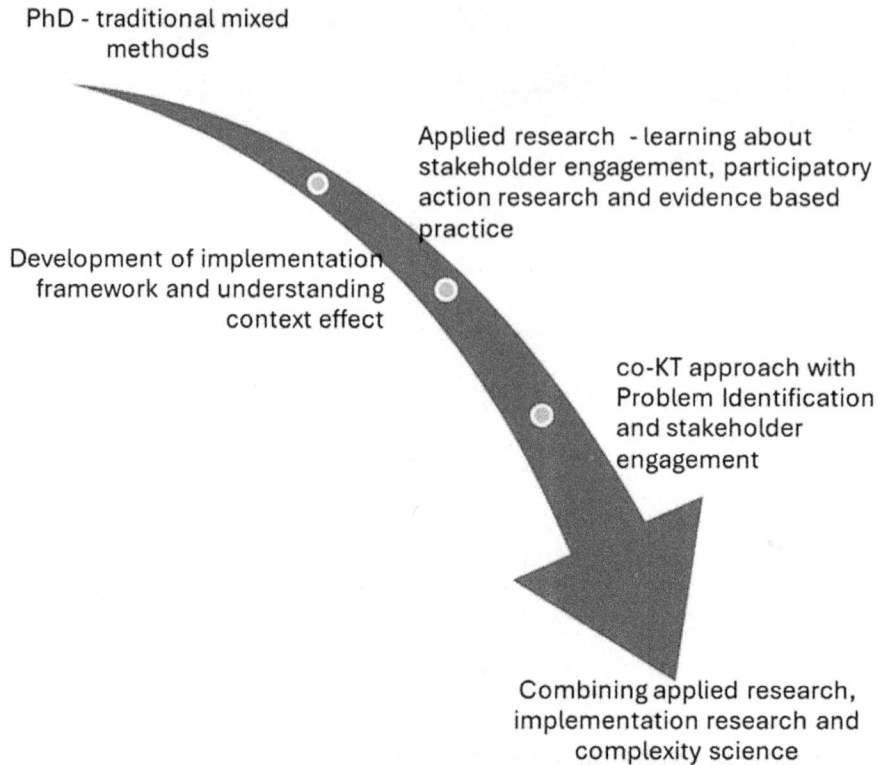

Figure 9.3 My research and integrated knowledge translation journey.
Source: https://doi.org/10.25451/flinders.29192828.v1

Leadership for integrated knowledge translation: from the perspective of the individual

There are at least three distinct but interrelated roles for individuals engaging in integrated knowledge translation activity. They can be, primarily or as their main focus, part of the 'research producer' group, part of the 'research user' group or someone who is recruited to be the 'link' between the two worlds. In the Caring Futures Institute, we have illustrated this connectivity by using the Knowledge Translation Complexity Network Model to illustrate how individuals, teams, networks and systems work synergistically together. Going back to the discussion on how individuals in systems respond to new knowledge and ideas (Chapter 4) we have used the language and terminology from complexity science. Individuals can act as 'nodes' within systems so they can become early adopters of new ideas or volunteer to be part of new projects. The individuals can influence others in the wider system by creating larger groups of interested individuals – 'nodes' become 'hubs' and when these groups reach a critical size, they are termed clusters – or sub-networks of individuals working collectively towards shared goals (Table 9.1).

Table 9.1 Definition of nodes, hubs, clusters and networks

Term	Explanation
Node	A single agent (individual, process or virtual system) that interacts with other single agents (nodes).
Hub	A single agent that interacts more extensively with other nodes and becomes the champion for collective actions, within and between clusters.
Cluster	A sub-network made up of nodes and hubs. The sub-network comprises a number of nodes, some of which act as hubs, pursuing the same goals. A cluster may be a sub-network involved with key areas of activity (such as PI) or a sub-network within a sector (such as a university health science research group).
Network	A collection of nodes, hubs, clusters and the connections between them.

Source: Reproduced from Kitson et al. (2018).

Figure 9.4 shows that in each of the research processes (problem identification, knowledge creation, knowledge synthesis, implementation, evaluation) there can be node, hub, cluster, and network activity happening as team members start to understand their roles in the research project and how they learn to interact with each other in their primary research space as well as start to explore other areas of research activity.

For example, in the project discussed earlier (on population health interventions for a rural community and understanding the nature of frailty (Kitson et al., 2013), it emerged that the success of the project rested on two major factors – one was aligning the population needs assessment with the government's policy and finance strategy and the other was linked to enabling general practitioners and allied health professionals to learn how to work more effectively together. Whilst there were local individuals who took on knowledge broker/facilitator roles to run the additional mobility clinics in the local area, the lack of translation of this commitment into wider system impact (individual nodes influencing hubs, leading to clusters and networks that could take the ideas generated in the research and move on them) meant that the implementation stalled. The project facilitator recruited to act as the local lead would feel that they had 'failed' because they weren't able to embed the changes needed to sustain the initiative. Research team members could conclude that collaborative approaches to integrated knowledge translation were not successful based on this experience. Yet, at another level of analysis, the fact that the whole interdisciplinary team learned about the interaction of context with policy and politics meant that individual researchers and others in the health and community systems had more of an appreciation of the levels of negotiation and engagement required to achieve lasting impact.

This means that the individual recruited into a research team needs to understand what role they are expected to perform and which of the research process pillars is their primary 'home'. They also need to understand the team's shared philosophy regarding working in partnership and integrating different types and sources of knowledge, as these will shape the nature of partner engagement and governance and accountability processes. As we saw in Chapters 6 and 7 the commitment to working authentically with community members and partners is time-consuming and expensive if done properly. It

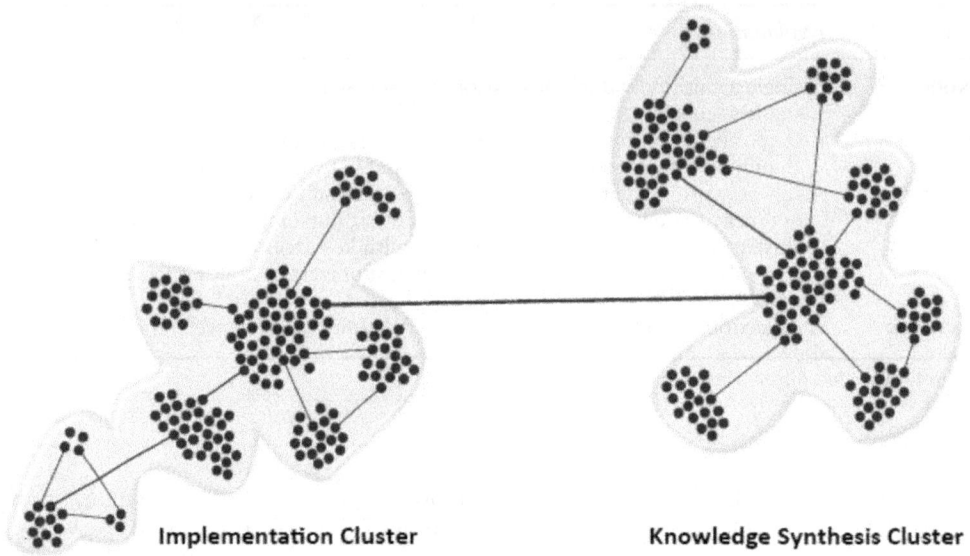

Implementation Cluster   **Knowledge Synthesis Cluster**

Figure 9.4 Representation of two clusters (sub-networks) within a knowledge translation complexity network.
Source: Kitson et al. (2018).

requires a shift in mindset from seeing knowledge producer, user, and linkage roles as separate to understanding the dynamic nature of each of these roles and how they are interdependent.

Research confirms (for example (Aarons, Ehrhart, Farahnak, et al., 2014)) that individual opinion leaders/local champions do influence the uptake of new knowledge into practice. Research into team science (Gagliardi & Dobrow, 2016) also indicates that it is important to nurture creative and inquiring minds if research leaders want to get the best results from their team members. Research into the effectiveness of organisational structures to bridge research production and research use divides also identified the importance of collaborative, respectful relationships with local level individuals being empowered to make their own decisions and problem solve (Kislov et al., 2018; Spyridonidis et al., 2015).

So, for the individual researcher, faced with working out where they belong in the research process, they need firstly to locate themselves into one of the pillars – is their project primarily about clarifying the problem, knowledge creation, synthesis, implementation, evaluation, or a mix of some or all? What are the key methodologies they are going to need to engage with partners, understand and review the evidence, work on generating an implementation and evaluation plan and then gather the right team to execute the task? What are the questions a novice researcher should be asking so they can appreciate the complex world they are entering?

The case studies in Chapter 5 illustrate the personal journeys several early, mid-career, and senior research leaders undertook to help them make sense of the integrated knowledge translation journey as it intersected with their research skill and competency development. The practical guidance in Chapter 8 is a start to helping individual researchers have guided conversations about **Connecting** the right people, **Clarifying** or making sure everyone is agreed on the problem(s) being investigated, adapting or **Customising** solutions or interventions to fit the setting, culture, and environment, collaborating closely with key partners to **Co-create** and test the proposed solutions and finally to check out or **Confirm** that what you intended to do has actually happened.

There will be some individual researchers who embrace the broader landscape of integrated knowledge translation more readily than others – they love engagement, partner involvement and working in the real-world. Others will work out this level of uncertainty and unpredictability is not for them, and they will gravitate to parts of the research process that requires and builds on their skills. What is important is that in the way of talking about and appreciating integrated knowledge translation we are starting to describe the range of skills and competencies required at an individual level and later we will be addressing some of the necessary skills for leaders in this applied field.

While integrated knowledge translation research has focused on the importance of partnerships between knowledge producers and users across different research processes, most of the focus has been on the implementation phase of research (Chapter 2). This means that while we might have some emerging understanding of how individual opinion leaders act as 'hubs' to shape the thinking of others around them and hence to influence wider social networks, we don't know whether these mechanisms work in other research processes. For example, in the problem identification phase – where research producers and users bring appropriate partners together to identify, and refine the problem – how should they target local influencers within systems so that these people can influence how the knowledge is generated and implemented?

In considering the individual in the context of integrated knowledge translation, and particularly the Knowledge Translation Complexity Network Model, it is important to understand their ability to make independent decisions, to influence those around them and to actively engage in creative problem solving. How research leaders recognise and use this in integrated knowledge translation activity in developing more shared understanding in and across teams is the next step.

How research leaders build team capacity and capability for integrated knowledge translation

We have acknowledged the importance of the individual researcher's ability to operate within complex adaptive systems across multiple research processes (see also Chapter 4). As they learn about knowledge creation and implementation, they will develop skills to respond to unexpected circumstances within and across the systems they work in and to do so in ways that engage other actors. These nodes, hubs and clusters create networks that are used to share knowledge and experiences. How this complexity thinking connects with our more conventional views of teams and how they get the work done is what we will focus on next.

Teamwork is essential to our working lives. There is almost nothing we can achieve without being reliant upon other individuals, teams, and groups to support us. Research leaders need to work out how they get their teams and their partners to operate effectively together. Some of the early challenges they face relate to the following:

- The length of time team members have worked together
- The dominant disciplinary orientation and the amount of diversity in the team
- Level of experience ranging from early-career to experienced researchers
- Views (often implicit) on the ontology/epistemology of knowledge and thus the hierarchy of opinions and decision making
- Views on methodological quality and appropriateness in terms of answering the research question
- Rationale and ways to engage partners, and consumers
- Understanding of and exposure to ideas around integrated knowledge translation and attitudes towards how a successful research career is determined.

All these factors are woven into a research program which creates its own timeframes, governance structures, accountability mechanisms, and success criteria. So, the question is why do we want to make the life of research leaders more complex by suggesting they need to be more aware of integrated knowledge translation and complexity theory approaches to add to the above list? The simple answer is that our research will not be effective in making changes if we don't learn how to embrace more integrated knowledge translation approaches and with the added focus on research impact in the real world, it is even more important that these competencies and new ways of thinking are embraced.

How did we go about creating such a culture within our research institute leadership team? Also, how did these leaders consider their own experiences of knowledge translation to inform their own teams in pursuing an integrated knowledge translation approach? This next section summarises the learning journeys of five research leaders and their exposure to knowledge translation ways of thinking.

How our research leaders learned about integrated knowledge translation

To get a sense of colleagues' experiences of integrated knowledge translation, I attended regular meetings involving five members of the Caring Futures Institute leadership team. I gained their permission to summarise their experiences of learning about and doing knowledge translation. Colleagues shared the impact of: prior experiences that they brought to their research leadership role; the mental models they had used to understand knowledge translation; strategies used to shape their teams' understanding of knowledge translation; how they shifted from monodisciplinary to interdisciplinary leadership perspectives; and their own reflections of the leadership skills they developed as a result of working in and thinking about knowledge translation.

Experience brought to the role

The research leadership experience within the group ranged from years to decades, representing a breadth of professional disciplines (physiotherapy, nursing, nutrition and dietetics, health service research, implementation science, and cancer care) across research-focussed, academic, joint appointment and management roles. Those with clinical backgrounds had been involved with implementation of new ideas, national clinical guideline development or delivery, clinical audit, or quality improvement methodologies.

Some had more traditional research approaches and acknowledged they had not been introduced to ways of thinking about knowledge translation that enabled them to consider broader individual and contextual variables. The focus had been very much on the quality and level of the evidence and ways to synthesise it (mostly via clinical guidelines).

Despite a lack of formal education or introduction, some identified early that they had a broader view of research and knowledge translation, and they actively explored opportunities to develop more integrated approaches and viewpoints. Some had extensive experience in whole-health-system thinking and improvement strategies and were already applying integrated approaches that included relationship-building, people and project management, clinical delivery, evaluation, and influencing policy.

Mental models used to understand knowledge translation

The research leaders identified a range of starting points. For some, learning about knowledge translation started with their doctoral studies. Guideline implementation was another experience several research leaders referred to; discovering the complexity of contextual factors that make implementation complex and challenges of scaling a successful intervention into a larger initiative.

Research leaders also mentioned learning about formal knowledge translation approaches when they developed research grants and had to describe how they were going to get research findings into practice. This was particularly the case for Centres of Research Excellence where the explicit aim of the scheme is to '…improve health outcomes and promote or improve translation of research outcomes into policy and/or practice' by way of supporting teams of researchers to work collaboratively and build research capacity (National Health and Medical Research Council, 2023).

Some research leaders mentioned how they found frameworks such as RE-AIM (Glasgow et al., 2019; Glasgow et al., 1999) and the Knowledge-to-Action framework (Graham et al., 2006) helpful in structuring their thinking. Other methodological approaches including Experience Based Co-Design (Bate & Robert, 2006), the i-PARIHS framework (Harvey & Kitson, 2016) and the Behavioural Change Wheel (Michie et al., 2011) were also used in discrete studies.

Research leaders shifted from implicit to explicit ways of describing knowledge translation, and their narratives moved from simple conceptual constructions or mental models to more nuanced understandings of the multiple factors that needed to be considered. For example, one research leader acknowledged that generating more understanding or new knowledge does not *per se* change anything – the important issue for the researcher is to understand how the user connects with the new knowledge and about the quality, accessibility and appropriateness of the content. This engagement with the end user was also reinforced by another research leader who described their engagement with Evidence Based Co-design (Bate & Robert, 2006) as one of the most 'obvious' ways to begin the necessary partner engagement work that shapes implementation.

Having that flexibility in one's own knowledge translation repertoire means that research leaders practising integrated knowledge translation can keep asking the right questions and can guide teams to construct the right questions, focus on the most appropriate methodologies and use existing frameworks in more deliberate ways.

Shaping the team's understanding of knowledge translation

Research leaders agreed that team members start at different points in their understanding of, interest in, and appreciation of knowledge translation. Deliberate strategies such as starting to talk about models and frameworks that helped team members move from simple steps to more complex constructs were described. However, a more overarching approach described by two research leaders was to generate team activity and cohesion around identifying and solving problems. By focusing on impact, solutions, and products research leaders described how they were then able to facilitate the team to work on problem solving and not necessarily rushing to solutions and closing off debate, inquiry, and discussion. This meant that knowledge translation theory did not necessarily 'drive' the way that teams began to understand what they were doing; it was used by research leads to explain what was happening at different levels of problem solving. Using integrated knowledge translation and co-design language and methods was seen as part of the continuous cycle of collaborative working necessary for influencing, implementing, and evaluating the impact of introducing new knowledge into systems, processes, and to partners.

Altogether, research leaders described their approaches to shaping team understanding of knowledge translation as emergent, facilitative, and guided by asking questions about the nature of the problem the team were exploring and then using knowledge translation theories, models, and frameworks to explain the underlying constructs.

From single discipline thinking to multiple perspectives – discovering transdisciplinary ways of thinking

Keeping team members focused on the problem and bringing diverse perspectives and skills to the process were skills that all research leaders talked about. Leaders did acknowledge that although discipline-specific knowledge may be needed – it also required the ability of team members to broaden their perspectives. These skills were seen as essential for leaders who had to engage in exploring their own perspectives, ways of thinking, knowing, and doing to demonstrate how they work across and beyond disciplinary boundaries. As one research leader observed, it was important to be able to work beyond health disciplines, embracing multiple perspectives to developing relevant products and services that meet consumer needs.

Research leaders also talked about 'democratising' knowledge, getting it to people who need it, and broadening it from the 'academic' mindset. This suggests that the knowledge translation skill set of engaging partners to identify the problem, co-design the solution(s), and then work together to implement and evaluate the proposed solutions would be intrinsic to effective leadership of interdisciplinary research teams.

What the literature says about a research leader's role in developing team understanding of knowledge translation

This reflective conversation with research leaders illustrates the challenges facing them in terms of where and how they developed their own competencies around integrated knowledge translation and then how in turn they facilitate that learning in their teams. The need to generate appropriate educational programs to equip research producers, users, and broker roles has been recognised with several significant programs being developed (Padek et al., 2015; Proctor et al., 2013) along with evaluations (Douglas et al., 2010) and emerging competency frameworks (Cassidy et al., 2021). However, the need for research leader support would seem still to be significant as described by (Thijsen et al., 2024).

Thijsen et al. (2024) undertook an international survey of researchers working in the specialism of transfusion medicine and found that although the researchers all agreed that knowledge translation was important and they felt responsible for doing it, they lacked the requisite skills and didn't know what to do. They tended to rely on traditional ways of knowledge sharing (dissemination at conferences and publications) although they knew these were not as effective as engaging more proactively with potential partners. Researchers who had experienced some level of knowledge translation training were more likely to design more tailored dissemination strategies and engage with end-users.

Proctor et al. (2013) work on developing and evaluating training for researchers in implementation science methods identified seven core elements to their program. Along with covering the theoretical basis of implementation science, selecting appropriate theories, models and frameworks, critiquing practice-change methodologies, and ensuring ethical approaches, they also acknowledged the need for training in context assessment, evaluating organisation support and engaging with key partners. What they also promoted was a strong mentoring and peer support approach between the research faculty (experienced research leads) and the program participants. This notion of learning from doing is also a common feature of several of the initiatives.

Attempts to describe core competencies for integrated knowledge translation have generated lists of generic skills and attributes targeted at both knowledge producers and knowledge users. Mallidou et al. (2018) identified 19 core competencies divided into three key categories of knowledge, skills and attitudes. Generic knowledge competencies across relevant groups (knowledge producers and knowledge users) included the ability to understand context, know about research processes and knowledge sharing, know how to generate and use evidence resources, be familiar with implementation approaches. Under skills Mallidou et al. (2018) identified the ability to work effectively in teams, assume leadership positions, share knowledge appropriately, know how to synthesise, disseminate and use research as well as be familiar with innovation and knowledge brokering skills. Attitudinal competences included confidence, trust, valuing research, lifelong learning and valuing teamwork. They recommended the generation and use of tools that could train and evaluate competencies as they developed. What they didn't discuss was who was responsible for making sure the competencies were developed and how they would then contribute to the success (or otherwise) of the proposed projects.

Yeung et al. (2021) looked at the knowledge producer and knowledge user competencies separately and under three common themes they identified a total of 48 competencies, 28 attributed to researchers and research teams and 18 for knowledge users. Table 9.2 summarises these competencies illustrating the distinct competencies for researchers, the areas of overlap and what distinct competencies are expected from knowledge users.

What is becoming increasingly clear is that embracing an integrated knowledge translation approach as a research leader requires very distinct and deliberate ways to embed this philosophy as well as understand how to begin the learning journey. The research leaders' own learning journeys were experiential; therefore, they (apart from one expert knowledge translation researcher) were not familiar with the structured learning required. It is also the case that the expertise across and within research institutions to undertake

Table 9.2 Overview of knowledge producer and knowledge user competencies

Knowledge producer competencies	Knowledge user competencies
Technical (evidence) domain	
1. Understand how different types of knowledge are generated and used 2. Apply appropriate research methodologies accounting for settings and groups 3. Design appropriate plans for evaluation, impact, effectiveness and sustainability 4. Respond to partners regarding evidence to inform decision making 5. Incorporate partner perspectives into research and implementation cycle 6. Select appropriate theory, framework or model 7. Help transform clinical/managerial/policy questions into research questions	1. Apply different types of knowledge to inform decision making. 2. Identify needs and priorities 3. Understand impact of local system factors that inform decisions (context)
Teamwork	
1. Use effective communication strategies within context 2. Use effective strategies to set priorities, manage conflict 3. Evaluate impact of knowledge brokers and connect evidence to impact 4. Promote appropriate behaviours and attitudes working with marginalised groups 5. Promote sustainable working relationships 6. Advocate for appropriate change/action 7. Form collaborative networks 8. Implement actionable strategies	1. Healthy teamworking relations 2. Foster productive networks within research and knowledge user groups 3. Promote formal and informal knowledge sharing 4. Role model appropriate behaviours with diverse group 5. Value/contribute to knowledge sharing 6. Advocate for knowledge user inclusivity
Knowledge translation activities	
1. Identify most appropriate approach to promoting effective knowledge to action in context 2. Develop/prioritise steps in dissemination plan within research design 3. Consider individual, organisational and system barriers and enablers 4. Develop a knowledge translation plan 5. Incorporate patient values into knowledge translation plans 6. Conduct partner analysis to gauge interest 7. Collaborate with policy/practice decision makers – synthesising/tailoring messages 8. Develop way to package evidence successfully 9. Identify knowledge translation roles and responsibilities 10. Design knowledge translation strategies that include program/organisational level knowledge translation 11. Use appropriate tools to support knowledge production processes	1. Address barriers and enablers in knowledge application 2. Interact with knowledge brokers/facilitators to increase implementation success 3. Identify evidence/practice gaps 4. Identify inconsistencies in practice 5. Involve patient perspectives 6. Appropriate patient involvement 7. Effective use of outcome data for evaluation/improvement activity 8. Adapt evidence to local context 9. Understand resource implications

Source: Adapted from Yeung et al. (2021).

this training is often not sufficient to meet the need (Thijsen et al., 2024). This means that from a team capacity building perspective research leaders ought to think about using knowledge translation projects as case studies from which to learn about effective knowledge translation activity and team learning.

This is why we have included a range of short case studies in Chapter 5 to illustrate how researchers at various career stages, along with their partners, learned on the job. Each of the case studies tells a story of hypothesis testing, reflection, retesting, data collection, synthesis, and then checking to see whether the outcome was achieved as expected. The challenges in negotiating practice change, managing the multiple partners and taking account of the context and culture are all essential dimensions for even novice applied researchers to consider. What is important is that they develop a confidence to describe these behavioural and contextual factors in ways that enrich and shed light onto the social and interpersonal processes at work in any knowledge translation enterprise.

Both the planning template in the implementation chapter (Chapter 2) and the partner template used in Chapter 3 provide structured ways for early and mid-career researchers, and all team members, to hone their assessment and engagement skills just in the same way as they are refining their research methods and systematic reviewing skills. It would seem that foundational knowledge translation skills are around understanding who the key partners are and know how best to engage them (**Connect**); the local and broader system context and its impact on the evidence/innovation being introduced (**Customise**); how to bring diverse voices together to come up with solutions to shared problems (**Co-create**); knowing how to choose the right implementation model or framework that will increase chances of successful implementation (**Clarify**); and finally making sure that there are appropriate process and evaluation mechanisms to provide credible feedback on the activity (**Confirm**). these five core elements are described in Chapter 8.

What research and implementation teams are keen to achieve is that any improvements are not only sustained, but that there are mechanisms that help teams, units, organisations, and system build on and spread the innovation. This leads to a dynamic reaction to the original engagement. This objective connects back to our description of integrated knowledge translation being linked to complexity science thinking: considering the active engagement of the nodes, hubs, clusters, networks and systems, one can begin to imagined the synergistic effects of different actors coming together to generate a shared understanding of how to tackle a problem, how to get everyone involved and understanding their role and then to continuously test out in small cycles of improvement how things might get better.

What and how early and mid-career applied researchers and team members learn about knowledge translation is still a bit of a 'hit and miss' experience. We have tried to illustrate in this book – and unpack further in this chapter – that if we are able to use the research processes from the Knowledge Translation Complexity Network Model, we will be able to identify the skill and competencies needed to combine good research with good integrated knowledge translation approaches. This endeavour requires that the research leaders understand the contribution integrated knowledge translation makes to research impact and that engaging different partners applies as much to internal research teams and disciplines, as it does to external partners. The next part of this chapter is on how research leaders champion integrated knowledge translation at organisational level and how they align integrated knowledge translation approaches to embracing more explicit transdisciplinary research leadership skills.

Integrated knowledge translation and transdisciplinary leadership

Embedding integrated knowledge translation into the research culture

Before research leaders can effectively champion an integrated knowledge translation agenda in their own work and in their organisation, there needs to be an alignment between the values and vision of the research enterprise and the philosophy of integrated knowledge translation. This often takes the shape of clear vision and mission statements of an organisation, linked to a set of values that promote diversity, inclusivity, and impact. One example of this is the way the Caring Futures Institute established its Knowledge Translation Platform as one of the key platforms of the Institute and used the Knowledge Translation Complexity Network Model as the organising framework to illustrate how teams work together to improve networking and learning opportunities. Figure 9.5 summarises what we did.

Other studies of how knowledge translation approaches are best enabled between organisational partners have focused on two major initiatives. One is the exploration of how effective transdisciplinary research teams are established and operate to ensure better impact because the partners are all working together bringing diverse skills and perspectives to the problem(s) under investigation (Choi & Pak, 2006; Emmons et al., 2008; Hall et al., 2008). This field of enquiry was embraced by the National Institutes of Health in the US from the early 2000s and a lot of investment went into understanding how research teams shift from single, to multidisciplinary to interdisciplinary perspectives, and then how in turn they learn to understand what it means to move from interdisciplinary working to embracing an integrative transdisciplinary approach.

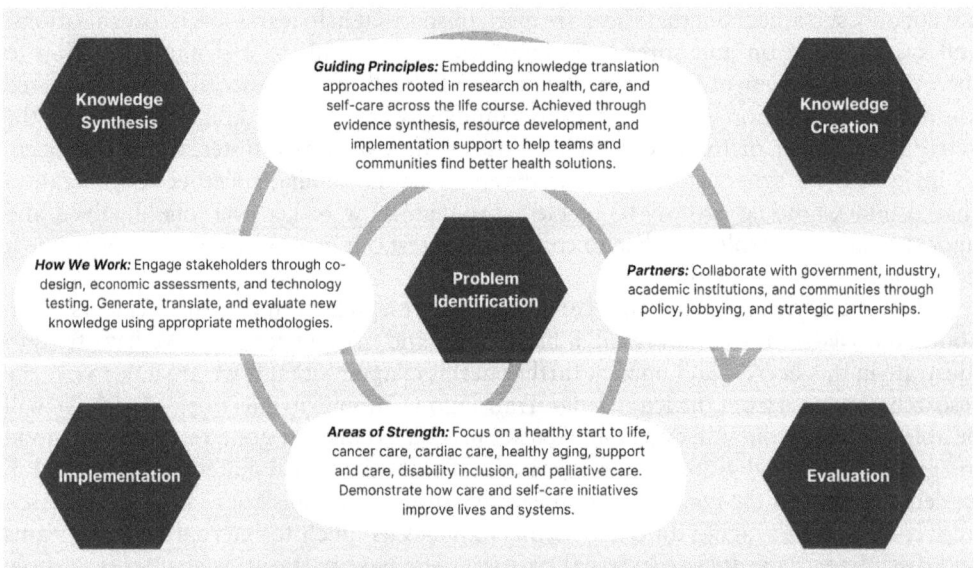

Figure 9.5 How the Caring Futures Institute is establishing its knowledge translation platform.
Source: https://doi.org/10.25451/flinders.29192837.v1

The other trend in the research literature has been the national evaluations of strategies such as the Collaborations for Leadership in Applied Health Research and Care programs, which were funded by National Institute of Health Research in England in 2008 and 2014. This initiative was generated to test how bringing knowledge producers (academic and research institutions) together with knowledge users (health service providers across acute, sub-acute and community services) could improve collaborations, and improve the uptake of research evidence into practice. In an early analysis Kislov et al. (2014) found that such partnerships needed to adopt an intentional capacity development approach if they were to be successful and adopting a practice-based, multi-level approach to capacity building, developing new competencies, and helping partners understand and work with complexity. They generated four working principles which they argued led to more productive collaboration between individuals, teams and groups that had not worked together before. These included embracing a continuous learning and development approach to capacity building; promoting active, continuous, and engaged learning rather than passive, rote, and didactic approaches; focusing on what the authors termed 'higher order' adaptation, absorption, and innovation skills rather than passive, transactional skills; and, finally, understanding the transitions or mechanisms between individual, group (team), and organisational learning. They promoted the idea of knowledge mobilisation experts as individuals who know how to move knowledge across boundaries. Their role would be to provide resources, facilitate learning, create opportunities for exchange, provide mentorship and support, be expert in knowledge translation activities, and be knowledgeable about theories, frameworks, and models that help staff integrate old and new knowledge. They suggested that three ways to enhance effectiveness was to use improvement methodologies to generate change; to support how knowledge shifts from 'new' to 'routine' in organisations; and to help make sense and manage different contexts.

A further review conducted by the same team focused on describing and exploring the early partnerships, vision, values, structures, and processes of the Collaboration for Leadership in Applied Health Research and Care programs; the nature and role of boundaries; how knowledge brokers and hybrid roles supported knowledge mobilisation; how patient and the public were involved; and capacity building (Kislov et al., 2018). They found that despite the significant investment evidence was lacking on the impact of the Collaboration for Leadership in Applied Health Research and Care programs particularly in relation to the knowledge mobilisation processes and practices adopted. Another review (Lockett et al., 2014) investigated identified five different archetypal models that the researchers observed in the ways that research producers and users interacted with one another. These ranged on a continuum from purposeful and deliberate integration of multidisciplinary teams to centralised command and control of activity and engagement.

What these two bodies of work tell us is that knowing how to effectively move knowledge across organisations and between partners is a complex activity. It's also deeply social, interactive, requiring engagement at multiple levels of organisations. Approaches need to be flexible to accommodate different contexts and cultures, power dynamics, and values. This also means that the research leaders who are going to be responsible for generating such programs need to have a deep understanding of some of the skills and competencies they will need to lead their teams and engage diverse groups.

This is where our final case study can be shared. It was the study undertaken by a knowledge translation team embedded in a National Health and Medical Research Council-funded Centre of Research Excellence in Frailty and Healthy Ageing, which I mentioned before (Ambagtsheer et al., 2022). In addition to the actual work of helping consumers and research staff come to a shared understanding of the problem being explored, the knowledge translation team also undertook a longitudinal evaluation of how the transdisciplinary research team learnt how to work together and how they embraced concepts of knowledge translation (Archibald et al., 2023). The ability to become an effective transdisciplinary research leader was found to relate to three key dimensions: general leadership capacity and capability; being a facilitative leader; and embracing the principles of integrated knowledge translation. These three dimensions were further refined in the research to show how effective transdisciplinary research leadership could be done. Figure 9.6 summarises what the research found.

Effective transdisciplinary leaders showed high level capability and competence in knowing how to navigate, negotiate and mobilise the networks they were operating in. Put simply, transdisciplinary research leaders seemed to be embracing many of the integrated knowledge translation techniques we have talked about in this book. Certainly, the journey the leaders and team members described showed that they matured in their

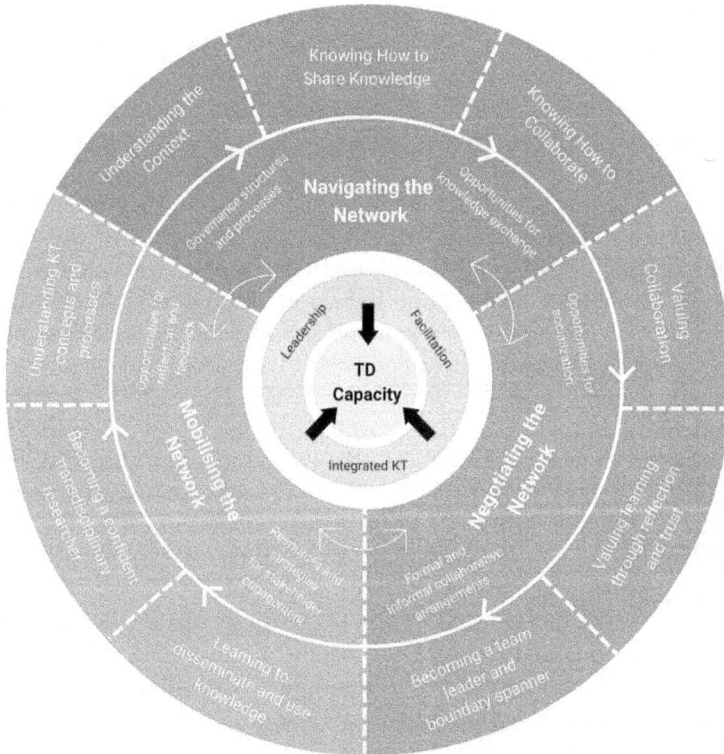

Figure 9.6 How transdisciplinary teams learn how to do knowledge translation; TD = transdisciplinary; KT = knowledge translation.
Source: Archibald et al. 2023.

understanding of both transdisciplinary leadership skills as well as an appreciation of how these skills could be used in knowledge translation activities.

They were using the formal governance and structure processes of their research program to facilitate a greater understanding of the context, embracing partner diversity and multiple ways of communicating the problems and ways to solve them, as well as creating open and respectful ways to collaborate. This was identified as their ability to '**navigate the network**'.

Transdisciplinary research leaders also knew how to '**negotiate the network**' which entailed them facilitating and influencing multiple formal and informal collaboration arrangements, role modelling how to work across discipline, geographic and other boundaries, as well as encouraging skills around reflection, critical thinking, and developing trusting relationships.

The ability of transdisciplinary research leaders to actively and consciously manage individual and social relationships as represented in networks we referred to as '**mobilise their networks**'. This mobilisation work involved them using resources and strategies for proactive partner engagement and for continuous reflection and learning for all members of the research team and those involved in the research activity. This meant that the products of the research enterprise were not just the 'results' but that the whole research process was one of productivity in that it shaped, moulded, and changed research teams' understanding of and ability to respond to the problem they were exploring.

The challenges of leading high-performing transdisciplinary research teams who embrace the concepts inherent in integrated knowledge translation (including problem identification, partner involvement, co-design, appropriate product development and implementation and evaluation) should not be underestimated. The good news is that we have demonstrated that research leaders from a series of diverse backgrounds can come together and share common experiences around how they moved from implicit to explicit ways of understanding and talking about knowledge translation. They were able to use different knowledge translation models and frameworks to help in their own conceptualisation, often moving from linear, directive models to models that were more multidimensional and attempted to describe the complexity of knowledge generation and implementation.

What has become clear is that effective leadership for integrated knowledge translation occurs at multiple, interconnected levels. Figure 9.7 distils the findings from recent studies (Archibald et al., 2023; Lawless et al., 2024; Mallidou et al., 2018; Yeung et al., 2021) illustrating three overlapping domains of leadership competencies required for integrated knowledge translation at the individual, team/organisational, and system levels. Effective research leaders combine skills like reflexivity, relational and adaptive leadership, draw on systems thinking to navigate uncertainty, foster inclusive and productive teams, and influence change within and across systems.

Summary: bringing the leadership threads together

This has been a complex story. It has started with the proposition that much of our own understanding of knowledge translation approaches as they relate to research leadership is based on our own experiences – the discipline we come from, our beliefs about how knowledge is generated and who should be involved, our formal and informal experiences and training, and our track record of successes and failures in attempting to get new knowledge into policy and practice. My own experiential journey and its impact

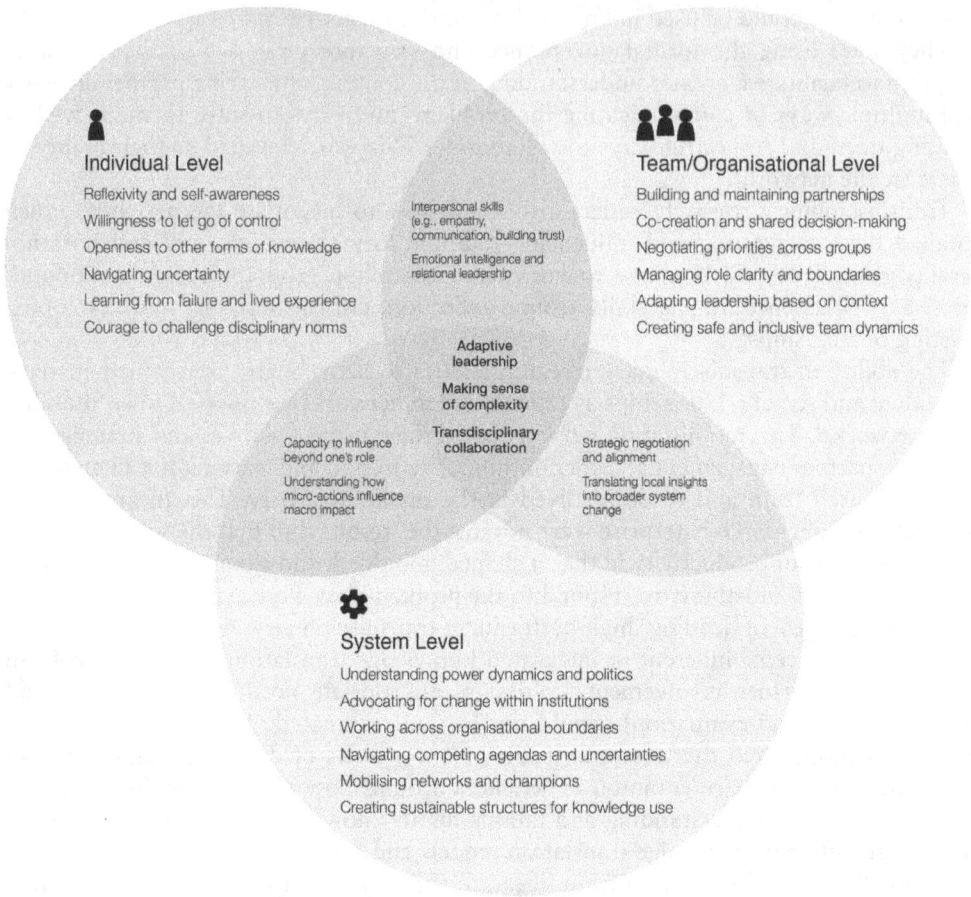

Individual Level

Reflexivity and self-awareness
Willingness to let go of control
Openness to other forms of knowledge
Navigating uncertainty
Learning from failure and lived experience
Courage to challenge disciplinary norms

Interpersonal skills
(e.g., empathy,
communication, building trust)

Emotional intelligence and
relational leadership

Team/Organisational Level

Building and maintaining partnerships
Co-creation and shared decision-making
Negotiating priorities across groups
Managing role clarity and boundaries
Adapting leadership based on context
Creating safe and inclusive team dynamics

Adaptive
leadership

Making sense
of complexity

Capacity to influence
beyond one's role

Transdisciplinary
collaboration

Strategic negotiation
and alignment

Understanding how
micro-actions influence
macro impact

Translating local insights
into broader system
change

System Level

Understanding power dynamics and politics
Advocating for change within institutions
Working across organisational boundaries
Navigating competing agendas and uncertainties
Mobilising networks and champions
Creating sustainable structures for knowledge use

Figure 9.7 Leadership competencies for integrated knowledge translation across system levels.
Source: https://doi.org/10.25451/flinders.29192840.v1

on me was confirmed by the conversations I had with research leader colleagues who also shared how their understanding of knowledge translation and the way they subsequently supported their teams was based on their experiences.

What was less clear from the literature was how research leaders are being supported to embrace this important dimension in their skill and competence repertoire. Much work has been done to describe what integrated knowledge translation is (Gagliardi et al., 2017), how it is associated with other research approaches, and particular with co-design, participatory action research, and engaged scholarship (Nguyen et al., 2020), and the range of competencies and skill sets for knowledge producers and users. But less information is available to guide and support the research leaders. We have acknowledged the contribution of team science and transdisciplinary work as well as larger evaluations of whole systems partnerships. Still the evidence is equivocal – we're not sure how we can move this complex but necessary leadership agenda forward. What we are proposing in this book is that by consciously and deliberately stating that our way of conceptualizing integrated knowledge translation through the lens of the Knowledge Translation Complexity Network Model that we can begin to evaluate the elements that are needed to build and develop more explicit learning materials, better mentoring and networking processes, better tools and evaluation processes.

These would include that shift from a discipline dominated way of thinking to sharing a common vision, defining, and solving a problem and making an impact. Looking for rich diversity in team members, making sure the problem is understood from multiple perspectives and holding people back from thinking they know the solution to the problem were all leadership characteristics that were identified. The focus on impact is essential, making sure that the new knowledge does not sit within a disciplinary boundary. Research leaders who champion integrated knowledge translation need to be multitalented interpreters of networks, nuances, and negotiations. They need to be pragmatic, flexible, strategic, and facilitative. They need to be able to train teams to be mentally agile, receptive to multiple ideas, and be great at diagnosing what's important and what's not. They need to role model how to work across boundaries and be clear about how they articulate impact in any research endeavour to all parties involved. They need to be able to **Connect, Clarify, Customise, Co-Create** and **Confirm** intentions and actions across complex adaptive systems (Chapter 8).

We have intentionally embedded knowledge translation as an enabling theme into the structure of our research institute. We are role modelling research leadership practices that celebrate diversity and challenge in teams. We are working on education programs that build on the scaffolding of this book. We are taking a principle and inquiry-based approach to learning; as well as completing the research tasks, novice researchers are encouraged to think outside the box, to feel comfortable with not knowing the answer and to be okay that multiple partners may provide them with conflicting interpretations of the problem.

Our research culture is vibrant and dynamic, in no small part due to our leadership commitment to navigate this knowledge translation pathway. We hope that by sharing our journey you will be inspired to continue your journey towards research leadership for knowledge translation leadership excellence. In the final chapter of the book, we will identify some additional challenges to the field of integrated knowledge translation.

References

Aarons, G. A., Ehrhart, M. G., & Farahnak, L. R. (2014). The implementation leadership scale (ILS): Development of a brief measure of unit level implementation leadership. *Implementation Science, 9*(1), 45. https://doi.org/10.1186/1748-5908-9-45

Aarons, G. A., Ehrhart, M. G., Farahnak, L. R., & Sklar, M. (2014). Aligning leadership across systems and organizations to develop a strategic climate for evidence-based practice implementation. *Annual Review of Public Health, 35*(2014), 255–274. https://doi.org/10.1146/annurev-pub lhealth-032013-182447

Aarons, G. A., Reeder, K., Miller, C. J., & Stadnick, N. A. (2020). Identifying strategies to promote team science in dissemination and implementation research. *Journal of Clinical and Translational Science, 4*(3), 180–187. https://doi.org/10.1017/cts.2019.413

Ambagtsheer, R., Archibald, M. M., Lawless, M., Mills, D., Yu, S., & Beilby, J. J. (2019). General practitioners' perceptions, attitudes and experiences of frailty and frailty screening. *Australian Journal of General Practice, 48*(7), 426–433. https://doi.org/10.31128/ajgp-11-18-4757

Ambagtsheer, R., Visvanathan, R., Cesari, M., Yu, S., Archibald, M., Schultz, T., Karnon, J., Kitson, A., & Beilby, J. (2017). Feasibility, acceptability and diagnostic test accuracy of frailty screening instruments in community-dwelling older people within the Australian general practice setting: A study protocol for a cross-sectional study. *BMJ Open*, 7(8), e016663. https://doi.org/10.1136/bmjopen-2017-016663

Ambagtsheer, R. C., Casey, M. G., Lawless, M., Archibald, M. M., Yu, S., Kitson, A., & Beilby, J. J. (2022). Practitioner perceptions of the feasibility of common frailty screening instruments within general practice settings: A mixed methods study. *BMC Primary Care*, 23(1), 160. https://doi.org/10.1186/s12875-022-01778-9

Archibald, M., Ambagtsheer, R., Beilby, J., Chehade, M. J., Gill, T. K., Visvanathan, R., & Kitson, A. L. (2017). Perspectives of frailty and frailty screening: Protocol for a collaborative knowledge translation approach and qualitative study of stakeholder understandings and experiences. *BMC Geriatrics*, 17(1), 87. https://doi.org/10.1186/s12877-017-0483-7

Archibald, M., Kitson, A., Frewin, D., & Visvanathan, R. (2017). Transdisciplinary research in frailty: Knowledge translation to inform new models of care. *Journal of Frailty & Aging*, 6(2), 62–64. https://doi.org/10.14283/jfa.2017.6

Archibald, M., Lawless, M., Ambagtsheer, R. C., & Kitson, A. (2020). Older adults' understandings and perspectives on frailty in community and residential aged care: An interpretive description. *BMJ Open*, 10(3), e035339. https://doi.org/10.1136/bmjopen-2019-035339

Archibald, M., Lawless, M., Gill, T. K., & Chehade, M. J. (2020). Orthopaedic surgeons' perceptions of frailty and frailty screening. *BMC Geriatrics*, 20(1), 17. https://doi.org/10.1186/s12877-019-1404-8

Archibald, M., Lawless, M., Harvey, G., & Kitson, A. L. (2018). Transdisciplinary research for impact: Protocol for a realist evaluation of the relationship between transdisciplinary research collaboration and knowledge translation. *BMJ Open*, 8(4), e021775. https://doi.org/10.1136/bmjopen-2018-021775

Archibald, M., Lawless, M. T., de Plaza, M. A. P., & Kitson, A. L. (2023). How transdisciplinary research teams learn to do knowledge translation (KT), and how KT in turn impacts transdisciplinary research: A realist evaluation and longitudinal case study. *Health Research Policy and Systems*, 21(1), 20–20. https://doi.org/10.1186/s12961-023-00967-x

Baloh, J., Zhu, X., & Ward, M. M. (2018). Types of internal facilitation activities in hospitals implementing evidence-based interventions. *Health Care Management Review*, 43(3). https://journals.lww.com/hcmrjournal/fulltext/2018/07000/types_of_internal_facilitation_activities_in.6.aspx

Bate, P., & Robert, G. (2006). Experience-based design: From redesigning the system around the patient to co-designing services with the patient. *Quality and Safety in Health Care*, 15(5), 307. https://doi.org/10.1136/qshc.2005.016527

Begerowski, S. R., Traylor, A. M., Shuffler, M. L., & Salas, E. (2021). An integrative review and practical guide to team development interventions for translational science teams: One size does not fit all. *Journal of Clinical and Translational Science*, 5(1), e198, Article e198. https://doi.org/10.1017/cts.2021.832

Bergström, A., Ehrenberg, A., Eldh, A. C., Graham, I. D., Gustafsson, K., Harvey, G., Hunter, S., Kitson, A., Rycroft-Malone, J., & Wallin, L. (2020). The use of the PARIHS framework in implementation research and practice-a citation analysis of the literature. *Implementation Science*, 15(1), 68. https://doi.org/10.1186/s13012-020-01003-0

Bidassie, B., Williams, L. S., Woodward-Hagg, H., Matthias, M. S., & Damush, T. M. (2015). Key components of external facilitation in an acute stroke quality improvement collaborative in the Veterans Health Administration. *Implementation Science*, 10(1), 69. https://doi.org/10.1186/s13012-015-0252-y

Birken, S. A., DiMartino, L. D., Kirk, M. A., Lee, S.-Y. D., McClelland, M., & Albert, N. M. (2016). Elaborating on theory with middle managers' experience implementing healthcare innovations in practice. *Implementation Science*, 11(1), 2. https://doi.org/10.1186/s13012-015-0362-6

Bowen, S., Botting, I., Graham, I. D., MacLeod, M., de Moissac, D., Harlos, K., Leduc, B., Ulrich, C., & Knox, J. (2019). Experience of health leadership in partnering with university-based researchers in Canada – A Call to "Re-imagine" Research. *International Journal of Health Policy and Management*, 8(12), 684–699. https://doi.org/10.15171/ijhpm.2019.66

Brook, A. H., Liversidge, H. M., Wilson, D., Jordan, Z., Harvey, G., Marshall, R. J., & Kitson, A. L. (2016). Health research, teaching and provision of care: Applying a new approach based on complex systems and a knowledge translation complexity network model. *International Journal of Design & Nature and Ecodynamics*, 11(4), 663–669. https://doi.org/10.2495/DNE-V11-N4-663-669

Bucknall, T. K., Considine, J., Harvey, G., Graham, I. D., Rycroft-Malone, J., Mitchell, I., Saultry, B., Watts, J. J., Mohebbi, M., Bohingamu Mudiyanselage, S., Lotfaliany, M., & Hutchinson, A. (2022). Prioritising Responses Of Nurses To deteriorating patient Observations (PRONTO): A pragmatic cluster randomised controlled trial evaluating the effectiveness of a facilitation intervention on recognition and response to clinical deterioration. *BMJ Quality & Safety*, 31(11), 818. https://doi.org/10.1136/bmjqs-2021-013785

Cassidy, C. E., Shin, H. D., Ramage, E., Conway, A., Mrklas, K., Laur, C., Beck, A., Varin, M. D., Steinwender, S., Nguyen, T., Langley, J., Dorey, R., Donnelly, L., & Ormel, I. (2021). Trainee-led research using an integrated knowledge translation or other research partnership approaches: A scoping review. *Health Research Policy and Systems*, 19(1), 135. https://doi.org/10.1186/s12961-021-00784-0

Chan, R. J., Knowles, R., Hunter, S., Conroy, T., Tieu, M., & Kitson, A. (2023). From Evidence-based practice to knowledge translation: What is the difference? What are the roles of nurse leaders? *Seminars in Oncology Nursing*, 39(1), 151363. https://doi.org/10.1016/j.soncn.2022.151363

Choi, B. C., & Pak, A. W. (2006). Multidisciplinarity, interdisciplinarity and transdisciplinarity in health research, services, education and policy: 1. Definitions, objectives, and evidence of effectiveness. *Clinical and Investigative Medicine*, 29(6), 351–364.

Dent, E., Hoon, E., Kitson, A., Karnon, J., Newbury, J., Harvey, G., Gill, T. K., Gillis, L., & Beilby, J. (2016). Translating a health service intervention into a rural setting: Lessons learned. *BMC Health Services Research*, 16(1), 62. https://doi.org/10.1186/s12913-016-1302-0

Dogherty, E. J., Harrison, M. B., & Graham, I. D. (2010). Facilitation as a role and process in achieving evidence-based practice in nursing: A focused review of concept and meaning. *Worldviews on Evidence-Based Nursing*, 7(2), 76–89. https://doi.org/https://doi.org/10.1111/j.1741-6787.2010.00186.x

Douglas, F. C., Gray, D. A., & van Teijlingen, E. R. (2010). Using a realist approach to evaluate smoking cessation interventions targeting pregnant women and young people. *BMC Health Services Research* , 10, 49. https://doi.org/10.1186/1472-6963-10-49

Emmons, K. M., Viswanath, K., & Colditz, G. A. (2008). The role of transdisciplinary collaboration in translating and disseminating health research: Lessons learned and exemplars of success. *American Journal of Preventive Medicine*, 35(2, Supplement), S204–S210. https://doi.org/https://doi.org/10.1016/j.amepre.2008.05.009

Fasugba, O., Cheng, H., Dale, S., Coughlan, K., McInnes, E., Cadilhac, D. A., Cheung, N. W., Hill, K., Page, K., Menendez, E. S., Neal, E., Pollnow, V., Slark, J., Gilder, E., Ranta, A., Levi, C., Grimshaw, J. M., & Middleton, S. (2025). Finding the right dose: A scoping review examining facilitation as an implementation strategy for evidence-based stroke care. *Implementation Science*, 20(1), 4. https://doi.org/10.1186/s13012-025-01415-w

Gagliardi, A. R., & Dobrow, M. J. (2016). Identifying the conditions needed for integrated knowledge translation (IKT) in health care organizations: Qualitative interviews with researchers and research users. *BMC Health Services Research*, 16(1), 256. https://doi.org/10.1186/s12913-016-1533-0

Gagliardi, A. R., Kothari, A., & Graham, I. D. (2017). Research agenda for integrated knowledge translation (IKT) in healthcare: What we know and do not yet know. *Journal of Epidemiology and Community Health (1979)*, 71(2), 105–106. https://doi.org/10.1136/jech-2016-207743

Glasgow, R. E., Harden, S. M., Gaglio, B., Rabin, B., Smith, M. L., & Porter, G. C. (2019). RE-AIM planning and evaluation framework: Adapting to new science and practice with a 20-year review. *Frontiers in Public Health* , 7, 64. https://doi.org/10.3389/fpubh.2019.00064

Glasgow, R. E., Vogt, T. M., & Boles, S. M. (1999). Evaluating the public health impact of health promotion interventions: The RE-AIM framework. *American Journal of Public Health (1971)*, 89(9), 1322–1327. https://doi.org/10.2105/AJPH.89.9.1322

Graham, I. D., Logan, J., Harrison, M. B., Straus, S. E., Tetroe, J., Caswell, W., & Robinson, N. (2006). Lost in knowledge translation: Time for a map? *The Journal of Continuing Education in the Health Professions*, 26(1), 13–24. https://doi.org/10.1002/chp.47

Greenhalgh, T., & Wieringa, S. (2011). Is it time to drop the 'knowledge translation' metaphor? A critical literature review. *Journal of the Royal Society of Medicine*, 104(12), 501–509. https://doi.org/10.1258/jrsm.2011.110285

Hall, K. L., Feng, A. X., Moser, R. P., Stokols, D., & Taylor, B. K. (2008). Moving the science of team science forward: Collaboration and creativity. *American Journal of Preventive Medicine*, 35(2 Suppl), S243–249. https://doi.org/10.1016/j.amepre.2008.05.007

Harvey, G., Collyer, S., McRae, P., Barrimore, S. E., Demmitt, C., Lee-Steere, K., Nolan, B., & Mudge, A. M. (2023). Navigating the facilitation journey: A qualitative, longitudinal evaluation of 'Eat Walk Engage' novice and experienced facilitators. *BMC Health Services Research*, 23(1), 1132. https://doi.org/10.1186/s12913-023-10116-3

Harvey, G., Gifford, W., Cummings, G., Kelly, J., Kislov, R., Kitson, A., Pettersson, L., Wallin, L., Wilson, P., & Ehrenberg, A. (2019). Mobilising evidence to improve nursing practice: A qualitative study of leadership roles and processes in four countries. *International Journal of Nursing Studies*, 90, 21–30. https://doi.org/10.1016/j.ijnurstu.2018.09.017

Harvey, G., & Kitson, A. (2016). PARIHS revisited: From heuristic to integrated framework for the successful implementation of knowledge into practice. *Implementation Science: IS*, 11(1), 33–33. https://doi.org/10.1186/s13012-016-0398-2

Harvey, G., & Kitson, A. L. (2015). *Implementing Evidence-based Practice in Healthcare: A Facilitation Guide*. Routledge. https://doi.org/10.4324/9780203557334

Harvey, G., Marshall, R. J., Jordan, Z., & Kitson, A. L. (2015). Exploring the hidden barriers in knowledge translation: A case study within an academic community. *Qualitative Health Research*, 25(11), 1506–1517. https://doi.org/10.1177/1049732315580300

Hoekstra, F., Mrklas, K. J., Khan, M., McKay, R. C., Vis-Dunbar, M., Sibley, K. M., Nguyen, T., Graham, I. D., Anderson, K., Anton, H., Athanasopoulos, P., Chernesky, J., Forwell, S., Maffin, J., Martin Ginis, K., McBride, C. B., Mortenson, B., Willms, R., Gainforth, H. L., & Panel, S. C. I. G. P. C. (2020). A review of reviews on principles, strategies, outcomes and impacts of research partnerships approaches: A first step in synthesising the research partnership literature. *Health Research Policy and Systems*, 18(1), 51. https://doi.org/10.1186/s12961-020-0544-9

Hoon-Leahy, C. E., Newbury, J., Kitson, A., Whitford, D., Wilson, A., Karnon, J., Baker, J., Jamrozik, K., & Beilby, J. (2012). The LINKIN Health Census process: Design and implementation. *BMC Health Services Research*, 12(1), 321. https://doi.org/10.1186/1472-6963-12-321

Hunter, S. C., Kim, B., & Kitson, A. L. (2020). Interactive workshop to develop implementation framework (i-PARIHS) resources to support practice facilitation. *Implementation Science Communication*, 1, 56. https://doi.org/10.1186/s43058-020-00046-0

Hunter, S. C., Kim, B., & Kitson, A. L. (2023). Mobilising implementation of i-PARIHS (Mi-PARIHS): Development of a facilitation planning tool to accompany the Integrated Promoting Action on Research Implementation in Health Services framework. *Implementation Science Communication*, 4(1), 2. https://doi.org/10.1186/s43058-022-00379-y

Hunter, S. C., Kim, B., Mudge, A., Hall, L., Young, A., McRae, P., & Kitson, A. L. (2020). Experiences of using the i-PARIHS framework: A co-designed case study of four multi-site implementation projects. *BMC Health Services Research*, 20(1), 573–573. https://doi.org/10.1186/s12913-020-05354-8

Hunter, S. C., Morgillo, S., Kim, B., Bergström, A., Ehrenberg, A., Eldh, A. C., Wallin, L., & Kitson, A. L. (2025). Combined use of the integrated-Promoting Action on Research Implementation in Health Services (i-PARIHS) framework with other implementation frameworks: A systematic review. *Implementation Science Communications*, 6(1), 25. https://doi.org/10.1186/s43058-025-00704-1

Kislov, R., Waterman, H., Harvey, G., & Boaden, R. (2014). Rethinking capacity building for knowledge mobilisation: Developing multilevel capabilities in healthcare organisations. *Implementation Science*, 9(1), 166. https://doi.org/10.1186/s13012-014-0166-0

Kislov, R., Wilson, P. M., Knowles, S., & Boaden, R. (2018). Learning from the emergence of NIHR Collaborations for Leadership in Applied Health Research and Care (CLAHRCs): A systematic review of evaluations. *Implementation Science*, 13(1), 111. https://doi.org/10.1186/s13012-018-0805-y

Kitson, A. (1986). Indicators of quality in nursing care — an alternative approach. *Journal of Advanced Nursing*, 11(2), 133–144. https://doi.org/10.1111/j.1365-2648.1986.tb01231.x

Kitson, A. (1987). A comparative analysis of lay-caring and professional (nursing) caring relationships. *International Journal of Nursing Studies*, 24(2), 155–165. https://doi.org/10.1016/0020-7489(87)90057-5

Kitson, A. (1991). *Therapeutic Nursing and the Hospitalized Elderly*. Scutari.

Kitson, A., Ahmed, L. B., Harvey, G., Seers, K., & Thompson, D. R. (1996). From research to practice: One organizational model for promoting research-based practice. *Journal of Advanced Nursing*, 23(3), 430–440. https://doi.org/10.1111/j.1365-2648.1996.tb00003.x

Kitson, A., Brook, A., Harvey, G., Jordan, Z., Marshall, R., O'Shea, R., & Wilson, D. (2018). Using complexity and network concepts to inform healthcare knowledge translation. *International Journal of Health Policy and Management*, 7(3), 231–243. https://doi.org/10.15171/ijhpm.2017.79

Kitson, A., Harvey, G., Gifford, W., Hunter, S. C., Kelly, J., Cummings, G. G., Ehrenberg, A., Kislov, R., Pettersson, L., Wallin, L., & Wilson, P. (2021). How nursing leaders promote evidence-based practice implementation at point-of-care: A four-country exploratory study. *Journal of Advanced Nursing*, 77(5), 2447–2457. https://doi.org/10.1111/jan.14773

Kitson, A., Harvey, G., Hyndman, S., Sindhu, F., & Yerrell, P. (1994). *A Study of the Impact of Nursing Quality Assurance Package, the Dynamic Standard Setting System (DySSSy) on Nursing Practice and Patient Outcomes,* National Institute for Nursing reports. no. 4,vol.3,, 1–21..

Kitson, A., Harvey, G., Hyndman, S., & Yerrell, P. (1994). Criteria formulation and application: An evaluative framework. *International Journal of Nursing Studies*, 31(2), 155–167. https://doi.org/10.1016/0020-7489(94)90042-6

Kitson, A., Harvey, G., & McCormack, B. (1998). Enabling the implementation of evidence based practice: A conceptual framework. *Quality in Health Care*, 7(3), 149–158. https://doi.org/10.1136/qshc.7.3.149

Kitson, A., Powell, K., Hoon, E., Newbury, J., Wilson, A., & Beilby, J. (2013). Knowledge translation within a population health study: How do you do it? *Implementation Science: IS*, 8(1), 54–54. https://doi.org/10.1186/1748-5908-8-54

Kitson, A. L., & Harvey, G. (2016). Methods to succeed in effective knowledge translation in clinical practice. *Journal of Nursing Scholarship*, 48(3), 294–302. https://doi.org/10.1111/jnu.12206

Lawless, M., Archibald, M., Pinero de Plaza, M. A., Drioli-Phillips, P., & Kitson, A. (2020). Peer-to-peer health communication in older adults' online communities: Protocol for a qualitative netnographic study and co-design approach. *JMIR Research Protocol*, 9(9), e19834. https://doi.org/10.2196/19834

Lawless, M., Archibald, M. M., Ambagtsheer, R. C., & Kitson, A. L. (2020). Factors influencing communication about frailty in primary care: A scoping review. *Patient Education and Counseling*, 103(3), 436–450. https://doi.org/10.1016/j.pec.2019.09.014

Lawless, M., Drioli-Phillips, P., Archibald, M. M., & Kitson, A. L. (2020). Engaging older adults in self-management talk in healthcare encounters: A systematic review protocol. *Systematic Review, 9*(1), 15. https://doi.org/10.1186/s13643-020-1276-1

Lawless, M., Tieu, M., Archibald, M. M., Pinero De Plaza, M. A., & Kitson, A. L. (2024b). From promise to practice: How health researchers understand and promote transdisciplinary collaboration. *Qualitative Health Research, 35*(1), 3–16. https://doi.org/10.1177/10497323241235882

Lockett, A., El Enany, N., Currie, G., Oborn, E., Barrett, M., Racko, G., Bishop, S., & Waring, J. (2014). Health services and delivery research. In *A formative evaluation of Collaboration for Leadership in Applied Health Research and Care (CLAHRC): Institutional Entrepreneurship for Service Innovation.* NIHR Journals Library. https://pubmed.ncbi.nlm.nih.gov/25642535/

Lynch, E. A., Mudge, A., Knowles, S., Kitson, A. L., Hunter, S. C., & Harvey, G. (2018). "There is nothing so practical as a good theory": A pragmatic guide for selecting theoretical approaches for implementation projects. *BMC Health Services Research, 18*(1), 857–857. https://doi.org/10.1186/s12913-018-3671-z

Mallidou, A. A., Atherton, P., Chan, L., Frisch, N., Glegg, S., & Scarrow, G. (2018). Core knowledge translation competencies: A scoping review. *BMC Health Services Research, 18*(1), 502–502. https://doi.org/10.1186/s12913-018-3314-4

Michie, S., van Stralen, M. M., & West, R. (2011). The behaviour change wheel: A new method for characterising and designing behaviour change interventions. *Implementation Science, 6*(1), 42. https://doi.org/10.1186/1748-5908-6-42

National Health and Medical Research Council. (2023). *Centres of Research Excellence.* National Health and Medical Research Council. Retrieved 14 June from www.nhmrc.gov.au/funding/find-funding/centres-research-excellence

Nguyen, T., Graham, I. D., Mrklas, K. J., Bowen, S., Cargo, M., Estabrooks, C. A., Kothari, A., Lavis, J., MacAulay, A. C., MacLeod, M., Phipps, D., Ramsden, V. R., Renfrew, M. J., Salsberg, J., & Wallerstein, N. (2020). How does integrated knowledge translation (IKT) compare to other collaborative research approaches to generating and translating knowledge? Learning from experts in the field. *Health Research Policy and Systems, 18*(1), 35–35. https://doi.org/10.1186/s12961-020-0539-6

Padek, M., Colditz, G., Dobbins, M., Koscielniak, N., Proctor, E. K., Sales, A. E., & Brownson, R. C. (2015). Developing educational competencies for dissemination and implementation research training programs: An exploratory analysis using card sorts. *Implementation Science, 10*(1), 114. https://doi.org/10.1186/s13012-015-0304-3

Proctor, E. K., Landsverk, J., Baumann, A. A., Mittman, B. S., Aarons, G. A., Brownson, R. C., Glisson, C., & Chambers, D. (2013). The implementation research institute: Training mental health implementation researchers in the United States. *Implementation Science, 8*(1), 105. https://doi.org/10.1186/1748-5908-8-105

Ritchie, M. J., Parker, L. E., & Kirchner, J. E. (2021). From novice to expert: Methods for transferring implementation facilitation skills to improve healthcare delivery. *Implementation Science Communications, 2*(1), 39. https://doi.org/10.1186/s43058-021-00138-5

Spyridonidis, D., Hendy, J., & Barlow, J. (2015). Leadership for knowledge translation: The case of CLAHRCs. *Qualitative Health Research, 25*(11), 1492–1505. https://doi.org/10.1177/1049732315583268

Stetler, C. B., Legro, M. W., Rycroft-Malone, J., Bowman, C., Curran, G., Guihan, M., Hagedorn, H., Pineros, S., & Wallace, C. M. (2006). Role of "external facilitation" in implementation of research findings: A qualitative evaluation of facilitation experiences in the Veterans Health Administration. *Implementation Science, 1*(1), 23. https://doi.org/10.1186/1748-5908-1-23

Thijsen, A., Masser, B., Davison, T. E., & Williamson, A. (2024). Researchers' views on and practices of knowledge translation: An international survey of transfusion medicine researchers. *Implementation Science Communications, 5*(1), 9. https://doi.org/10.1186/s43058-024-00546-3

Ward, M. F., Titchen, A., Morrell, C., McCormack, B., & Kitson, A. (1998). Using a supervisory framework to support and evaluate a multiproject practice development programme. *Journal of Clinical Nurse*, 7(1), 29–36. https://doi.org/10.1046/j.1365-2702.1998.00135.x

Yeung, E., Scodras, S., Salbach, N. M., Kothari, A., & Graham, I. D. (2021). Identifying competencies for integrated knowledge translation: A Delphi study. *BMC Health Services Research*, 21(1), 1181. https://doi.org/10.1186/s12913-021-07107-7

Zych, M. M., Berta, W. B., & Gagliardi, A. R. (2020). Conceptualising the initiation of researcher and research user partnerships: A meta-narrative review. *Health Research Policy and Systems*, 18(1), 24. https://doi.org/10.1186/s12961-020-0536-9

10 Future proofing knowledge translation for policy and practice

Alison Kitson and Gill Harvey

Introduction

In this final chapter we shift from an institutional case study perspective to considering the potential trends shaping and influencing the art and science of integrated knowledge translation. We argue that future success in knowledge translation investment will require more transdisciplinary research leadership capability, more diversity in team composition and skill, and more capability around identifying and working with partners at each point of the research process. Underpinning such developments will be new research governance and accountability structures. Investment in much more training and development programs for knowledge producers, users and roles that connect the two worlds will be needed together with more diverse and fit-for-purpose designs that can accommodate complexity in both the interventions under investigation, as well as the contexts into which they are being introduced. This shift will require a move away from thinking of knowledge translation as a linear, logical flow of knowledge from one set of developers to others who will use it to, understanding the complex ebb and flow of knowledge within systems, and between individuals and teams in those systems.

Although stated many times, this reality has still to be acknowledged and accepted by many partners, and particularly those whose power and influence in systems may be challenged by more democratic ways of co-designing, testing, and using knowledge. Taking account of knowledge flow also requires deliberate consideration of new technological advances and at the same time taking account of equity and sustainability factors. These arguments are presented in the form of ten short propositions together with proposed actions for future consideration.

We are all familiar with the lag time between the generation of clinical evidence in the form of best practice guidelines and the time it takes for such evidence to get into practice. In fact, the evidence-practice gap has remained largely static over the last 25 years. A seminal study in the US in 1998 indicated that 30%–50% of health care delivery was not in line with best available evidence (Schuster et al., 1998); subsequent studies, undertaken in Europe in primary care (Grol, 2001), in acute care and in children's and aged care facilities in Australia (Braithwaite et al., 2018; Hibbert et al., 2024; Runciman et al., 2012) and in Canada (Squires et al., 2022) reached similar conclusions. This suggests that a 30–40% gap between the best available evidence and clinical practice persists, despite the investment that has gone into building a deeper understanding of the knowledge to practice gaps (Braithwaite et al., 2020).

Other lags have been identified but not discussed. Thus, there have been consistent exhortations for researchers to embrace new paradigms to help them to understand the

DOI: 10.4324/9781003245995-13

complex structures and systems within which they operate, and which will shape the way evidence is applied in practice. Across a similar timespan of 25 years, there has been a growing number of calls to embrace complexity science (Plsek & Greenhalgh, 2001), to understand concepts of innovation and improvement, and how these could shape evidence implementation (Edmondson, 2000; Greenhalgh et al., 2004; Van de Ven, 2007), and calls to extend the ontological and epistemological boundaries shaping knowledge generation and testing in health care (Greenhalgh & Papoutsi, 2018; Greenhalgh & Wieringa, 2011). And despite the increase in evidence that shows that the way we undertake implementation science needs to embrace broader paradigms regarding our thinking and understanding of the impact of systems and people in those systems, we are still wedded to old ways of thinking and doing implementation research.

For example, Harvey, Rycroft-Malone, et al. (2023) demonstrated that implementation strategies have tended to emphasize questions of effectiveness, with a corresponding focus on experimental studies, rather than take account of the other variables influencing the adoption of new evidence into practice. They cite the findings of a number of large robust implementation trials that report null outcomes and demonstrate through embedded process evaluations the contextual variables that contributed to these results. The question Harvey and colleagues ask is that if we know that implementation is complex, non-linear, and heavily context-dependent then why aren't these characteristics taken account of in the research design and conduct rather than described in a post-hoc process evaluation way? Furthermore, when considering implementation studies, there are likely to be broader questions of interest than simply the effectiveness of an implementation intervention, including recognised implementation outcomes such as acceptability, appropriateness, affordability, practicability, unintended consequences, equity, and feasibility (Proctor et al., 2011). Harvey et al. (2023) make the case for re-thinking implementation research and implementation practice, highlighting the need to become better at working with context throughout the entire research process, from planning to doing, analysing, interpretation, and sharing of results, whilst maintaining relevance and rigour at all stages.

The propositions

The question we have to ask ourselves as we look to the future is why given what we know – getting (or implementing) new knowledge into practice is a hard job – do we continue to think and research in traditional ways? It requires multiple partners to be involved at multiple levels in a system for it to be effective. So, why haven't our research leadership and methodological innovation capabilities matched the need for such changes in the way we think about and do this sort of research? In order to promote debate and to attempt to move the paradigm forward we have put forward ten propositions with short rationales as to why we think these are key challenges – or opportunities – facing us in the future if we want to really see transformations in new knowledge uptake and impact. We've also suggested actions that will keep us talking and moving forward.

BOX 10.1 Proposition 1
We need to continue to innovate in the knowledge translation space and proactively develop and test structures and collaborations between organisations that have a stake in improving the uptake of new knowledge into practice

We have seen significant experimentation with organisational structures (Academic Health Science Centres/ Research Translation Centres in Australia; Collaborations for Leadership in Applied Health Research and Care, and more recent iterations in the United Kingdom) to improve the partnerships between academic researchers and service providers. The idea was relatively simple – incentivise academic institutions to work more closely with service delivery systems and there will be greater synergy and collaboration. Evaluations of the Collaborations for Leadership in Applied Health Research and Care initiatives (Kislov et al., 2018) have been equivocal in terms of success – indicators of success consistently tell stories of the importance of existing relationships across boundaries and systems to enhance new ways of working. Where incentives and timescales across the different systems did not align, there were often tensions between a push for a more decentralised approach to decision making versus a centralised approach. Old hierarchies and power structures, in other words, were being challenged by this more engaged, democratic, and innovative way of enabling decision making to happen at the point of care delivery (Lockett et al., 2014).

Descriptions of the development of Academic Health Science Centres (also termed Research Translation Centres) in Australia indicate that they developed several years after the initiatives in the UK. Studies would seem to indicate that the Australian system did not learn from the evaluations undertaken in the UK and the work of the Research Translation Centres have come up against the same challenges, namely confusion over governance arrangements (Edelman et al., 2022), challenges with collaboration (Ferlie, 2022), and lack of clarity over the investment in roles such as 'knowledge brokers', and how these discrete roles can impact large organisational change (Jorm & Piper, 2022).

What sadly seems to happen with national initiatives is that traditional organisational structures are encouraged to collaborate from a top-down policy perspective without due attention being paid to the motivation and 'what's-in-it-for-me' incentivisation at local level (Rycroft-Malone et al., 2016). Until or unless decision-makers at national and local level align with their views of why such initiatives matter and how they will improve lives and work experiences, such investments will fail to achieve desired results.

Proposed action:
Commit to undertaking evaluations of top-down national policy driven initiatives that engage key partners at all levels of the systems involved from the start and commit to learning from evaluation results, so the same mistakes are not replicated, and that money is not wasted.

	BOX 10.2 Proposition 2 We need to invest in research leadership capability to embrace transdisciplinary research activity and to role model excellence in transdisciplinary research leadership

We know that in order to manage the complexity of the interventions and the contexts within with we work and do our research, we need to develop a set of research leadership skills that also embrace complexity and uncertainty. Our own research (Archibald et al., 2023; Lawless et al., 2025) indicates that characteristics of effective transdisciplinary research leadership relate to the leader's ability to negotiate, navigate, and mobilise the multiple networks in which they operate. This means that in addition to understanding the rigour around research design and running projects, transdisciplinary leaders need to know how to recognise and engage various partners, know how to build diverse teams and ensure they all know how to work together as well as actively manage all range of relationships.

Proposed action:
Align what we know from the Team Science literature (Begerowski et al., 2021; Hall et al., 2019) and the growing evidence from initiatives such as the Swiss Arts and Science Academy, which provides advice to policymakers and society on science and socially relevant issues, so we can modernise our ways of thinking about research teams and how they interface with the 'real-world'.

	BOX 10.3 Proposition 3
	We need to proactively think about how we educate our future research leaders to embrace a transdisciplinary approach

One of the great things about taking a knowledge translation lens to the entire research process is that whether you are working to identify and refine the research question with key partners or whether you are considering the most appropriate research design, you will be required to think holistically in terms of future impact, and how what you are producing could, should, and will be used. This conscious consideration is vital for effective design and testing of experiments. If we embrace a pragmatic approach to real world testing (Greenhalgh & Engebretsen, 2022b) then this approach offers great opportunities not only for better science but for better implementation success. Organisations such as the Swiss Academies of Arts and Science (https://swiss-academies.ch/) have generated a range of transdisciplinary toolbox profiles which provide tools and approaches that can be used to engage different disciplines to problem solve together as well as working with different groups to agree on what the actual research problem is.

Experience of working in high performing transdisciplinary research teams should be the norm for early and mid-career researchers as well as for consumers, knowledge users, and other key partners. That there is still confusion over the distinctions between disciplinary, multidisciplinary, interdisciplinary, and transdisciplinary activity means that we have still work to do to help team members feel comfortable and know where they fit in undertaking this work. Lawless et al. (2025) also found that proactive approaches to engaging team members and role modelling effective 'networking' capabilities were important elements to start to generate such a culture of development and learning.

Proposed action:
Build transdisciplinary research leadership skills and competency development into every early and mid-career research development program.

	Box 10.4 Proposition 4
	We need to understand how to more easily conduct ongoing 'experiments' in the real world that involve and engage our partners, our consumers and our multiple systems

Whole system problems need to be studied in all their richness and complexity rather than oversimplifying them into sets of relationships that we have the current knowledge and capacity to recognise and control. This means that any set of complex intervention and context studies, whether it's introducing improved oral care to elderly patients in an acute hospital setting (Murray et al., 2023) or finding solutions to childhood obesity (Hunter et al., 2022) will require multiple perspectives being brought to bear not only on what we currently know about what does and does not work but how this knowledge can then be tested out in real life. By engaging partners – if we take the childhood obesity example, we will be involving families, communities, multiple systems, researchers, food companies – then how we break down these discrete activities into manageable small scale but robust experiments that aggregate together to begin to provide us with a more integrated picture is an exciting thought for the future. Taking such an inclusive approach means that we will be working in partnership; a partnership described by Greenhalgh and Engebretsen as 'participatory democracy through citizen education' (Greenhalgh & Engebretsen, 2022a). Such an approach to research design and methodological innovation needs to embrace the fallibility of us knowing about things – there will always be uncertainty and the need for individuals to make informed decisions and doing research doesn't necessarily fill this gap. We need to challenge tendencies toward reductionist thinking and instead focus on concrete and practical experimentation in the real world, documenting experiences and impacts so that they can help shed light on what's really happening in our systems. The consequence of us embracing these approaches means there is less desire to think in linear, reductionist ways and less need to hold on to exclusive epistemologies that create a narrow interpretation of the world in which we live.

Proposed action:
Develop training programs that teach researchers how to think ontologically – reflecting on their assumptions about reality and the nature of knowledge – while also learning how to manage uncertainly and appreciate other disciplines' worldviews so they can be creative problem solvers and innovators rather than prescriptive rule followers.

> **Box 10.5 Proposition 5**
> **We need to embrace a more inclusive approach to understanding the nature of knowledge generation, testing, and use to combat a 'post-truth' movement**

Knowledge translation approaches are important to society as they offer ways to introduce scientific evidence into the public discourse. They need to do this because of the wider forces happening in society, culture, politics, and market forces that challenge traditional notions of scientific evidence and its dominance (Tieu et al., 2023). The notion of consensus on what a problem is, and a commitment to democratic participation in knowledge generation, and testing, is axiomatic to an engaged knowledge translation process. However, particularly after the pandemic (Greenhalgh & Engebretsen, 2022a) different groups have challenged how knowledge is generated and used and have shown distrust and discord in accepting rules and directives, particularly when they challenge perceived freedom of choice. Such activity can then fuel existing and emerging political and cultural divisions leading to further distrust, misinformation, and a loss of faith in key institutions. Our experience with COVID and the vaccine debate illustrates how interconnected our research and policy and practice worlds are, and it does not take much to create conditions for counterforces to take control of arguments. With the rapid rise of multiple communication channels with their different perspectives on what constitutes truth in a post-truth era, the challenges for knowledge translation research teams should not be underestimated.

Proposed action:
Explore the construct 'participatory democracy through citizen education' and encourage research teams to debate what this means to the ways they engage and involve partners and share knowledge.

	Box 10.6 Proposition 6
	We need to understand how best to use existing routine data sets as well as start to generate quality data sets fit for artificial intelligence utilization

There is no such thing as a perfect data set. Our challenge is not that there isn't sufficient data that is collected but that we often don't know or have forgotten why it has been collected, and that those who could benefit from using it to improve services don't have the time or have not been encouraged to use it in an interpretative, quality improvement way. In addition, a lot of routinely collected data is perceived as inferior and insufficiently robust for academic research use and therefore left unused. This was the situation (Wolpert & Rutter, 2018) found themselves in when they tried to use routinely collected data from services that were part of a national service transformation initiative in child mental health. They found the routinely collected data was flawed, due to missing or erroneously recorded entries; uncertain, due to differences in how data items were rated or conceptualised; proximate, in that data items were a proxy for key issues of concern; and sparse, in that a low volume of cases within key subgroups may limit the possibility of statistical inference. They coined the term 'FUPS' to describe these flawed, uncertain, proximate, and sparse datasets. They went on to use the FUPS dataset to support meaningful dialogue between key partners, including service providers, funders, and users, in relation to outcomes of services with a particular focus on the potential for service improvement and learning.

What their research showed was that paying attention to and improving existing data collection systems was in itself an important scientific exercise that enhanced learning and understanding across teams and service delivery boundaries. They also raised more philosophical questions about the nature of a quality data set arguing that most data sets are flawed, uncertain, proximate, and sparse and part of our capacity is to fill in the gaps and look for patterns that help us improve what we do. Such a piece of innovative work could help other health communities address the gap between the ideal of comprehensive clear data used in complicated, but not complex, contexts, and the reality of FUPS data in the context of complexity.

At the other end of the data use spectrum is the growing debate about how implementation science and knowledge translation approaches can more effectively use technology and particularly artificial intelligence. Trinkley et al. (2024) have identified the fact that artificial intelligence can already be used for predicting disease outbreaks, enhancing medical imaging, refining patient communication using technology such as Chatbots to influence change at individual and staff organisational level. The next logical step is to ask whether these technologies could speed up the adoption and use of new complex interventions into everyday practice. Trinkley et al. (2024) identify six potential benefits in starting to adopt artificial intelligence use – increasing the speed of adoption, more sustainable solutions, greater equity and generalisability, and more accuracy in assessing context and context-related outcomes, together with assessing causality and underlying mechanisms influencing and driving change. Their aspirations are of course predicated on the strength of their own mental models and conceptual frameworks which lead them to select what data they are going to use, how they are going to engage their many and various partners and how they are going to overcome the evidence generated by teams such as (Greenhalgh et al., 2017) who found that most technological innovations were underwhelming in their ability to improve patient outcomes and system enhance effectiveness. Perhaps it is a question of reflecting on how best to use this technology. Trinkley et al. (2024) indeed provide a list – build effective transdisciplinary teams; have a creative mindset, be audacious, humble and persistent, insist on and monitor quality, be iterative and conduct rapid learning cycles.

Proposed action:
Generate ways to improve the use of routinely collected data in knowledge translation research, improve its quality and generate better links between what frontline staff are collecting and how these data can be harnessed using AI and other technologies.

Box 10.7 Proposition 7
We need to understand how research leaders enable effective 'boundary spanning' activity and roles as part of the complex intervention research process

---

There is general acceptance that in addition to research producer and research user roles there is a need for linkage and exchange roles whose job it is to work across producer and user boundaries both at an individual and organisational level (Bornbaum et al., 2015). What is less clear is agreement on what these roles are called (knowledge and exchange, linkage, knowledge broker, facilitator, etc.), how they are trained and mentored, and whether and how they work (Kislov et al., 2017; Rycroft-Malone et al., 2018).

In addition, little attention has been given to this enabling or facilitative role within the research team. For example, is the expert knowledge translation researcher someone who has a deep understanding of the three distinct roles – knowledge producer, knowledge user, and knowledge broker? And if they need to understand how these roles work in order to design appropriate partner events, work with partner organisations and design complex interventions using some sort of knowledge brokering process, how do they know which ones to use, how do they select and train potential knowledge brokers and how do they know that the knowledge brokers have been successful?

These questions have already generated a lot of debate (for example see (Bucknall et al., 2022; Harvey, Collyer, et al., 2023; Harvey et al., 2018) but we still aren't any closer to understanding the underlying mechanisms (Kilbourne et al., 2023) that enable such roles to facilitate shifts and changes in people's behaviour and attitudes, if in fact they do. It is the contention in this book that the active ingredient for local behaviour and attitude change is the individual who responds positively to innovation or new knowledge coming into a system and then uses their own agency and influence to encourage other people to adopt the new ideas. In Rogers' (Rogers, 2003) language, these individuals are called 'local champions'; and in network theory they are called 'hubs' who connect with 'nodes' creating 'clusters' to form 'networks' that generate change (Kitson et al., 2018). The question would then be how do newly introduced roles (such as knowledge brokers or facilitators) into the local networked system recognise and work with these local champions and how does the relationship start to generate dynamic change within the system?

Some systems have generated a whole new role called practice facilitators (Baskerville et al., 2012) and this has seemed to work effectively within primary care settings. Other systems (Ritchie et al., 2020) have also explored the notion that certain systems are so deficient in contextual factors that even large 'doses' of knowledge broker or facilitation intervention would not be successful. So, we are beginning to get some sense of what needs to be studied in this complex area.

Proposed action:
Generate new integrated research programs around the concept of 'knowledge broker' roles incorporating learnings from organisational theory, facilitation, and complexity science.

	Box 10.8 Proposition 8 **We need to ensure appropriate governance and accountability processes**

The failures of large organisational knowledge translation collaborative efforts may be due in part to the fact that we have not paid sufficient attention to how our local research teams are set up and run with a view to incorporating a knowledge translation lens onto their work. Themes across the previous propositions point to the need for research leaders to demonstrate ability to negotiate, navigate, and mobilise all sorts of networks for effective impact. But these activities need to be represented within appropriate governance and accountability structures. One study that proactively addressed this issue was the work of Keefe et al (Keefe et al., 2020) who described the way that their research governance structures had to change to accommodate the complex interdependencies and teamwork required to address ways to enhance quality of life in long term care settings. They describe how they had to establish what they called a 'team of teams' that oversaw the multiple programs of work, each one of which had its own partners and methodological approaches, but which had to align in order to generate an integrated understanding of the whole picture. To what extent this narrative is novel or whether transdisciplinary research teams are generating the sophisticated governance and accountability structures that maintain control but also ensure appropriate involvement and leaning is a moot question. The fact may be that many of our structures are still holding on to old paradigms of thinking as it is easier – or more comfortable and certainly rewarded – to embrace linear, logical, ways of doing research rather than embrace pragmatic experimentation in the real world.

Proposed action:
Ensure governance and accountability structures for knowledge translation research programs are fit-for-purpose.

⚖	**Box 10.9 Proposition 9** **We need to ensure that equity is a central consideration in all knowledge translation efforts**

Failure to consider issues of equity in knowledge translation can unintentionally result in unequal benefits of health interventions between societal groups with differing levels of advantage or disadvantage (Gustafson et al., 2023). This is a topic that is receiving growing attention within global health, in part due to the current political climate, including changes in the foreign policies of high-income countries (The Lancet Global Health, 2025). Whilst challenging and concerning, this is also seen by some commentators to present a timely opportunity for addressing health inequities and decolonising global health by empowering communities and community members (The Lancet Global Health, 2025). However, to achieve this, it will be essential to position equity considerations at every stage of the knowledge translation process, embracing knowledge co-production, participatory approaches, inclusive research leadership, and equity-informed knowledge translation theories and frameworks. We have highlighted the importance of many of these principles throughout the preceding chapters, emphasising the participatory nature of knowledge translation from problem identification, knowledge generation and synthesis through to implementation and evaluation. What then are the additional considerations and actions needed to fully position equity front and centre in our knowledge translation endeavours?

Whilst there is increasing discussion in the literature, for example, within the implementation science community, about the need to give health equity a higher priority (Brownson et al., 2021) and examples of initiatives to do this (Aschbrenner et al., 2023), an international review of knowledge translation models suggested that few implicitly or explicitly acknowledged issues of health equity (Davison et al., 2015). This was evident, for example, by the under-representation of issues of power and power imbalances in most knowledge translation frameworks. Others have commented on the marginalisation of community members in knowledge production and the challenge of integrating tacit and indigenous knowledge with more traditional scientific evidence (The Lancet Global Health, 2025). Additionally, the choice of outcome measures for evaluation needs to embrace partner engagement and community preferences, alongside the more commonly used measures such as feasibility and fidelity (The Lancet Global Health, 2023).

Responding to concerns related to power and wealth imbalances, the Canadian Coalition of Global Health Research proposed a set of principles that could act as a framework to guide consideration of equity within everyday research, knowledge translation and practice (Plamondon & Bisung, 2019). These six principles with a focus on the importance of authentic partnering, inclusion, shared benefits, commitment to the future, responsiveness to causes of inequity, and humility, provide a useful lens through which to encourage equity-focused reflection and dialogue, examining assumptions, decisions and choices.

Proposed action:
Commit to a careful and systematic focus and reflection on issues of equity at all stages of the knowledge translation process.

	Box 10.10 Proposition 10
	We need to address issues of sustainability and ensure that translational initiatives are embedded in practice and policy

Knowledge translation initiatives can often happen within the context of a grant-funded research project, where a proportion of the budget is allocated to translation and dissemination activities. However, when the research funding ends and dedicated resources are no longer available, promising initiatives may start to decline, evaporate, or disappear altogether. This highlights the importance of building sustainability into a project from the outset and requires attention to several strategies that can be optimised during the design and conduct of the knowledge translation project. Firstly, ensuring that the intended research is focused on questions that matter from a partner perspective is key to ensuring that the knowledge generated is practical, context-relevant, and accessible (The Lancet Global Health, 2025). This increases the likelihood that it will be sustainably adopted by the communities that need it and is a central tenet of integrated knowledge translation. The knowledge translation strategies also need to be designed and selected with sustainability in mind, including clarity about components such as dose, frequency, adaptations, and cost (Flynn et al., 2023). The use of established sustainability planning tools can assist in this process (see, for example, the Program and Clinical Sustainability tools; https://sustaintool.org/).

Clearly understanding the costs and return on investment of knowledge translation and implementation is important in terms of making a business case for sustainment (Eisman et al., 2020). This is a growing focus within the field of implementation science, with new practical costing instruments being developed to making costing information available to decision makers faced with competing demands on finite resources (Donovan et al., 2025; Knocke & Wagner, 2022).

A further consideration relates to environmental sustainability. On the one hand, there is potential for knowledge translation and implementation science to help guide climate-related health research (Neta et al., 2022), improve environmental sustainability (Davies et al., 2024), and solve big problems such as pandemics (Fisher et al., 2025). On the reverse side, it is also important to take note of the potential unintended consequences of knowledge translation (Dadich et al., 2023), including activities that can incur environmental costs, for example, related to travel and communication.

Proposed action:
Pay attention to sustainability in the broadest sense when planning, conducting and evaluating knowledge translation initiatives, including designing and applying strategies that optimise sustainability and take account of both economic and environmental factors.

Summary

These ten propositions have outlined an agenda for the future that will continue to make integrated knowledge translation relevant and appropriate. It relies upon acknowledging a set of values guiding knowledge generation and use, namely, involvement and engagement with key partners, embracing principles of equity, inclusion, sustainability, and value for money. The future also relies upon investing in our knowledge translation researchers, equipping them with the appropriate leadership and interpersonal skills required to bring whole teams and systems to new ways understanding and working together. These leadership skills can then be supported by better governance models, and better utilisation of data, technology, and artificial intelligence. What is crucial to remember is that doing knowledge translation is a deeply social and interactive process requiring ongoing reflection and active learning for all participants, whether you are a knowledge producer, knowledge user or knowledge broker or someone who moves between each of these roles at different times depending on the research need and the context. This interdependency and recognition of collaborative action leading to effective knowledge translation is key to success.

References

Archibald, M. M., Lawless, M. T., de Plaza, M. A. P., & Kitson, A. L. (2023). How transdisciplinary research teams learn to do knowledge translation (KT), and how KT in turn impacts transdisciplinary research: A realist evaluation and longitudinal case study. *Health Research Policy and Systems, 21*(1), 20–20. https://doi.org/10.1186/s12961-023-00967-x

Aschbrenner, K. A., Oh, A. Y., Tabak, R. G., Hannon, P. A., Angier, H. E., Moore, W. T., Likumahuwa-Ackman, S., Carroll, J. K., Baumann, A. A., Beidas, R. S., Mazzucca-Ragan, S., Waters, E. A., Sadasivam, R. S., & Shelton, R. C. (2023). Integrating a focus on health equity in implementation science: Case examples from the national cancer institute's implementation science in cancer control centers (ISC(3)) network. *Journal of Clinical and Translation Science, 7*(1), e226. https://doi.org/10.1017/cts.2023.638

Baskerville, N. B., Liddy, C., & Hogg, W. (2012). Systematic review and meta-analysis of practice facilitation within primary care settings. *Annals of Family Medicine, 10*(1), 63–74. https://doi.org/10.1370/afm.1312

Begerowski, S. R., Traylor, A. M., Shuffler, M. L., & Salas, E. (2021). An integrative review and practical guide to team development interventions for translational science teams: One size does not fit all. *Journal of Clinical and Translational Science, 5*(1), e198, Article e198. https://doi.org/10.1017/cts.2021.832

Bornbaum, C. C., Kornas, K., Peirson, L., & Rosella, L. C. (2015). Exploring the function and effectiveness of knowledge brokers as facilitators of knowledge translation in health-related settings: A systematic review and thematic analysis. *Implementation Science, 10*(1), 162. https://doi.org/10.1186/s13012-015-0351-9

Braithwaite, J., Glasziou, P., & Westbrook, J. (2020). The three numbers you need to know about healthcare: The 60-30-10 Challenge. *BMC Medicine, 18*(1), 102–102. https://doi.org/10.1186/s12916-020-01563-4

Braithwaite, J., Hibbert, P. D., Jaffe, A., White, L., Cowell, C. T., Harris, M. F., Runciman, W. B., Hallahan, A. R., Wheaton, G., Williams, H. M., Murphy, E., Molloy, C. J., Wiles, L. K., Ramanathan, S., Arnolda, G., Ting, H. P., Hooper, T. D., Szabo, N., Wakefield, J. G., ... Muething, S. (2018). Quality of Health Care for Children in Australia, 2012–2013. *JAMA: The Journal of the American Medical Association, 319*(11), 1113–1124. https://doi.org/10.1001/jama.2018.0162

Brownson, R. C., Kumanyika, S. K., Kreuter, M. W., & Haire-Joshu, D. (2021). Implementation science should give higher priority to health equity. *Implementation Science, 16*(1), 28. https://doi.org/10.1186/s13012-021-01097-0

Bucknall, T. K., Considine, J., Harvey, G., Graham, I. D., Rycroft-Malone, J., Mitchell, I., Saultry, B., Watts, J. J., Mohebbi, M., Bohingamu Mudiyanselage, S., Lotfaliany, M., & Hutchinson, A.

(2022). Prioritising Responses Of Nurses To deteriorating patient Observations (PRONTO): A pragmatic cluster randomised controlled trial evaluating the effectiveness of a facilitation intervention on recognition and response to clinical deterioration. *BMJ Quality & Safety*, 31(11), 818. https://doi.org/10.1136/bmjqs-2021-013785

Dadich, A., Vaughan, P., & Boydell, K. (2023). The unintended negative consequences of knowledge translation in healthcare: A systematic scoping review. *Health Sociology Review*, 32(1), 75–93. https://doi.org/10.1080/14461242.2022.2151372

Davies, J. F., Ikin, B., Francis, J. J., & McGain, F. (2024). Implementation approaches to improve environmental sustainability in operating theatres: A systematic review. *British Journal of Anaesthesia*, 133(6), 1383–1396. https://doi.org/10.1016/j.bja.2023.05.017

Davison, C. M., Ndumbe-Eyoh, S., & Clement, C. (2015). Critical examination of knowledge to action models and implications for promoting health equity. *International Journal for Equity in Health*, 14(1), 49. https://doi.org/10.1186/s12939-015-0178-7

Donovan, T., Abell, B., McPhail, S. M., & Carter, H. E. (2025). Development of an instrument (Cost-IS) to estimate costs of implementation strategies for digital health solutions: A modified e-Delphi study. *Implementation Science*, 20(1), 13. https://doi.org/10.1186/s13012-025-01423-w

Edelman, A., Clay-Williams, R., Fischer, M., Kislov, R., Kitson, A., McLoughlin, I., Scouter's, H., & Harvey, G. (2022). Academic health science centres as vehicles for knowledge mobilisation in Australia? A qualitative study. *International Journal of Health Policy and Management*, 11(6), 840–846. https://doi.org/10.34172/ijhpm.2020.247

Edmondson, A. C. (2000). "The Innovation Journey," by Andrew Van de Ven, Douglas E. Polley, Raghu Garud, and Sankaran Venkataraman (Book Review). In (Vol. 25, pp. 885). Ada, Ohio, etc: Academy of Management.

Eisman, A. B., Kilbourne, A. M., Dopp, A. R., Saldana, L., & Eisenberg, D. (2020). Economic evaluation in implementation science: Making the business case for implementation strategies. *Psychiatry Research*, 283, 112433. https://doi.org/10.1016/j.psychres.2019.06.008

Ferlie, E. (2022). AHSCs as Health Policy Transfer: Some emergent evidence from Australia Comment on "Academic Health Science Centres as Vehicles for Knowledge Mobilisation in Australia? A Qualitative Study". *International Journal of Health Policy and Management*, 11(6), 862–864. https://doi.org/10.34172/ijhpm.2022.6284

Fisher, G., Smith, C. L., Pagano, L., Spanos, S., Zurynski, Y., & Braithwaite, J. (2025). Leveraging implementation science to solve the big problems: A scoping review of health system preparations for the effects of pandemics and climate change. *Lancet Planet Health*, 9(4), e326–e336. https://doi.org/10.1016/s2542-5196(25)00056-7

Flynn, R., Cassidy, C., Dobson, L., Al-Rassi, J., Langley, J., Swindle, J., Graham, I. D., & Scott, S. D. (2023). Knowledge translation strategies to support the sustainability of evidence-based interventions in healthcare: A scoping review. *Implementation Science*, 18(1), 69. https://doi.org/10.1186/s13012-023-01320-0

Greenhalgh, T., & Engebretsen, E. (2022a). The science-policy relationship in times of crisis: An urgent call for a pragmatist turn. *Social Science & Medicine*, 306, 115140. https://doi.org/10.1016/j.socscimed.2022.115140

Greenhalgh, T., & Engebretsen, E. (2022b). The science-policy relationship in times of crisis: An urgent call for a pragmatist turn. *Social Science & Medicine (1982)*, 306, 115140–115140. https://doi.org/10.1016/j.socscimed.2022.115140

Greenhalgh, T., & Papoutsi, C. (2018). Studying complexity in health services research: Desperately seeking an overdue paradigm shift. *BMC Medicine*, 16(1), 95–95. https://doi.org/10.1186/s12916-018-1089-4

Greenhalgh, T., Robert, G., Macfarlane, F., Bate, P., & Kyriakidou, O. (2004). Diffusion of innovations in service organizations: Systematic review and recommendations. *The Milbank Quarterly*, 82(4), 581–629. https://doi.org/10.1111/j.0887-378X.2004.00325.x

Greenhalgh, T., Wherton, J., Papoutsi, C., Lynch, J., Hughes, G., A'Court, C., Hinder, S., Fahy, N., Procter, R., & Shaw, S. (2017). Beyond adoption: A new framework for theorizing and evaluating Nonadoption, abandonment, and challenges to the scale-up, spread, and sustainability of health and care technologies. *Journal of Medical Internet Research, 19*(11), e367. https://doi.org/10.2196/jmir.8775

Greenhalgh, T., & Wieringa, S. (2011). Is it time to drop the 'knowledge translation' metaphor? A critical literature review. *Journal of the Royal Society of Medicine, 104*(12), 501–509. https://doi.org/10.1258/jrsm.2011.110285

Grol, R. (2001). Successes and failures in the implementation of evidence-based guidelines for clinical practice. *Medical Care, 39*(8), II46–II54. https://doi.org/10.1097/00005650-200108002-00003

Gustafson, P., Abdul Aziz, Y., Lambert, M., Bartholomew, K., Rankin, N., Fusheini, A., Brown, R., Carswell, P., Ratima, M., Priest, P., & Crengle, S. (2023). A scoping review of equity-focused implementation theories, models and frameworks in healthcare and their application in addressing ethnicity-related health inequities. *Implementation Science, 18*(1), 51. https://doi.org/10.1186/s13012-023-01304-0

Hall, K. L., Vogel, A. L., & Croyle, R. T. (2019). *Strategies for Team Science Success: Handbook of Evidence-Based Principles for Cross-Disciplinary Science and Practical Lessons Learned from Health Researchers* (1st ed. 2019. ed.). Springer International Publishing. https://doi.org/10.1007/978-3-030-20992-6

Harvey, G., Collyer, S., McRae, P., Barrimore, S. E., Demmitt, C., Lee-Steere, K., Nolan, B., & Mudge, A. M. (2023). Navigating the facilitation journey: A qualitative, longitudinal evaluation of 'Eat Walk Engage' novice and experienced facilitators. *BMC Health Services Research, 23*(1), 1132. https://doi.org/10.1186/s12913-023-10116-3

Harvey, G., McCormack, B., Kitson, A., Lynch, E., & Titchen, A. (2018). Designing and implementing two facilitation interventions within the 'Facilitating Implementation of Research Evidence (FIRE)' study: A qualitative analysis from an external facilitators' perspective. *Implementation Science, 13*(1), 141. https://doi.org/10.1186/s13012-018-0812-z

Harvey, G., Rycroft-Malone, J., Seers, K., Wilson, P., Cassidy, C., Embrett, M., Hu, J., Pearson, M., Semenic, S., Zhao, J., & Graham, I. D. (2023). Connecting the science and practice of implementation – applying the lens of context to inform study design in implementation research. *Frontier Health Services, 3*, 1162762. https://doi.org/10.3389/frhs.2023.1162762

Hibbert, P. D., Molloy, C. J., Cameron, I. D., Gray, L. C., Reed, R. L., Wiles, L. K., Westbrook, J., Arnolda, G., Bilton, R., Ash, R., Georgiou, A., Kitson, A., Hughes, C. F., Gordon, S. J., Mitchell, R. J., Rapport, F., Estabrooks, C., Alexander, G. L., Vincent, C., . . . Braithwaite, J. (2024). The quality of care delivered to residents in long-term care in Australia: An indicator-based review of resident records (CareTrack Aged study). *BMC Medicine, 22*(1),15–22. https://doi.org/10.1186/s12916-023-03224-8

Hunter, K. E., Johnson, B. J., Askie, L., Golley, R. K., Baur, L. A., Taylor, R. W., Wolfenden, L., Wood, C. T., Mihrshahi, S., Hayes, A. J., Rissel, C., Robledo, K. P., O'Connor, D. A., Espinoza, D., Staub, L. P., Barba, A., Libesman, S., Smith, W. A., Sue-See, M., . . . Widen, E. (2022). Transforming Obesity Prevention for CHILDren (TOPCHILD) Collaboration: Protocol for a systematic review with individual participant data meta-analysis of behavioural interventions for the prevention of early childhood obesity. *BMJ Open, 12*(1), e048166–e048166. https://doi.org/10.1136/bmjopen-2020-048166

Jorm, C., & Piper, D. (2022). When health systems consider research to be beyond the scope of healthcare delivery, research translation is crippled comment on "Academic Health Science Centres as Vehicles for Knowledge Mobilisation in Australia? A Qualitative Study". *International Journal of Health Policy and Management, 11*(6), 855–858. https://doi.org/10.34172/ijhpm.2021.104

Keefe, J., Hande, M. J., Aubrecht, K., Daly, T., Cloutier, D., Taylor, D., Hoben, M., Stajduhar, K., Cook, H., Bourgeault, I. L., MacDonald, L., & Estabrooks, C. A. (2020). Team-based integrated knowledge translation for enhancing quality of life in long-term care settings: A Multi-method, multi-sectoral research design. *International Journal of Health Policy Management*, 9(4), 138–142. https://doi.org/10.15171/ijhpm.2019.123

Kilbourne, A. M., Geng, E., Eshun-Wilson, I., Sweeney, S., Shelley, D., Cohen, D. J., Kirchner, J. E., Fernandez, M. E., & Parchman, M. L. (2023). How does facilitation in healthcare work? Using mechanism mapping to illuminate the black box of a meta-implementation strategy. *Implementation Science Communications*, 4(1), 53–12. https://doi.org/10.1186/s43058-023-00435-1

Kislov, R., Wilson, P., & Boaden, R. (2017). The 'dark side' of knowledge brokering. *Journal of Health Services Research & Policy*, 22(2), 107–112. https://doi.org/10.1177/1355819616653981

Kislov, R., Wilson, P. M., Knowles, S., & Boaden, R. (2018). Learning from the emergence of NIHR Collaborations for Leadership in Applied Health Research and Care (CLAHRCs): A systematic review of evaluations. *Implementation Science*, 13(1), 111. https://doi.org/10.1186/s13012-018-0805-y

Kitson, A., Brook, A., Harvey, G., Jordan, Z., Marshall, R., O'Shea, R., & Wilson, D. (2018). Using complexity and network concepts to inform healthcare knowledge translation. *International Journal of Health Policy and Management*, 7(3), 231–243. https://doi.org/10.15171/ijhpm.2017.79

Knocke, K., & Wagner, T. W. (2022). The evolving economics of implementation. *BMJ Quality & Safety*, 31(8), 555. https://doi.org/10.1136/bmjqs-2021-014411

Lawless, M. T., Tieu, M., Archibald, M. M., Pinero De Plaza, M. A., & Kitson, A. L. (2025). From promise to practice: How health researchers understand and promote transdisciplinary collaboration. *Qualitative Health Research*, 35(1), 3–16. https://doi.org/10.1177/10497323241235882

Lockett, A., El Enany, N., Currie, G., Oborn, E., Barrett, M., Racko, G., Bishop, S., & Waring, J. (2014). A formative evaluation of Collaboration for Leadership in Applied Health Research and Care (CLAHRC): Institutional entrepreneurship for service innovation. *Health Services and Delivery Research*, 2(31), 1–124. https://doi.org/10.3310/hsdr02310

Murray, J., Hunter, S. C., Splawinski, Z., & Conroy, T. (2023). Lessons learned from the preimplementation phase of an oral health care project. *JDR Clinical and Translational Research*, 8(3), 299–301. https://doi.org/10.1177/23800844221083966

Neta, G., Pan, W., Ebi, K., Buss, D. F., Castranio, T., Lowe, R., Ryan, S. J., Stewart-Ibarra, A. M., Hapairai, L. K., Sehgal, M., Wimberly, M. C., Rollock, L., Lichtveld, M., & Balbus, J. (2022). Advancing climate change health adaptation through implementation science. *The Lancet Planetary Health*, 6(11), e909–e918. https://doi.org/10.1016/S2542-5196(22)00199-1

Plamondon, K. M., & Bisung, E. (2019). The CCGHR Principles for Global Health Research: Centering equity in research, knowledge translation, and practice. *Social Science & Medicine*, 239, 112530. https://doi.org/10.1016/j.socscimed.2019.112530

Plsek, P. E., & Greenhalgh, T. (2001). Complexity science: The challenge of complexity in health care. *BMJ*, 323(7313), 625–628. https://doi.org/10.1136/bmj.323.7313.625

Proctor, E., Silmere, H., Raghavan, R., Hovmand, P., Aarons, G., Bunger, A., Griffey, R., & Hensley, M. (2011). Outcomes for implementation research: Conceptual distinctions, measurement challenges, and research agenda. *Administration Policy Mental Health*, 38(2), 65–76. https://doi.org/10.1007/s10488-010-0319-7

Ritchie, M. J., Parker, L. E., & Kirchner, J. E. (2020). From novice to expert: A qualitative study of implementation facilitation skills. *Implementation Science Communications*, 1(1), 25. https://doi.org/10.1186/s43058-020-00006-8

Rogers, E. M. (2003). *Diffusion of innovations* (5th ed.). Free Press.

Runciman, W. B., Coiera, E. W., Day, R. O., Hannaford, N. A., Hibbert, P. D., Hunt, T. D., Westbrook, J. I., & Braithwaite, J. (2012). Towards the delivery of appropriate health care in Australia. *Medical Journal of Australia*, 197(2), 78–81. https://doi.org/10.5694/mja12.10799

Rycroft-Malone, J., Burton, C. R., Wilkinson, J., Harvey, G., McCormack, B., Baker, R., Dopson, S., Graham, I. D., Staniszewska, S., Thompson, C., Ariss, S., Melville-Richards, L., & Williams, L.

(2016). Collective action for implementation: A realist evaluation of organisational collaboration in healthcare. *Implementation Science: IS, 11*(1), 17–17. https://doi.org/10.1186/s13 012-016-0380-z

Rycroft-Malone, J., Seers, K., Eldh, A. C., Cox, K., Crichton, N., Harvey, G., Hawkes, C., Kitson, A., McCormack, B., McMullan, C., Mockford, C., Niessen, T., Slater, P., Titchen, A., van der Zijpp, T., & Wallin, L. (2018). A realist process evaluation within the Facilitating Implementation of Research Evidence (FIRE) cluster randomised controlled international trial: An exemplar. *Implementation Science: IS, 13*(1), 138–115. https://doi.org/10.1186/s13012-018-0811-0

Schuster, M. A., McGlynn, E. A., & Brook, R. H. (1998). How good is the quality of health care in the United States? *The Milbank Quarterly, 76*(4), 517–563. https://doi.org/10.1111/1468-0009.00105

Squires, J. E., Cho-Young, D., Aloisio, L. D., Bell, R.., Bornstein, S., Brien, S. E., Decary, S., Varin, M.D., Dobrow, M.., Estabrooks, C. A., Graham, I. D., Greenough, M., Grinspun, D., Hillmer, M., Horsley, T.., Hu, J.., Katz, A, Krause, C., Lavis, J., ... Grimshaw, J. M. (2022). Inappropriate use of clinical practices in Canada: A systematic review. *Canadian Medical Association Journal (CMAJ), 194*(8), E279–E296. https://doi.org/10.1503/cmaj.211416

The Lancet Global Health. (2023). Implementing implementation science in global health. *The Lancet Global Health, 11*(12), e1827. https://doi.org/10.1016/S2214-109X(23)00523-5

The Lancet Global Health. (2025). Redefining implementation science for global health decolonisation. *The Lancet Global Health, 13*(4), e599. https://doi.org/10.1016/s2214-109x(25)00116-0

Tieu, M., Lawless, M., Hunter, S. C., Pinero de Plaza, M. A., Darko, F., Mudd, A., Yadav, L., & Kitson, A. (2023). Wicked problems in a post-truth political economy: A dilemma for knowledge translation. *Humanities & Social Sciences Communications, 10*(1), 280–280. https://doi.org/10.1057/s41599-023-01789-6

Trinkley, K. E., An, R., Maw, A. M., Glasgow, R. E., & Brownson, R. C. (2024). Leveraging artificial intelligence to advance implementation science: Potential opportunities and cautions. *Implementation Science, 19*(1), 17. https://doi.org/10.1186/s13012-024-01346-y

Van de Ven, A. H. (2007). *Engaged scholarship: A guide for organizational and social research.* Oxford University Press.

Wolpert, M., & Rutter, H. (2018). Using flawed, uncertain, proximate and sparse (FUPS) data in the context of complexity: Learning from the case of child mental health. *BMC Medicine, 16*(1), 82–82. https://doi.org/10.1186/s12916-018-1079-6

Index

Note: Page numbers in **bold** indicate tables, and those in *italics* indicate figures.

For Product Safety Concerns and Information please contact our EU
representative GPSR@taylorandfrancis.com
Taylor & Francis Verlag GmbH, Kaufingerstraße 24, 80331 München, Germany

www.ingramcontent.com/pod-product-compliance
Lightning Source LLC
Chambersburg PA
CBHW081101220326
41598CB00038B/7186